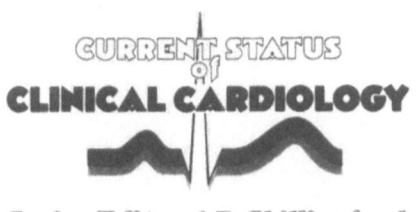

Series Editor J.P. Shillingford

HEART MUSCLE DISEASE

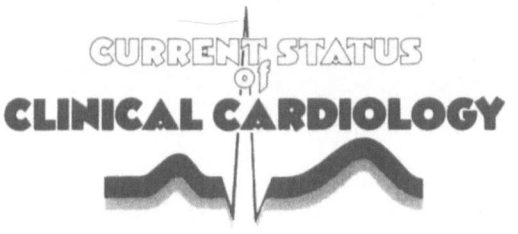

CURRENT STATUS of CLINICAL CARDIOLOGY

Series Editor J. P. Shillingford

HEART MUSCLE DISEASE

Edited by
J.F.Goodwin

Emeritus Professor of Clinical Cardiology
Royal Postgraduate Medical School
London

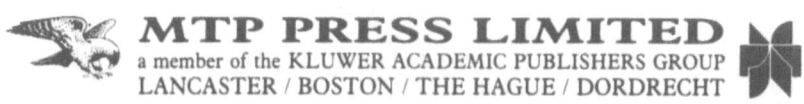

MTP PRESS LIMITED
a member of the KLUWER ACADEMIC PUBLISHERS GROUP
LANCASTER / BOSTON / THE HAGUE / DORDRECHT

Published in the UK and Europe by
MTP Press Limited
Falcon House
Lancaster, England

British Library Cataloguing in Publication Data
Heart muscle disease.—(Current status of
clinical cardiology).
1. Heart—Muscle—Diseases
I. Goodwin, J.F.   II. Series
616.1'24   RC685.M9

Published in the USA by
MTP Press
A division of Kluwer Boston Inc
190 Old Derby Street
Hingham, MA 02043, USA

Library of Congress Cataloging in Publication Data

Main entry under title:

Heart muscle disease.

(Current status of clinical cardiology)
Includes bibliographies and index.
1. Heart—Muscle—Diseases. I. Goodwin, John F.
II. Series. [DNLM: 1. Myocardial Diseases.
WG 280 H437]
RC685.M9H38 1985   616.1'24   85-7121

ISBN-13: 978-94-010-8657-8   e-ISBN-13: 978-94-009-4874-7
DOI: 10.1007/978-94-009-4874-7

Contents

CONTENTS

Preface

Twenty five years ago, cardiomyopathies or myocardopathies as they were sometimes called, were in very small print, and often the terms myocarditis and cardiomyopathy were used interchangeably. Now definition and classification can be precise and terminology has been refined.

Although a great deal still has to be learnt about the heart muscle diseases, they have now achieved the status of an important group of cardiovascular disorders. Their importance is out of proportion to their frequency because the cardiomyopathies so often attack young otherwise active and healthy people, and are notable for sudden unexpected death, and for intractable congestive heart failure. They are especially a meance in age groups younger than those most commonly effected by coronary heart disease.

This book presents an analysis and review by many experts of the present knowledge about heart muscle diseases and employs the approach to classification and terminology now generally, though not universally, agreed. It will be apparent that much fundamental research must be done now that the clinical problems have been defined. In the future, the collaboration of molecular biologists and other basic scientists will be needed to illuminate the dark places of our ignorance.

Knowledge is promoted by the stimulus of argument and counter-argument over controversial issues, and so, because of the importance of certain differing viewpoints on causation and function, the last two chapters deal with the significance of outflow tract gradients in hypertrophic cardiomyopathy and with the infectious/immune theory of causation of dilated cardiomyopathy, respectively. The preface to the last two chapters (p. 155) will attempt to justify this selection.

J.F. Goodwin

List of Contributors

H.-D. Bolte
Zentral Klinikum Augsburg
D-8900 Augsberg
West Germany

R.O. Brandenburg
Cardiovascular Division
The Mayo Clinic
Rochester, MN 55905
USA

J.M. Criley
Division of Cardiology
Harbor – UCLA Medical Center
1000 West Carson Street
Torrance, CA 90509
USA

J. Davies
Department of Cardiology
Royal Gwent Hospital
Newport
Gwent, South Wales
UK

J.F. Goodwin
Department of Clinical Cardiology
Royal Postgraduate Medical School
Hammersmith Hospital
Ducane Road
London W12 0HS
UK

M. Henderson
Division of Cardiology
12 Eaton N, Room 217B
Toronto General Hospital
101 College Street
Toronto, Ontario
CANADA M5G 1L7

H. Kuhn
Stadtische Krankenanstalten
Bielefeld Mitte
Medizinische Klinik II
Akademisches Lehrkrankenhaus der
    Universität Munster
D-4800 Bielefeld 1
West Germany

W.A. Littler
Department of Cardiovascular
    Medicine
University of Birmingham
East Birmingham Hospital
Bordesley Green East
Birmingham B9 5ST
UK

P.J. Lowry
Department of Cardiovascular
    Medicine
University of Birmingham
East Birmingham Hospital
Bordesley Green East
Birmingham B9 5ST
UK

W.J. McKenna
Department of Clinical Cardiology
Royal Postgraduate Medical School
Ducane Road
London W12 0HS
Uk

J.W. Miller
US Army Medical Corps
Cardiology Service
Department of Medicine
Brooke Army Medical Center
Fort Sam Houston
TX 78234-6200
USA

J.P. Murgo
US Army Medical Corps
Cardiology Service
Department of Medicine
Brooke Army Medical Center
Fort Sam Houston
TX 78234-6200
USA

C. Oakley
Department of Medicine
Hammersmith Hospital and
   The Royal Postgraduate Medical
   School
Ducane Road
London W12 0HS
UK

E.G.J. Olsen
Department of Morbid Anatomy
   and Histopathology
National Heart and Chest Hospitals
Westmorland Street
London W1M BA
UK

J.K. Perloff
Division of Cardiology RM 47–123
   Departments of Medicine and
   Pediatrics
Center for the Health Sciences

University of California
Los Angeles, CA90024
USA

C. Pollick
Division of Cardiology
12 Eaton N, Room 217B
Toronto General Hospital
101 College Street
Toronto, Ontario
Canada M5G 1L7

H.R. Rakowski
Division of Cardiology
12 Eaton N, Room 217B
Toronto General Hospital
101 College Street
Toronto, Ontario
Canada M5G 1L7

W.C. Roberts
Division of Cardiology
Departments of Medicine and
   Pediatrics
Center for the Health Sciences
University of California
Los Angeles
California
USA

Z. Sasson
Division of Cardiology
12 Eaton N, Room 217B
Toronto General Hospital
101 College Street
Toronto, Ontario
Canada M5G 1L7

R.J. Siegel
Division of Cardiology
Harbor – UCLA Medical Center
1000 West Carson Street
Torrance, CA 90509
USA

D.D. Sugrue
Department of Cardiovascular
  Disease
Mayo Clinic
Rochester, MN 55904
USA

N.K. Wenger
Department of Medicine
  (Cardiology)
Emory University School of
  Medicine

69 Butler Street, SE
Atlanta, GA 30303
USA

E.D. Wigle
Division of Cardiology
12 Eaton N, Room 217B
Toronto General Hospital
101 College Street
Toronto, Ontario
Canada M5G 1L7

Current Status of Clinical Cardiology Series

Drugs in the Management of Heart Disease
Edited by A. Breckenridge

Heart Muscle Disease
Edited by J. F. Goodwin

Congenital Heart Disease
Edited by F.J. Macartney

Invasive and Non-Invasive Diagnosis of Heart Disease
Edited by A. Maseri

Ischaemic Heart Disease
Edited by K. Fox

Immunology and Heart Disease
Edited by C.J.F. Spry

Series Editor's Note

The last few decades have seen an explosion in our knowledge of cardio-vascular disease as a result of research in many disciplines. The tempo of research is ever increasing, so that it is becoming more and more difficult for one person to encompass the whole spectrum of the advances taking place on many fronts.

Even more difficult is to include the advances as they affect clinical practice in one textbook of cardiovascular disease. Fifty years ago all that was known about cardiology could be included in one textbook of moderate size and at that time there was little research so that a textbook remained up to date for several years. Today all this has changed, and books have to be updated at frequent intervals to keep up with the results of research and changing fashions.

The present series has been designed to cover the field of cardiovascular medicine in a series of, initially, eight volumes which can be updated at regular intervals and at the same time give a sound basis of practice for doctors looking after patients.

The future volumes will include the following subjects: heart muscle disease; congenital heart disease, invasive and non-invasive diagnosis; ischaemic heart disease; immunology and heart disease; irregularities of the heart beat; and each is edited by a distinguished British author with an international reputation, together with an international panel of contributors.

The series will be mainly designed for the consultant cardiologist as reference books of manageable size to assist him in his day-to-day practice and keep him up to date in the various fields of cardiovascular medicine.

J.P. Shillingford
British Heart Foundation

1
Cardiomyopathies and specific heart muscle diseases: definition, terminology and classification

J.F. GOODWIN

In the last three decades, cardiomyopathies have emerged from the fog of inprecision and uncertainty into the light of scientific scrutiny. Progress in understanding of this group of diseases was hindered by lack of consensus on terminology and definition. In the 1950s, in the USA, Mattingly, Burch and Proctor Harvey were selecting and studying cases, while in 1957, in London, Brigden published his St Cyres Lecture on 'Uncommon myocardial diseases – the non-coronary cardiomyopathies'[1]. In 1961, Goodwin et al.[2] proposed a definition and classification based on disorders of structure and function[3]. Subsequently, the definition of cardiomyopathies was shortened to 'a disorder of cardiac muscle of unknown cause'[4]. Myocardial diseases that were part of a general system disease were defined as '(rare) specific heart muscle diseases'. The classification based on structural and functional disorders introduced by Goodwin et al. in 1961[2] and Goodwin in 1964[3] was modified to: hypertrophic obstructive, congestive, restrictive, and obliterative[4-7].

This classification was sanctioned and approved by the World Health Organization/International Society and Federation of Cardiology Task Force on the definition and classification of cardiomyopathies[8] with the proviso that the congestive type should be renamed 'dilated' – this being a more accurate and descriptive term than 'congestive'. Growing realization that obstruction is not the main feature of hypertrophic obstructive cardiomyopathy led to the word 'obstructive' being omitted. The term 'obliterative' was dropped from the classification as it represented essentially the advanced stage of restrictive cardiomyopathy due to endomyocardial fibrosis.

Although a member of the WHO/ISFC Task Force and a party to its report[8], the present writer prefers to retain the word 'congestive' in the definition of dilated cardiomyopathy, because 'congestive' has become an

1

accepted and understood term, even though 'dilated' is more appropriate. The retention of the 'obliterative' group is clearly now not warranted.

The separation of the cardiomyopathies, as defined, from the specific heart muscle diseases is important, because it avoids unwieldy lists of heart diseases due to systemic causes, and allows concentration on the important aspects of the cardiomyopathies, which are causation and treatment.

As with all classifications of biological phenomena and systems, exceptions occur. Although amyloid disease, for example, affects only the muscle of the heart, it is difficult to fit into the definitions. Sometimes the heart may be the only organ affected, in which case amyloid comes into the definition of cardiomyopathy. But when, as is not infrequent, amyloid disease affects several organs other than the heart, it comes into the group of specific heart muscle diseases. Furthermore, its functional disorder does not fit neatly into the classification either. For example, there are none of the systolic abnormalities found in *hypertrophic cardiomyopathy*, but ventricular hypertrophy undoubtedly occurs, and abnormality of filling of the ventricles is always present. Resistance to filling – due, in amyloid disease, to rigidity of the myocardium and in hypertrophic cardiomyopathy to myofibrillar disarray and fibrosis – is a feature common to both disorders, although detailed analysis of diastolic function reveals important differences (see Chapters 2.2 and 2.6). In addition, some of the diastolic features of amyloid disease resemble those of *restrictive cardiomyopathy* but, again, there are important differences (*see* Chapter 6). In the late stage of amyloid disease systolic pump failure is commonplace, and resembles that of dilated cardiomyopathy, but earlier in the disease systolic function may remain competent.

There are other conditions which do not lend themselves readily to any firm classification – and do not exactly meet the criteria for cardiomyopathy. These indeterminate diseases are: tachyarrhythmic syndromes with incessant repetitive arrhythmia leading to heart failure; localized conducting tissue disorder syndromes, such as the long QT disorder; and angina with 'normal' coronary arteries. Until more is understood about these conditions they must remain, as far as cardiomyopathies are concerned, an indeterminate group[9].

Hypertrophic cardiomyopathy is an inherited disorder characterized by massive ventricular hypertrophy, impaired diastolic function and overzealous ventricular contraction. It is notable for systolic pressure gradients in the left ventricle and for hypertrophy of the ventricular septum, which is often, but not always, asymmetrical in distribution. Hypertrophic cardiomyopathy is essentially a patchy disease involving both ventricles, but mainly the left. A notable feature is the large size and smooth bore of the coronary arteries. The cause of hypertrophic cardiomyopathy is unknown, but possibly a disorder of catecholamine handling by the fetal myocardium may be implicated[6,7,9,10].

Although initially the condition was thought to be mainly a disorder of systolic function, it is now accepted that the main disorder is in diastole, with impaired relaxation and filling of the ventricles. The validity of true obstruction to outflow is still debated, and will be discussed by proponents and opponents respectively in Chapter 10.

The main hazard of hypertrophic cardiomyopathy is sudden death, which is often unexpected as the disease tends to affect young, vigorous and active people. Sudden death is due, usually, to ventricular arrhythmias, but sometimes to hindrance to filling of the left ventricle (Chapter 2.2).

Dilated (congestive) cardiomyopathy is a completely different entity from hypertrophic cardiomyopathy, and is primarily a disease of systolic, not diastolic, function. The main disorder is impairment of contractility and effective pump action. Hypertrophy of the ventricles is slight or moderate, never massive, and dilatation of the ventricles is the cardinal feature. Congestive heart failure of unknown cause is the hallmark, and no evidence of causation emerges from any investigation; even tissue examination fails to reveal an answer. Of many possible causes, the most likely seems to be previous viral infection of the heart leading to an immunological disorder which progressively destroys the myocardium. Although a rare right ventricular type, notable for arrhythmia, has been described[11], dilated (congestive) cardiomyopathy usually affects both ventricles and is a diffuse process. The coronary arteries are normal and, except for rare cases, there is no familial incidence.

Contrary to views sometimes expressed, dialted (congestive) cardio-myopathy is not a late stage of hypertrophic cardiomyopathy but a completely separate entity[9].

Restrictive cardiomyopathy The main cause is endomyocardial fibrosis (EMF), of which there are two types: the tropical without hypereosinophilia and the temperate climate variety with considerable eosinophilia, originally described by Löffler. The characteristic lesion is fibrosis of the endomyocardium, with added thrombus and involvement of the atrioventricular valves. As the disease advances, the fibrosis obliterates the apices of the ventricles.

It is now thought that both types of EMF are basically the same disease; certainly the pathology is indistinguishable[12], though there are some aspects that differ – probably as a result of local environmental and, perhaps, genetic factors. The cause is thought to be an inflammatory response of the myocardium and the endocardium to irritant cationic proteins extruded from clones of disturbed eosinophils, which display immunological abnormalities. The tropical and temperate climate forms of EMF are collectively now known as 'eosinophilic endomyocardial disease'[8] (Chapter 4).

TERMINOLOGY

It is important to clarify certain terms that will be used in ensuing chapters[9].

Elimination refers to the disappearance of the ventricular cavity in systole by apposition and compression of its walls in hypertrophic cardiomyopathy.

Obstruction refers to organic physical obstruction to ventricular outflow.

Restriction refers to organic interference with filling from endomyocardial disease. As in constrictive pericarditis, early ventricular filling is rapid, but late ventricular filling is slow and much reduced.

Resistance refers to hindrance to ventricular filling caused by stiff, irregularly relaxing, poorly compliant ventricles as in hypertrophic cardiomyopathy and amyloid disease.

Obliteration refers to organic blockage of the ventricular cavities by fibrotic material, usually commencing at the apices, as typically in endomyocardial fibrosis with thrombosis.

Amyloid heart disease

As already noted, this has some characteristics of diastolic function similar to both restrictive and hypertrophic cardiomyopathies, and therefore needs to be considered separately (Chapter 6).

Specific heart muscle diseases

These will be covered in Chapter 8 and will be divided into granulomata (sarcoid); infectious causes; neurological and neuromuscular diseases; collagen vascular diseases; tumours; metabolic disorders; blood diseases; endocrine and nutritional causes; drugs, poisons and toxic causes; and miscellaneous groups[1,2].

Most specific heart muscle diseases produce a dilated form of cardiomyopathy with impaired systolic ventricular function, heart failure and often tachy- and bradyarrhythmias. Sometimes Friedreich's ataxia and Pompe's disease can produce a hypertrophic picture, while amyloid disease has some resemblance to both hypertrophic and restrictive cardiomyopathies. Sarcoid heart disease may produce some of the features of coronary heart disease and its complications, such as regional ventricular dyskinesia, ventricular aneurysm and papillary muscle damage.

CONCLUSION

The chapters dealing with the various types of cardiomyopathy will emphasize the recent advances, and will discuss the propositions that hypertrophic cardiomyopathy may be an endocrine disorder; that dilated congestive cardiomyopathy is probably a disorder of disturbed cellular immunity set up by previous viral infection; and that endomyocardial fibrosis is a disease of immunity of the eosinophil.

References

1. Brigden, W. (1957). Uncommon myocardial diseases – the non-coronary cardiomyopathies. *Lancet*, 2, 1179, 1243
2. Goodwin, J.F., Holman, A. and Bishop, M.B. (1961). Clinical aspects of cardiomyopathy. *Brit. Med. J.*, 1, 69–79

3. Goodwin, J.F. (1964). Cardiac function in primary myocardial disorders. *Brit. Med. J.*, 1, 1527, 1595
4. Goodwin, J.F. (1970). Congestive and hypertrophic cardiomyopathies – a decade of study. *Lancet*, 1, 731
5. Goodwin, J.F. and Oakley, C.M. (1972). Editorial: The cardiomyopathies. *Brit. Heart J.*, 34, 545
6. Goodwin, J.F. (1974). Prospects and predictions for the cardiomyopathies. *Circulation*, 50, 210
7. Goodwin, J.F. (1979). Cardiomyopathy: an interface between fundamental and clinical cardiology. In Hayasi, S. and Murao, S. (eds.) *Proceedings of the VIII World Congress of Cardiology*. (Excerpta Medica International Congress Series No. 470.) p. 103. (Amsterdam: Elsevier-North-Holland)
8. Report of the WHO/ISFC Task Force on the definition and classification of cardiomyopathies. (1980). *Brit. Heart J.*, 44, 672
9. Goodwin, J.F. (1982). The frontiers of cardiomyopathy. *Brit. Heart J.*, 48, 1
10. Perloff, J.K. (1981). Pathogenesis of hypertrophic cardiomyopathy: hypotheses and speculation. *Am. Heart J.*, 101, 219
11. Fitchett, D.H., Sagrue, D.D., MacArthur, C.G.C. and Oakley, C.M. (1984). Right ventricular dilated cardiomyopathy. *Br. Heart J.*, 51, 25
12. Olsen, E.G.J. and Spry, C.J.F. (1979). The pathogeneses of Löffler's endomyocardial disease, and its relationship to endomyocardial fibrosis. In Yu, P.N. and Goodwin, J.F. (eds.) *Progress in Cardiology*. Vol 8. p. 281. (Philadelphia: Lea & Febiger)
13. Goodwin, J.F. (1983). Terminology of disorders of cardiac muscle. In Symons, C., Evans, T. and Mitchell, A.G. (eds.) *Specific Heart Muscle Disease*. p. 1. (Bristol, London, Boston: Wright, P.S.G.)

2.1
Pathogenesis of hypertrophic cardiomyopathy

J.K. PERLOFF

In most patients, hypertrophic cardiomyopathy is genetic with an autosomal dominant pattern of inheritance[1-3]. In something less than half of the cases, the disease is sporadic[1]; an unknown number of these cases, probably in younger patients, may represent mutations. The remainder of the sporadic type probably reflect diverse aetiologies[1]. Genetic hypertrophic cardiomyopathy was defined in Chapter 1, and it is with this variety that I shall deal. The relationship between genetic hypertrophic cardiomyopathy and the non-genetic sporadic type is presently unclear.

In discussing pathogenesis, stress will be placed on *three anatomical points*: (1) ventricular septal thickness, (2) ventricular septal shape and (3) septal cellular disarray; *three physiological points*: (1) hypercontractile left ventricular free wall, (2) hypocontractile ventricular septum and (3) left ventricular cavity obliteration; and *three clinical points*: (1) occasional appearance of overt disease of birth, implying intrauterine presence, (2) more typically, occult disease at birth with gradual progression to the clinically overt state and (3) genetic transmission, implying a primary biochemical determinant. *Two basic questions* follow: (1) What initiates the intrauterine disease? (2) What is responsible for its subsequent progression?

NORMAL CARDIAC EMBRYOLOGY

Information from normal mammalian cardiac morphogenesis sheds light on certain features of ventricular septal architecture, on the development of the sympathetic nervous system external to the heart and within developing cardiac muscle (sympathetic nerve endings and receptor sites), and on early intrauterine sources of circulating (non-neuronal) catecholamines. The developing septum in embryos and young fetuses has been reported to be disproportionately thick relative to left ventricular free wall, with ratios reaching 2.0[4-8]. The septal/free wall ratio then diminishes in a curvilinear fashion and approximates unity in the full-term newborn[4]. Ratios greater than 1.5/1 are occasionally found in normal neonates, but serial

7

observations on these infants have shown that the increased ratios normalize within the first few months or year of life[9].

In embryonic chick ventricular myocardium, myofibres during early cardiac morphogenesis are randomly oriented[10]. A disorderly arrangement of cellular architecture is also found in certain primitive hearts (crustaceans)[11] and in organ cultures of beating salamander myocardium[12]. During these early stages of cellular disarray, the randomly oriented fibres are believed to contract antagonistically[10]. From a phylogenetic point of view, random cellular architecture might well be a feature of early mammalian cardiac embryogenesis, but evidence in this regard is lacking[12]. Small foci of cellular disarray are present in human embryonic hearts, but these foci are similar to those found in normal fetuses, infants, children and adults[4,8,13].

NEUROEMBRYOLOGY

The nervous system develops from a thickened area of embryonic ectoderm, the neural plate, which appears during developmental stage 8 (about 18 days)[5]. The neural plate gives rise to the neural tube, which ultimately differentiates into the central nervous system, and the neural crest which differentiates into most of the peripheral nervous system[5]. Neural crest derivatives include multipolar neurons from the autonomic ganglia, chromaffin cells of the paraganglia, the sympathetic cardiac plexus and cells of the adrenal medulla[5]. Each of these derivatives is a source of norepinephrine (noradrenaline). Catecholamines have been detected in the primary sympathetic chain of the chick embryo 3.5 days after fertilization, and are prominent by the 6-to-8 day stage when the secondary sympathetic trunk is formed. In addition, the human fetal heart is capable of synthesizing norepinephrine as early as the thirteenth week of gestation. Although there is uncertainty regarding precise timing of sympathetic innervation of specific regions of the mammalian heart and regarding the establishment of definitive neuromuscular relationships[16], a number of points have nevertheless been established[14–20]. The fetal myocardial receptor sites are supersensitive to circulating norepinephrine and to neuronal release of norepinephrine caused by stellate stimulation despite relatively fewer β-adrenergic receptor sites per cell[18,19,21–23]. Immature cardiac sympathetic nerve endings possess a reduced capacity to bind and inactivate circulating norepinephrine[20]; the reduced inactivation permits higher concentrations of the neurotransmitter to reach and stimulate myocardial receptors, providing the substrate for 'supersensitivity'[20]. Tyrosine hydroxylase and monoamine oxidase, for example, are important for norepinephrine biosynthesis and degradation, and are located in intracellular storage vesicles within terminations of sympathetic nerves[20,24]. Importantly, inheritance plays a significant role in the regulation of the catecholamine biosynthetic and metabolic enzymes[24]. Concentrations of these enzymes (and of norepinephrine) are lowest in the fetal heart, higher in the newborn, and highest in the adult heart[20].

Conversely, the adrenal gland has abundant stores of norepinephrine during developmental stages when the opposite is true for the heart[18,21]. Plasma catecholamine concentrations in the newborn are about thirtyfold greater than in the adult, while neonatal myocardial catecholamine content is one tenth of adult levels[18]. These data point to a dominant role for circulating catecholamines at birth and earlier, underscoring the importance of non-neural adrenergic amines in the maintenance of circulatory integrity in the young[18].

A glycoprotein, 'nerve growth factor', plays an indisputable role in the normal development of sympathetic ganglia and in the growth and maintenance of sympathetic innervation of the heart[25-28]. Administration of the glycoprotein to neonatal mice causes not only extensive ganglionic hypertrophy, but also causes a fivefold elevation in the specific activity of tyrosine hydroxylase and dopamine-β-hydroxylase in the superior cervical ganglion[28]. Regenerating central and peripheral norepinephrine neurons appear to be most sensitive to the action of nerve growth factor during the very early stages of the regeneration process[27].

In the light of this background on normal cardiac embryology and neuroembryology, let me now elaborate on the *anatomical, physiological* and *clinical points* posed earlier.

Three *anatomical features*, two gross and one histological (ultrastructural) must be considered, namely, ventricular septal mass (disproportionate septal thickness, asymmetric septal hypertrophy), ventricular septal configuration (catenoid), and extensive septal cellular disarray[2,3,11,29-32]. Teare's report of 'asymmetrical hypertrophy of the heart'[33] was formalized in 1973 as an important gross anatomic feature of genetic hypertrophic cardiomyopathy[2,30]. While asymmetric septal hypertrophy occurs in other cardiac diseases (both acquired and congenital)[2,8,32,34], and is not always present in hypertrophic cardiomyopathy[29], it nevertheless remains the most typical gross anatomical marker[35], with a specificity of 90%[29]. In the occasional infant born with clinically overt hypertrophic cardiomyopathy, asymmetric septal hypertrophy is present at birth and therefore *in utero*[36]. It is not known, however, whether a disproportionately thick septum is constantly present at birth in infants destined years or decades later to manifest the clinically overt disease.

It has been postulated that failure of regression and subsequent progression of the normal intrauterine disproportionate septal thickness (*see* Normal Cardiac Embryology, above) is fundamental in the pathogenesis of hypertrophic cardiomyopathy[32,37]. If this proposal is correct, what mechanism(s) might be responsible for failure of regression of the thick intrauterine septum? A causal role has been assigned to abnormal septal curvature (catenoid shape) at the time of septal formation[32]. This argument holds that the catenoid shape with its net zero curvature and inherently isometric contraction (adjacent fibre tracks with opposite curvatures would develop maximum tension but would not have motion) initiates both fibre disarray and local hypertrophy, setting the stage for disproportionate septal thickness[32]. An alternative proposal is that early and extensive intrauterine

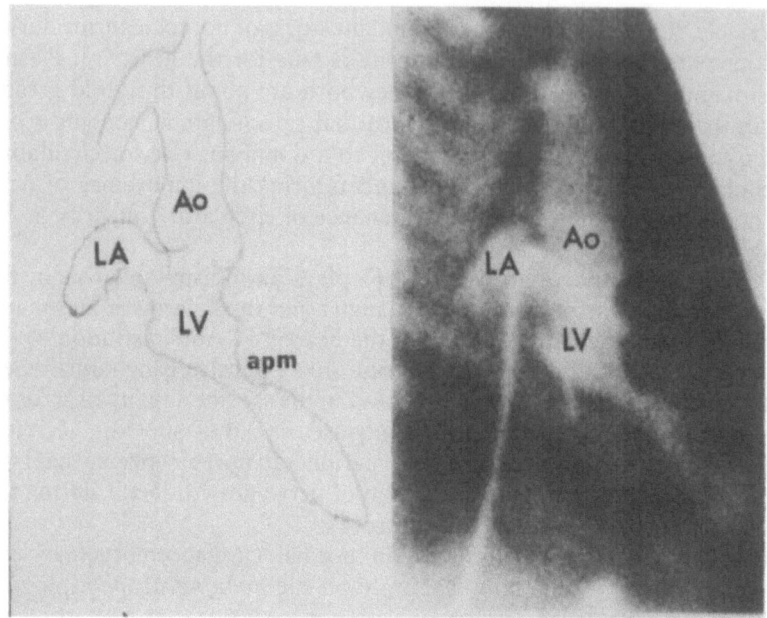

Figure 2.1.1 Left ventricular cineangiocardiogram (systolic frame, right anterior oblique) from an infant with genetic hypertrophic obstructive cardiomyopathy. There is typical cavity obliteration. Ao = aorta; LA = left atrium. (With kind permission, Dr David C. Schwartz, Cincinnati Children's Hospital, Cincinnati, Ohio)

septal cellular disarray initiates isometric contraction that in turn results in failure of regression of disproportionate septal thickness of the fetus[37].

The most characteristic microscopic feature of genetic hypertrophic cardiomyopathy is the cellular disarray described by Teare as 'a bizarre arrangement of bundles of muscle fibres running in diverse directions'[33]. The specificity of cellular disarray has been questioned, and there is little doubt that it occurs in hearts not afflicted with hypertrophic cardiomyopathy[3,4,8]. Maron *et al.*[13,38] sought to clarify this ambiguity by proposing that septal cellular disarray is significantly more common (95% of patients) and quantitatively considerably more extensive in hypertrophic cardiomyopathy than in other cardiac disorders or in normal subjects. Fibre disarray of the same extent occurs in other settings[39], but in its proper clinical and pathological context, extensive septal cellular disarray remains an important marker of genetic hypertrophic cardiomyopathy[39].

Three *physiological points* can now be stated, namely (1) the hypercontractile left ventricular free wall, (2) the relatively hypocontractile ventricular septum and (3) left ventricular cavity obliteration in latter systole. Normal ventricular contraction consists of an isovolumetric phase that occupies about 10% of systole, and an ejection phase with fibre shortening that occupies 80–90% of systole. In genetic hypertrophic cardiomyopathy, a third phase is added. Ejection is completed in the first 60–80% of systole; the cavity then obliterates and the myocardium contracts isometrically.

Thus, an important haemodynamic feature of hypertrophic cardio-myopathy is a prolonged and abnormally powerful isometric contraction phase accompanied by a relatively hypodynamic septum and hyperdynamic free wall[40].

Several clinical points must now be posed. The overt disease is sometimes manifest at birth (Figure 2.1.1) and therefore must have been present *in utero*[36]. However, the disease is usually clinically occult in the neonate and in early childhood, progressing over a decade or more to its overt state. What *initiates* genetic hypertrophic cardiomyopathy? Genetic transmission implies that the primary fault requires biochemical definition. The second basic question follows: What is responsible for progression of the initially occult disease to its clinically overt state a decade or more after birth?

ANATOMICAL AND PHYSIOLOGICAL POINTS ELABORATED

In its proper clinical and pathological context, extensive myocardial fibre disarray is an important morphological marker in hypertrophic cardiomyopathy[39,41]. The extensive cellular disarray in semilunar valve atresia with an intact ventricular septum, in the infundibulum of hearts with tetralogy of Fallot, and in the border zones of myocardial infarction should not obscure the potential importance of this ultrastructural feature in the pathogenesis of genetic hypertrophic cardiomyopathy[39].

What is responsible for extensive septal cellular disarray? Is this pattern 'primary', that is, does it precede the gross anatomical abnormalities of septal mass and configuration? Does the isometric contraction inherent in both the 'catenoid' shape and left ventricular cavity obliteration serve as an initiating cause or a later synergistic cause of cellular disarray, that is, do septal shape and cavity obliteration play primary or secondary roles in pathogenesis? Stated somewhat differently, does isometric contraction (catenoid shape and/or cavity obliteration) cause (initiate) cellular disarray, or does cellular disarray cause (initiate) isometric septal contraction? These questions should be addressed in the light of genetic transmission which implies a primary biochemical defect as the initiating pathogenetic abnormality.

A catenoid shape has the distinctive property of net zero curvature of every point on its surface[32]. The ventricular septum of hearts with genetic hypertrophic cardiomyopathy has a configuration that may resemble a catenoid[32,42]. If the configuration of the embryonic septum were catenoid, that shape could in turn account for both isometric contraction and cellular disarray[32]. Consideration must be given, however, to the observation that the entire septum is not always that extensively thickened in hypertrophic cardiomyopathy but, instead, the disproportionate hypertrophy (thickening) may selectively involve the basal, mid, or apical portions[43–45] without a catenoid shape.

That cavity obliteration with isometric contraction can be responsible for cellular disarray has been convincingly argued, using as models hearts with semilunar valve atresia and intact ventricular septum[39]. However, infants of diabetic mothers sometimes exhibit hypertrophic cardiomyopathy with typical cavity obliteration, but at necropsy there is no cellular disarray, and the hypertrophic cardiomyopathy with asymmetric septal hypertrophy consistently regresses[46–49]. Accordingly, cavity obliteration, even in the developing heart, does not necessarily provoke cellular disarray, and is therefore not likely to be the initiating cause of the fundamental ultrastructure abnormality in genetic hypertrophic cardiomyopathy.

Alternatively, intrauterine septal cellular disarray may be initiated by a disorder of catecholamines. In 1973, Goodwin[50] proposed and later reaffirmed[51] that an abnormality of catecholamines might be at the root of hypertrophic cardiomyopathy. He stated: 'If the catecholamine hypothesis has any validity, it is likely that the relationship is a complex one that exerts its effect on the growing myocardium, rather than a simple matter of excessive amounts of catecholamines acting on the heart over a prolonged period later in life'[51].

THE CATECHOLAMINE HYPOTHESIS: EXPERIMENTAL EVIDENCE

One line of reasoning that bears on this idea is experimental – observations on norepinephrine and on the glycoprotein 'nerve growth factor'. Norepinephrine, an endogenous catecholamine, is synthesized in intraneural granules and stored in sympathetic nerve endings of the myocardium. Stimulation of β-adrenergic receptor sites on myocardial cell surfaces results from activation of cardiac sympathetic nerve endings that release stored norepinephrine, and from circulating (non-cardiac) norepinephrine. Fetal myocardial adrenergic receptor sites are 'supersensitive' to norepinephrine (*see above*), which is available to the circulation from stores in the developing adrenal gland and extra-adrenal chromaffin tissue (the paraganglia and organs of Zukerkandl)[18,21,22]. The interaction between circulating norepinephrine and supersensitive myocardial receptor sites is finely balanced during normal intrauterine and cardiac development[19]. A pivotal question is whether and how this balance is disturbed *in utero* in subjects subsequently fated to develop overt genetic hypertrophic cardiomyopathy.

Norepinephrine appears to be important in the induction of myocardial cellular growth[52]. Chronic non-hypertensive infusions in mature dogs are capable of producing cardiac hypertrophy[53]. The left ventricular hypertrophy in systemic hypertension is sometimes out of proportion to the degree of afterload, and a link between hypertrophy and the autonomic nervous system has been proposed[54]. Basic information on the property of norepinephrine in inducing myocyte growth comes from observations in tissue cultures[55]. Cells maintained in a serum-free medium do not increase in size, but chronic exposure to isoproterenol or norepinephrine significantly stimulates cell hypertrophy[55]. Accordingly, myocardial cell hypertrophy can be induced in culture, and is regulated by variations in the culture medium

12

including catecholamines, serum hormones and growth factors[55]. These observations underscore the regulation of myocardial cell hypertrophy by non-haemodynamic factors[55]. Conversely, it is also relevant that long-term β-adrenergic blockade in young rabbits causes a reduction in the rate of cardiac growth[56].

Nerve growth factor, a naturally occurring glycoprotein, is necessary for growth and maintenance of sympathetic and certain sensory neurons[26-28] (see above), is present in human placental cotyledons[25], and elicits its maximum effect during embryogenesis[26]. Increased stimulation of receptor sites can result from a nerve growth hormone-induced increase in tyrosine hydroxylase, causing augmented biosynthesis of norepinephrine at the sympathetic nerve endings[28]. When nerve growth factor was administered to newborn puppies and to pregnant bitches, heart weights increased; the hypertrophy was either asymmetric or concentric with severely compromised left ventricular cavities[57]. On electron microscopy, myofibrillar disarray was the most characteristic abnormality[57]. Myocardial catecholamine content was increased[57]. Since myocardial catecholamine content directly reflects the degree of sympathetic innervation, these data imply that administration of nerve growth factor in that experimental setting resulted in an increase in sympathetic innervation of the heart[57]. The interaction between placental nerve growth factor and sympathetic innervation during normal intrauterine cardiac development must be a delicate one. An important unanswered question is whether this interaction is deranged in utero in subjects destined to develop clinically overt hypertrophic cardiomyopathy.

If extensive fibre disarray is the basic ultrastructural component in the pathogenesis of genetic hypertrophic cardiomyopathy, a fundamental question is: what initiates the fibre disarray? There is reason to believe that the primary cause may not be isometric contraction (cavity obliteration) or a catenoid-shaped septum, but instead a biochemical abnormality. This proposal is in accord with genetic transmission which presupposes a biochemical determinant. Important light was shed on these points in a study of overcontraction and excess actin elements in specimens from endomyocardial biopsies of the ventricular septum in patients with hypertrophic cardiomyopathy[58]. The purpose of that study was to define the relationship between overcontraction of the sarcomeres, the ensuing arrangements of actin filaments, and the effect on muscle fibres. The authors confirmed overcontraction of sarcomeres, with actin filaments irregularly distributed within a given hexagon[58]. Excessive shortening of sarcomeres was held responsible for overlap of actin filaments, and the overlap was believed to result in disarray of the actin filaments[58]. The ensuing ultrastructural derangement should influence sarcomere function, with forces within the sarcomere non-synergistic wherever maximal disarray is located[58]. The end result – a thick, hypocontractile muscle. If these observations are correct, overcontraction of the sarcomeres is a basic element of fibre disarray[58]. The stimulus to overcontraction (intensified shortening) of sarcomeres then becomes fundamental to our understanding of the pathogenesis of hypertrophic cardiomyopathy. It is here that the link with the autonomic nervous system (catecholamines) may be forged.

THE CATECHOLAMINE HYPOTHESIS: CLINICAL EVIDENCE

The second line of reasoning in the proposed link of genetic hypertrophic cardiomyopathy to norepinephrine and the adrenergic nervous system is clinical and admittedly largely circumstantial – observations on a group of otherwise unrelated diseases that have in common the occasional occurrence of hypertrophic cardiomyopathy together with disorders (or presumed disorders) of catecholamines and the sympathetic nervous system[37,50]. It is important to recognize that the majority of diagnoses of cardiomyopathy in these settings lack necropsy confirmation[37]. It must also be borne in mind that genetic hypertrophic cardiomyopathy is sufficiently prevalent to warn against assuming that its occasional coexistence with another disease represents sequence and not coincidence.

Lentiginosis is a genetic disorder in which cardiac involvement takes the form of hypertrophic cardiomyopathy confirmed at necropsy[59-61]. The pigmentary abnormalities of the skin and mucous membranes involve neural crest derivatives (melanoblasts, precursors of melanocytes)[59]. The relationship between catecholamines and melanocytes is reflected in a common embryological pathway as well as in presumed secretory activity of the naevoid lentigines[59]. Further to this point, pigmented naevi are occasionally profuse in patients with Noonan's syndrome (Turner phenotype with normal karyotype); hypertrophic cardiomyopathy has been described in this syndrome but without necropsy proof of both asymmetric septal hypertrophy and extensive septal cellular disarray[62-64]. Nor are the Noonan cases with hypertrophic cardiomyopathy clearly those with profuse pigmented naevi.

Clinical diagnoses of hypertrophic cardiomyopathy have been reported in von Recklinghausen's disease, which is characterized by pigmented skin lesions and multiple neurofibromas; a relationship with norepinephrine and the adrenergic nervous system has been proposed[50,65]. This relationship could rest on either or both of two assumptions: secretory activity of the pigmented lesions themselves, or the documented elevations of nerve growth factor[66]. The neuroproliferation in von Recklinghausen's disease might be a response to nerve growth factor, or the neurofibromas might secrete the glycoprotein[67]. Furthermore, there is an association between von Recklinghausen's disease and phaeochromocytoma, a norepinephrine-producing tumour, and attention has been called to patients with phaeochromocytoma and clinical diagnoses of hypertrophic cardiomyopathy[50,68] (Figure 2.1.2). There is also a connection between neurofibromatosis and tuberous sclerosis, and one report mentions a clinical diagnosis of hypertrophic cardiomyopathy in a patient with tuberous sclerosis[69].

In Friedreich's ataxia, the cardiomyopathy may express itself as either asymmetric or concentric left ventricular hypertrophy[70,71] (Figure 2.1.3). Plasma catecholamines are significantly elevated in some patients[72]. In-

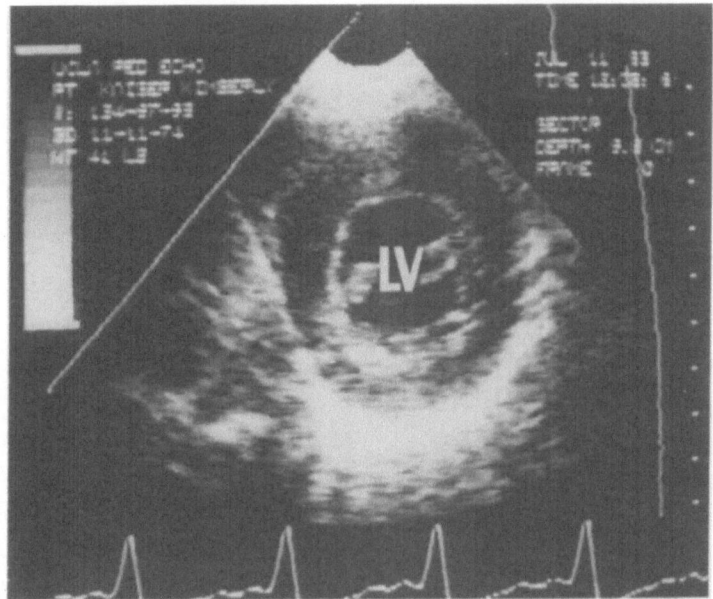

Figure 2.1.2 Two-dimensional echocardiogram (short axis) from a 9-year-old girl with phaeochromocytoma, intermittent hypertension and symmetrical left ventricular hypertrophy

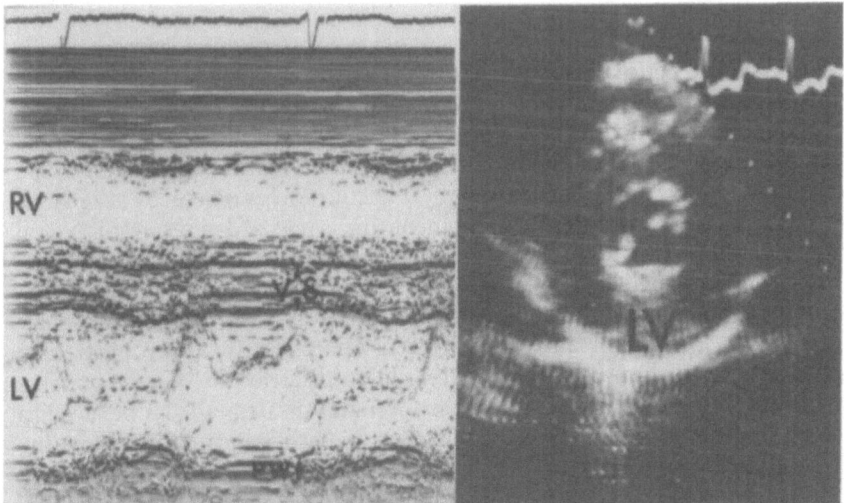

Figure 2.1.3 Echocardiograms from two patients with Friedreich's ataxia. The M-mode, from a 39-year-old man, shows a disproportionately thick ventricular septum (VS). PW = posterior wall, LV = left ventricle; RV = right ventricle. The 2D (short axis), from a 26-year-old man, shows concentric left ventricular hypertrophy

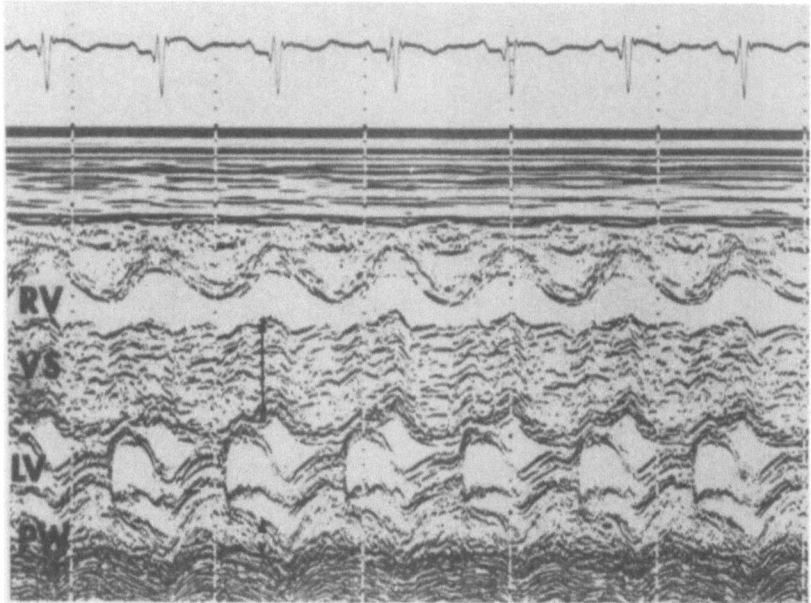

Figure 2.1.4 M-mode echocardiogram from an infant of a diabetic mother. There is hypertrophic cardiopathy with marked disproportionate septal thickening and systolic anterior motion of the anterior mitral leaflet. RV = right ventricle; LV = left ventricle; VS = ventricular septum; PW = posterior wall

creased sympathetic stimulation has been held responsible for inappropriate sinus tachycardia in Friedreich's ataxia[73] since early observations in 1938[74].

Infants of diabetic mothers sometimes exhibit typical echocardiographic (Figure 2.1.4), haemodynamic and angiographic features of hypertrophic cardiomyopathy[46,47,75]. The fetus of the diabetic mother is beset by adrenergic stimulation, since intrauterine norepinephrine is released in response to fetal hypoglycaemia caused by fetal hyperinsulinism and exogenous maternal insulin[76]. Nevertheless, this form of hypertrophic cardiomyopathy is transient with the disproportionate septal thickness resolving during early infancy[46,47,49,75]. Importantly, necropsied infants show disproportionate septal thickness but *not* significant cellular disarray[47,75]. These patients therefore lack the hallmark of extensive cellular disarray that is believed to be pathogenetically important in genetic hypertrophic cardiomyopathy. Resolution during early infancy is in accord with the view that marked cellular disorganization is required for the persistence and progression of asymmetric septal hypertrophy. The cause of disproportionate septal thickness in infants of diabetic mothers may therefore be related to fetal hyperinsulinism[49]. Interestingly, there is a distinct homology between nerve growth factor and insulin[28].

Pancreatic islet cell tumours and nesidioblastosis (hyperplasia of islets) are characterized metabolically by persistence of inappropriately high levels of circulating insulin during fasting hypoglycaemia. An association between these disorders and clinical hypertrophic cardiomoyopathy was identified in both adults[37] and infants[49].

Additional evidence of hormonal-induced cellular disarray and hypertrophic cardiomyopathy stems from observations on thyroid hormone. Three cases of clinical hypertrophic cardiomyopathy and hyperthyroidism have been described[77]. More to the point, when TRIAC (diethanolamine salt of triiodothyroacetic acid) was administered to pregnant female rats and to non-gravid adult animals, the offspring had hypertrophy and widespread cellular disarray, while the hearts of mothers and non-pregnant females given TRIAC showed cardiac hypertrophy but no cellular disarray[78]. These observations provide evidence of hormonal-induced cellular disarray, and underscore the vulnerability of the developing, immature heart in this regard.

PROPOSED PATHOGENETIC SEQUENCE

Phase one (Figure 2.1.5)

Intrauterine septal cellular disarray may be the primary pathogenetic *ultrastructural* abnormality. Overcontraction (intensified shortening) of sarcomeres may provoke overlap of actin filaments producing disarray of

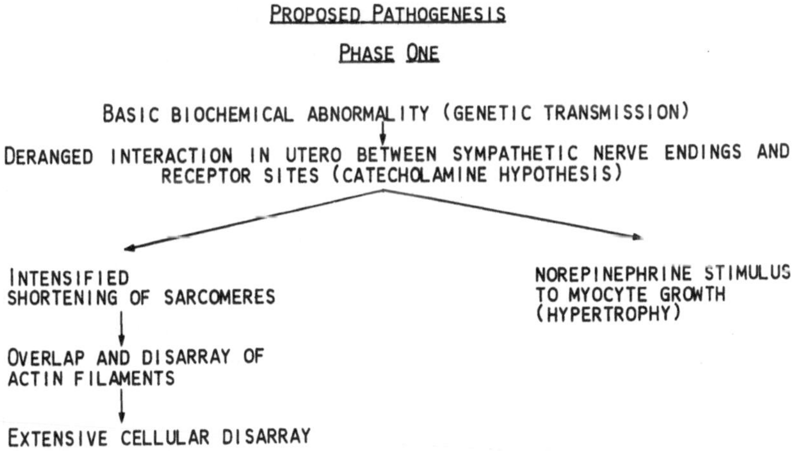

PROPOSED PATHOGENESIS

PHASE ONE

BASIC BIOCHEMICAL ABNORMALITY (GENETIC TRANSMISSION)

DERANGED INTERACTION IN UTERO BETWEEN SYMPATHETIC NERVE ENDINGS AND RECEPTOR SITES (CATECHOLAMINE HYPOTHESIS)

INTENSIFIED SHORTENING OF SARCOMERES

NOREPINEPHRINE STIMULUS TO MYOCYTE GROWTH (HYPERTROPHY)

OVERLAP AND DISARRAY OF ACTIN FILAMENTS

EXTENSIVE CELLULAR DISARRAY

Figure 2.1.5 Proposed pathogenesis – phase one

the filaments. The stimulus to over-contraction and cellular disarray is likely to originate as a biochemical abnormality that is genetically determined. The biochemical abnormality may express itself as deranged interaction of the cardiac sympathetic nerve endings and their receptor sites (catecholamine hypothesis).

Phase two (Figure 2.1.6)

Myocardial cellular disarray, irrespective of cause, is a powerful stimulus for hypertrophy. Onset of extensive septal disarray *in utero* could result in

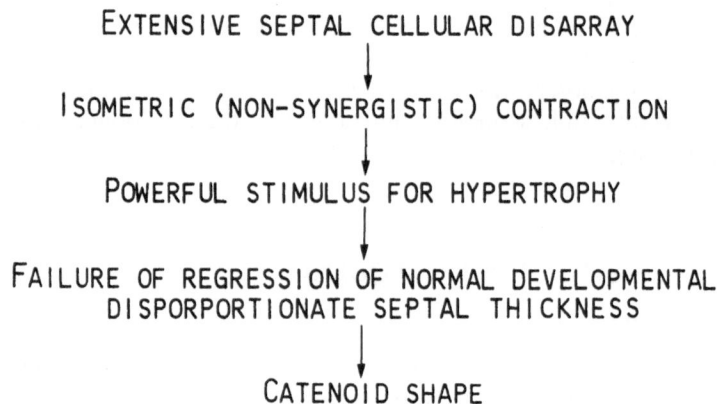

PHASE TWO

EXTENSIVE SEPTAL CELLULAR DISARRAY

ISOMETRIC (NON-SYNERGISTIC) CONTRACTION

POWERFUL STIMULUS FOR HYPERTROPHY

FAILURE OF REGRESSION OF NORMAL DEVELOPMENTAL DISPORPORTIONATE SEPTAL THICKNESS

CATENOID SHAPE

Figure 2.1.6   Proposed pathogenesis – phase two

failure of regression of the normal developmental disproportionate septal thickness, setting the stage for subsequent extrauterine progression to the clinically overt disease.

Phase three (Figure 2.1.7)

Extensive ventricular septal cellular disarray may be the primary cause of isometric contraction and of the relatively adynamic septum. Exaggerated contractility of the left ventricular free wall may in part be compensatory and in part a response to adrenergic stimulation acting synergistically to increase contractility still further. The hypercontractile left ventricular free wall is associated with cavity obliteration and a prolonged and abnormally powerful isometric contraction phase. Isometric contraction serves to promote additional cellular disarray. If the abnormally thick septum assumes a catenoid shape, either *in utero* or later, the isometric contraction caused by that shape may promote further cellular disarray.

Conclusions

This proposed pathogenetic sequence takes into account three anatomical points – ventricular septal cellular disarray, asymmetric septal hypertrophy and septal shape; three physiological points – adynamic septal contraction, hypercontractile left ventricular free wall, and cavity obliteration; and three

PATHOGENESIS OF HYPERTROPHIC CARDIOMYOPATHY

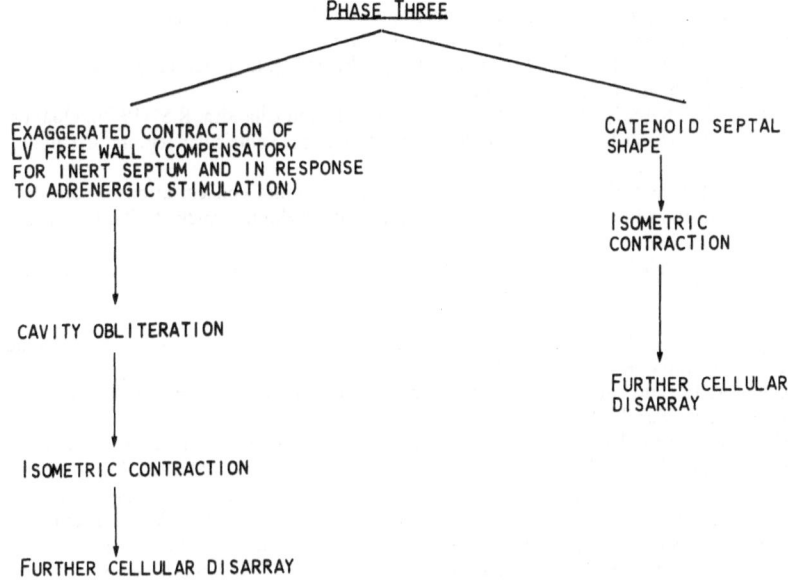

PHASE THREE

EXAGGERATED CONTRACTION OF
LV FREE WALL (COMPENSATORY
FOR INERT SEPTUM AND IN RESPONSE
TO ADRENERGIC STIMULATION)

CATENOID SEPTAL
SHAPE

↓

ISOMETRIC
CONTRACTION

↓

CAVITY OBLITERATION

↓

FURTHER CELLULAR
DISARRAY

↓

ISOMETRIC CONTRACTION

↓

FURTHER CELLULAR DISARRAY

Figure 2.1.7 Proposed pathogenesis – phase three

clinical points – presence of the disorder at birth and therefore *in utero*, subsequent extrauterine progression to the clinically overt disease, and the implication that the pathogenesis of a genetic disorder requires a primary biochemical definition.

References

1. Maron, B.J., Pickle, N.L.W. and Mulvihill, J.J. (1983). Echocardiographic assessment of patterns of inheritance in hypertrophic cardiomyopathies: a genetic disease or multiple etiologies. *Circulation*, 68, 111–62 (Abstract)
2. Henry, W.L., Clark, C.E. and Epstein, S.E. (1973). Asymmetric septal hypertrophy (ASH): Unifying link in the IHSS disease spectrum. *Circulation*, 47, 827
3. Maron, B.J., Ferrans, V.J., Henry, W.L., Clark, C.E., Redwood, D.R., Roberts, W.C., Morrow, A.G. and Epstein, S.E. (1974). Differences in distribution of myocardial abnormalities in patients with obstructive and nonobstructive asymmetric septal hypertrophy (ASH): light and electron microscopic findings. *Circulation*, 50, 436
4. Maron, B.J., Verter, J. and Kapur, S. (1978). Disproportionate ventricular septal thickening in the developing normal human heart. *Circulation*, 57, 520
5. Moore, A.L. (1977). *The Developing Human*. 2nd Edn. p. 348. (Philadelphia: Saunders)
6. Hamilton, W.J. and Mossman, H.W. (eds.) (1972). *Human Embryology*. 4th Edn. p. 250. (Baltimore: Williams & Wilkins)
7. Van Mierop, L.H.S. (1974). Embryology. In Netter, F.H. and Yonkman, F.Y. (eds.) *Heart*. (The CIBA Collection of Medical Illustrations, Vol. 5.) (Summit, NJ: CIBA Pharmaceutical)
8. Bulkley, B.H., Weisfeldt, M.L. and Hutchins, G.M. (1977). Asymmetric septal hypertrophy and myocardial fiber disarray. *Circulation*, 56, 292
9. Larter, W.E., Allen, H.D., Sahn, D.J. and Goldberg, S.J. (1976). The asymmetrically hypertrophied septum: further differentiation of its causes. *Circulation*, 53, 19
10. Manasek, F.J. (1970). Histogenesis of the embryonic myocardium. *Am. J. Cardiol.*, 25, 149

11. Ferrans, V.J., Morrow, A.G. and Roberts, W.C. (1972). Myocardial ultrastructure in idiopathic hypertrophic subaortic stenosis. *Circulation*, **45**, 769
12. Millhouse, E.W., Chiakulas, J.J. and Scheving, L.E. (1971). Long-term organ culture of the salamander heart. *J. Cell Biol.*, **40**, 1
13. Maron, B.J., Sato, N., Roberts, W.C., Edwards, J.E. and Chandra, R.S. (1979). Quantitative analysis of cardiac muscle cell disorganization in the ventricular septum. *Circulation*, **60**, 685
14. Ignarro, L.J. and Shideman, F.E. (1968). Appearance and concentrations of catecholamines and their biosynthesis in the embryonic and developing chick. *J. Pharmacol. Exp. Ther.*, **159**, 38
15. Enemar, A., Flick, B. and Hakanson, R. (1965). Observations on the appearance of norepinephrine in the sympathetic nervous system of the chick embryo. *Devel. Biol.*, **11**, 268
16. Pappano, A.J. (1977). Ontogenetic development of autonomic neuroeffector transmission and transmitter reactivity in embryonic and fetal hearts. *Pharmacol. Rev.*, **29**, 3
17. Gennser, G. and Studnitz, W. (1975). Noradrenaline synthesis in human fetal heart. *Experientia (Basel)*, **31**, 1422
18. Geis, W.P., Tatoales, C.J., Priola, D.V. and Friedman, W.F. (1975). Factors influencing neurohumoral control of the heart in the newborn dog. *Am. J. Physiol.*, **228**, 1685
19. Friedman, W.F. (1973). The actions of cardioactive drugs on developing myocardium. In Harmison, L.T. (ed.) *Research Animals in Medicine*. p. 735. DHEW Publication No. (NIH) 72–333, (Bethesda, MD: Department of Health, Education and Welfare)
20. Friedman, W.F. (1972). The intrinsic physiologic properties of the developing heart. In Friedman, W.F., Lesch, M. and Sonnenblick, E.H. (eds.) *Neonatal Heart Disease*, p. 21. (New York: Grune & Stratton)
21. Friedman, W.F., Pool, P.E., Jacobowitz, D., Seagren, S.C. and Braunwald, E. (1968). Sympathetic innervation of the developing rabbit heart. *Circ. Res.*, **23**, 25
22. Kralios, F.A. and Miller, C.K. (1978). Functional development of cardiac sympathetic nerves in newborn dogs. *Cardiovasc. Res.*, **12**, 547
23. Dempsey, P.J. and Cooper, T. (1968). Supersensitivity of the chronically denervated feline heart. *Am. J. Physiol.*, **215**, 1245
24. Weinshilboum, R.M. (1983). Biochemical genetics of catecholamines in humans. *Mayo Clin. Proc.*, **58**, 319
25. Goldstein, L.D., Reynolds, C.P. and Perez-Palo, J.R. (1978). Isolation of human nerve growth factor from placental tissue. *Neurochem. Res.*, **3**, 175
26. Mobley, W.C., Server, A.C., Ishii, D.N., Riopelle, R.J. and Shooter, E.M. (1977). Nerve growth factor. *N. Engl. J. Med.*, **297**, 1096
27. Kaye, M.P., Wells, D.J. and Tyce, G.M. (1979). Nerve growth factor-enhanced reinnervation of surgically denervated canine heart. *Am. J. Physiol.*, **236**, H624
28. Golde, D.W., Herschman, H.R., Lusis, A.J. and Groopman, J.E. (1980). Growth factors. *Ann. Intern. Med.*, **92**, 650
29. Maron, B.J. and Epstein, S.E. (1980). Hypertrophic cardiomyopathy. Recent observations regarding the specificity of three hallmarks of the disease: asymmetric septal hypertrophy, septal disorganization and systolic anterior motion of the anterior mitral leaflet. *Am. J. Cardiol.*, **45**, 141
30. Henry, W.L., Clark, C.E. and Epstein, S.E. (1973). Asymmetric septal hypertrophy. *Circulation*, **47**, 225
31. Wigle, E.D. and Silver, M.D. (1978). Myocardial fibre disarray and ventricular septal hypertrophy in asymmetrical hypertrophy of the heart. *Circulation*, **58**, 398
32. Hutchins, G.M. and Bulkley, B.H. (1978). Catenoid shape of the interventricular septum: possible cause of idiopathic hypertrophic subaortic stenosis. *Circulation*, **58**, 392
33. Teare, R.D. (1958). Asymmetrical hypertrophy of the heart. *Br. Heart J.*, **20**, 1
34. Maron, B.J., Edwards, J.E., Ferrans, V.J., Clark, C.E., Lebowitz, E.A., Henry, W.L. and Epstein, S.E. (1975). Congenital heart malformations associated with disproportionate ventricular septal thickening. *Circulation*, **52**, 926
35. Roberts, W.C. and Ferrans, V.J. (1975). Pathologic anatomy of the cardiomyopathies. *Hum. Pathol.*, **6**, 287

36. Maron, D.J., Edwards, J.E., Henry, W.L., Clark, E.C., Bingle, G.J. and Epstein, S.E. (1974). Asymmetric septal hypertrophy (ASH) in infancy. *Circulation*, 50, 809
37. Perloff, J.K. (1981). Pathogenesis of hypertrophic cardiomyopathy: hypotheses and speculations. *Am. Heart J.*, 101, 219
38. Maron, B.J. and Roberts, W.C. (1979). Quantitative analysis of cardiac muscle cell disorganization in the ventricular septum in patients with hypertrophic cardiomyopathy. *Circulation*, 59, 698
39. Bulkley, B.H., D'Amico, B. and Taylor, A.L. (1983). Extensive myocardial fiber disarray in aortic and pulmonary atresia. *Circulation*, 67, 191
40. Wyne, J. and Braunwald, E. (1980). The cardiomyopathies and myocarditides. In Braunwald, E. (ed.) *Heart Disease*, p. 1437. (Philadelphia: Saunders)
41. Maron, B.J. (1983). Myocardial disorganization in hypertrophic cardiomyopathy. *Br. Heart J.*, 50, 1
42. Silverman, K.J., Hutchins, G.M., Weiss, J.L. and Moore, G.W. (1982). Catenoidal shape of the interventricular septum in idiopathic hypertrophic subaortic stenosis: two dimensional echocardiographic confirmation. *Am. J. Cardiol.*, 49, 27
43. Yamaguchi, H., Ishimura, T., Nishiyama, S., Negasaki, F., Takatsu, F., Nakanishi, S., Nishijo, T., Umeda, T. and Machii, K. (1979). Hypertrophic nonobstructive cardiomyopathy with giant negative T waves (apical hypertrophy). *Am J. Cardiol.*, 44, 401
44. Maron, B.J., Bonow, R.O., Seshagiri, T.N.R., Roberts, W.C. and Epstein, S.E. (1982). Hypertrophic cardiomyopathy with ventricular septal hypertrophy localized to the apical region of the left ventricle (apical hypertrophic cardiomyopathy). *Am. J. Cardiol.*, 49, 1838
45. Maron, B.J., Gotdiener, J.S., and Epstein, S.E. (1981). Patterns and significance of the distribution of left ventricular hypertrophy in hypertrophic cardiomyopathy. *Am. J. Cardiol.*, 48, 418
46. Way, G.L., Wolfe, R.R. Eshaghpour, E., Bender, R.L., Jaffee, R.B. and Ruttenberg, H.D. (1979). The natural history of hypertrophic cardiomyopathy in infants of diabetic mothers. *J. Pediatr.*, 95, 1020
47. Breitweser, J.A., Meyer, R.A., Sperling, M.A., Tsang, R.C. and Kaplan, S. (1980). Cardiac septal hypertrophy in hyperinsulinemic infants. *J Pediatr.*, 96, 535
48. Gutgesell, H.P., Speer, M.E. and Rosenberg, H.S. (1980). Characterization of the cardiomyopathy in infants of diabetic mothers. *Circulation*, 61, 441
49. Gutgesell, H.P., Mullins, C.E., Gillette, P.C., Speer, M., Rudolph, A.J. and McNamara, D.G. (1976). Transient hypertrophic subaortic stenosis in infants of diabetic mothers. *J. Pediatr.*, 89, 120
50. Goodwin, J.F. (1974). Prospects and predictions for the cardiomyopathies. *Circulation*, 50, 210
51. Goodwin, J.F. (1979). Cardiomyopathy: an interface between fundamental and clinical cardiology. In Hayasi, S. and Murao, S. (eds.) *Proceedings of the VIII World Congress of Cardiology*, p. 103. (Excerpta Medica International Congress Series No. 470.) (Amsterdam: Elsevier-North-Holland)
52. Laks, M.M. and Morady, F. (1976). Norepinephrine – the myocardial hypertrophy hormone? *Am. Heart J.*, 91, 674
53. Laks, M.M., Morady, F. and Swan, H.J.C. (1973). Myocardial hypertrophy produced by chronic infusion of subhypertensive doses of norepinephrine in the dog. *Chest*, 64, 75
54. Ostman-Smith, I. (1981). Cardiac sympathetic nerves as the final common pathway in the induction of adaptive cardiac hypertrophy. *Clin. Sci.*, 61, 265
55. Simpson, P., McGrath, A. and Savion, S. (1982). Myocyte hypertrophy in neonatal rat heart cultures and its regulation by serum and by catecholamines. *Circ. Res.*, 51, 787
56. Vaughan Williams, E.M., Tasgal, J. and Raine, A.E.G. (1977). Morphometric changes in rabbit ventricular myocardium produced by long-term beta-adrenoceptor blockade. *Lancet*, 2, 850
57. Kaye, M.P., Witzke, D.J., Wells, D.J. and Fuster, V. (1982). Cardiac effects of nerve growth factor in dogs. In Kaltenbach, M. and Epstein, S.E. (eds.) *Hypertrophic Cardiomyopathy*. p. 88. (Berlin, Heidelberg: Springer)

58. Harmjanz, D. and Reale, E. (1981). Overcontraction and excess actin filaments. Basic elements of hypertrophic cardiomyopathy. *Br. Heart J.*, **45**, 494
59. Polani, P.E. and Moynahan, E.J. (1972). Progressive cardiomyopathic lentigenosis. *Q. J. Med.*, **41**, 295
60. Somerville, J. and Bonham-Carter, R.E. (1972). The heart in lentiginosis. *Br. Heart J.*, **34**, 58
61. Moynahan, E.J. (1970). Progressive cardiomyopathic lentiginosis. *Proc. R. Soc. Med.*, **63**, 448
62. Hirsh, H.D., Gelband, H., Garcia, O., Tottlieb, S. and Tamer, D.M. (1975). Hypertrophic obstructive cardiomyopathy in Noonan's syndrome. *Circulation*, **52**, 1161
63. Ehler, K.H., Engle, M.A., Levin, A.R. and Deely, W.J. (1972). Eccentric ventricular hypertrophy and sporadic instances of 46XX,XY Turner phenotype. *Circulation*, **45**, 639
64. Phornphutkul, C., Rosenthal, A. and Nadas, A.S. (1973). Cardiomyopathy in Noonan's syndrome. *Br. Heart J.*, **35**, 99
65. Elliott, C.M., Tajik, A.J., Giuliani, E.R. and Gordon, H. (1976). Idiopathic hypertrophic subaortic stenosis associated with cutaneous neurofibromatosis. *Am. Heart J.*, **92**, 368
66. Schenkein, I., Bueker, E.D., Helson, L., Axelrod, R. and Dancis, J. (1974). Increased nerve-growth-stimulating activity in disseminated neurofibromatosis. *N. Engl. J. Med.*, **290**, 613
67. Snyder, S.H. (1974). Nerve growth in neurofibromatosis. *N. Engl. J. Med.*, **290**, 626
68. Shub, C., Williamson, D., Tajik, A.J. and Eubanks, D.R. (1981). Dynamic left ventricular outflow tract obstruction associated with pheochromocytoma. *Am. Heart J.*, **102**, 286
69. Brandenburg, R.O., Tajik, A.J., Giuliani, E.R., Weidman, W.H., Ritter, D.G., Davis, G.D. and McGoon, D.C. (1972). Congenital cardiovascular lesions associated with idiopathic hypertrophic subaortic stenosis. *Circulation*, **46**, (suppl. II) 134
70. Smith, E.R., Sangalang, V.E., Hefferman, L.P., Welch, J.P. and Flemington, C.S., (1977). Hypertrophic cardiomyopathy: the heart disease of Friedreich's ataxia. *Am. Heart J.*, **94**, 428
71. Bach, P.M., Child, J.S., Perloff, J.K., Wolfe, A. and Kark, R.A.P. (1983). *Circulation*, **68**, III–334 (Abstr.)
72. Pasternac, A., Wagniart, P., Olivenstein, R., Petitclerc, R., Krol, R., Andermann, E., Melancon, S., Geoffroy, G., de Champlain, J. and Barbeau, A. (1982). Increased plasma catecholamines in patients with Friedreich's ataxia. *Can. J. Neurol. Sci.*, **9**, 195
73. Thoren, C. (1964). Cardiomyopathy in Friedreich's ataxia. *J. Acta Paediatr.*, **153**, (Suppl.), 1
74. Hartman, J., Booth, R.W. (1960). Friedreich's ataxia: a neurocardiac disease. *Am. Heart J.*, **60**, 716
75. Halliday, H.L. (1981). Hypertrophic cardiomyopathy in infants of poorly controlled diabetic mothers. *Arch. Dis. Child.*, **56**, 258
76. Stern, L., Ramos, A. and Leduc, J. (1968). Urinary catecholamine excretion in infants of diabetic mothers. *Pediatrics*, **42**, 598
77. Symons, C., Richardson, P.J. and Feizi, O. (1974). Hypertrophic cardiomyopathy and hyperthyroidism: a report of three cases. *Thorax*, **29**, 713
78. Olsen, E.G.J., Symons, C. and Hawkey, C. (1977). Effect of triac on the developing heart. *Lancet*, **2**, 221

2.2
Clinical aspects and investigations

J.F. GOODWIN

SYMPTOMS

Dyspnoea, chest pain, palpitations, dizziness and syncope are the principal symptoms, but extreme tiredness has been noted in severe patients.

Dyspnoea

This is due to the raised left atrial pressure consequent upon the high end-diastolic pressure on the left ventricle and is most marked on effort.

Chest pain

This often closely resembles angina and may well be due to cardiac ischaemia. The exact mechanism is uncertain; probably compression of the arterial arcade in the subendocardium by the greatly hypertrophied but poorly relaxing ventricular muscle is the cause. However, prolonged attacks of pain, or even myocardial infarction, may occur in the presence of normal coronary arteries. But in 5–15% of patients atherosclerotic coronary artery disease does accompany hypertrophic cardiomyopathy, and readily explains anginal pain and infarction.

Palpitations

Palpitations may be produced by tachycardia, by powerful pulsation of the overactive ventricles, or by ectopic rhythm. Atrial fibrillation occurs in around 15%[1], and usually produces severe symptoms due to hypotension and pulmonary congestion especially if the ventricular rate is rapid. The reduced diastolic filling period and loss of atrial drive add to the circulatory embarrassment.

Supraventricular tachycardia and ectopic beats are also causes of palpitations. Occasionally, bradycardia may occur as a result of sinus node disease or other conduction defects, and the large stroke volume results in powerful beats which occasion a sensation of palpitation. Ventricular arrhythmias are very common; 30% of patients have multiform and frequent ventricular ectopic contractions or runs of ventricular tachycardia. The patients are usually virtually unaware of these arrhythmias.

Dizziness and syncope, or near-syncope

These warn of severe prognosis. Syncope is due usually to arrhythmias, notably ventricular tachycardia; but it may be due to insufficient filling of the stiff left ventricle and elimination of the left ventricular cavity in systole (Figure 2.2.1).

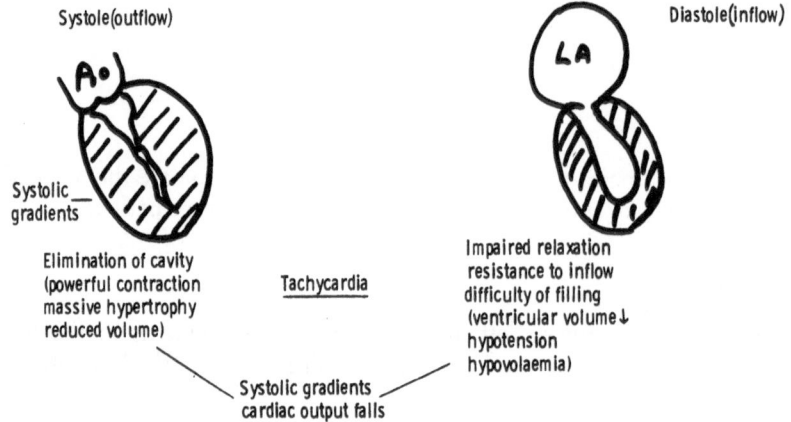

Systole(outflow)

Diastole(inflow)

Systolic gradients

Elimination of cavity (powerful contraction massive hypertrophy reduced volume)

Tachycardia

Impaired relaxation resistance to inflow difficulty of filling (ventricular volume↓ hypotension hypovolaemia)

Systolic gradients cardiac output falls

Figure 2.2.1 Diagram to show interaction between systolic and diastolic function in hypertrophic cardiomyopathy in relation to sudden death

Other observations

Despite the number of symptoms and their frequent severity, patients are often well developed, athletic and tend to underplay their symptoms. A family history of the disease or of sudden death at an early age occurs in at least 50% of patients.

CLINICAL EXAMINATION

The clinical picture has a broad spectrum ranging from normality to characteristic physical signs, depending on the extent and severity of the disease, and the presence of an intraventricular pressure gradient in systole. In typical cases with a gradient, there are three characteristic signs: the arterial pulse, the systolic murmur and the cardiac impulse[2].

The pulse has a rapid upstroke and rapid collapse; it is ill-sustained, but of normal volume. Its character is due to the powerful rapid contraction of the left ventricle and the sudden collapse occurs when the blood has left the left ventricle.

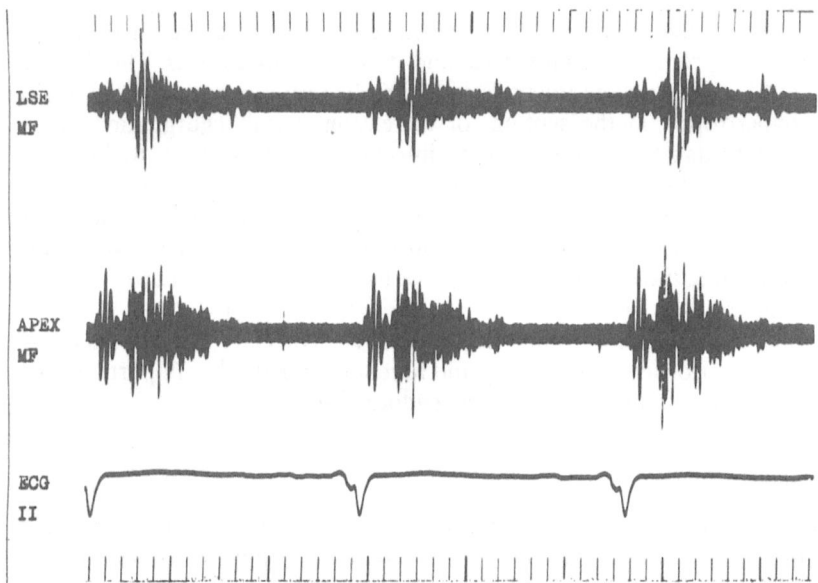

Figure 2.2.2 Ejection systolic murmur of late onset, ill-sustained arterial pulse and atrial beat shown on impulse cardiogram in hypertrophic cardiomyopathy

The cardiac impulse indicates left ventricular hypertrophy without dilatation; it is a powerful, localized ill-sustained thrust, often outside the left midclavicular line, and is preceded by a less powerful thrust, the atrial beat, due to the left atrium contracting powerfully to fill the stiff left ventricle (Figure 2.2.2)[3].

The systolic murmur is of late onset, there being a short silent period in early systole after the first heart sound. The murmur is ejection in type and extends up to aortic valve closure, which is usually normal. There may be reversed splitting of the second heart sound due to the delayed closure of the aortic valve. The murmur may vary from grade 1 to grade 4 in intensity, and is heard at the left sternal edge and apex, but rarely at the base of the heart. The systolic murmur is due to three factors: outflow pressure gradient, turbulence and mitral regurgitation. The powerful, rapidly contracting left ventricle, which expels much of its contents in the first half of systole, eliminates the mid-apical portion of the left ventricle, and creates noisy eddies, while the apposition to the mitral valve apparatus to the hypertrophied septum augments the pressure gradients produced in the body of the left ventricle. Mitral regurgitation occurs when the anterior apparatus of the mitral valve stripes the septum in systole, and is usually mild.

Occasionally an apical mid-diastolic murmur may be heard – due to slow filling of the stiff left ventricle, or to projection of the hypertrophied upper ventricular septum into the inflow tract of the left ventricle.

A third heart sound is heard in those patients whose left ventricle fills rapidly, but in others is absent. The fourth heart sound is usually too low pitched for audibility.

Murmurs may change during the course of the disease, and these changes may have prognostic significance and differing implications. The development of, or increase in intensity of, a systolic murmur suggests progression of hypertrophy in the septum, or increasing mitral regurgitation due to secondary damage to the valve by infection or calcification. Reduction in intensity of the murmur, or its disappearance, suggests that the powerful contraction of the left ventricle is waning owing to the spread of the disease process (the myofibrillar disarray and fibrosis) throughout the ventricular myocardium, indicating increasing severity that may be followed by congestive heart failure, especially if atrial fibrillation develops.

But the change in murmurs does not always correlate with the haemodynamics or disordered physiology and function, and another important cause of a change in murmur is infective endocarditis.

Electrocardiogram

The electrocardiogram may be normal, though rarely so in older adults. Typically it shows severe left ventricular hypertrophy, with deep T wave inversion and increased QRS voltage; Q waves are often seen in anterior chest leads as a result of hypertrophy and fibrosis in the septum. Broad bifid P waves indicate left atrial enlargement, and the PR interval inclines to the short range of normal. Very severe electrocardiographic changes may be seen in symptomless patients with few, if any, physical signs. These changes may occasion unwarranted fear that a silent massive heart attack has occurred[4].

Radiography

The chest radiograph is often unhelpful, but may show slight left atrial enlargement, interstitial oedema, and reduced calibre of vessels to the lower zones (flow diversion), resembling mitral stenosis. Striking cardiomegaly is unusual, but occasionally the left border of the heart may show a bulge or shelf due to massive hypertrophy.

Calcification of the mitral valve occurs in perhaps 5–10% of patients and heightens the radiological similarity to rheumatic mitral valve disease.

Echocardiography

M-mode echocardiography may show many abnormalities: notably disproportionate thickness of the interventricular septum which may be up to 1.5 times that of the posterior wall; reduction of dimension of the left ventricular cavity; decreased diastolic closure slope of the mitral valve; systolic anterior motion of the mitral valve; mid-systolic closure of the aortic valve. The ventricular septum may appear to be immobile, but this may be for technical reasons rather than a true finding.

Only when all the features are present can a definite diagnosis be made on M-mode echocardiography. When hypertrophy is asymmetrical, M-mode echocardiography may miss the diagnosis because the hypertrophied area of the septum is not traversed by the beam. Our recent work[5] has shown that, in 89 patients proven to have the disease, hypertrophy may be symmetrical (31%), asymmetrical (55%) or distal ventricular (14%). In the distal type with marked papillary muscle thickening, only one patient could be diagnosed by M-mode echocardiography.

Two-dimensional echocardiography is much more valuable, for it scans the whole of the heart and can detect asymmetrical hypertrophy. When reviewed in real time it can show the elimination of the ventricular cavity in systole by the massive septum. Thickening and calcification of the mitral valve may be represented by bright echoes and restricted movement of the valve, but usually the mitral valve appears normal.

In severe systemic hypertension, the appearances may closely resemble hypertrophic cardiomyopathy – certainly asymmetric hypertrophy can occur in hypertension, but mid-systolic closure of the aortic valve[6] and systolic anterior movement of the mitral valve are unusual in personal experience.

DIFFERENTIAL DIAGNOSIS

From the history

The most important differential diagnosis is coronary heart disease, but attacks of syncope may suggest conditions causing arrhythmia or obstruction to the blood flow through the heart or lesser circulation, such as valvar aortic stenosis, idiopathic primary pulmonary hypertension or atrial myxoma.

From the physical signs

The differential diagnosis will vary according to the presence or absence of pressure gradients in systole within the left ventricle. When these are appreciable there will be a loud systolic murmur and other characteristic signs, but a loud systolic murmur may occur in the absence of gradients. When there is a loud systolic murmur, valvar aortic stenosis, discrete subvalvar aortic stenosis, ventricular septal defect and mitral regurgitation may be suggested. The jerky arterial pulse can suggest aortic regurgitation, while the left atrial beat preceding the localized powerful ill-sustained thrust of the left ventricle may suggest severe systemic hypertension.

However, the peculiar character of the systolic murmur, with its late onset, is highly suggestive of hypertrophic cardiomyopathy, and is only closely resembled by murmurs of subvalvar mitral lesions, such as prolapsing mitral valve. When the ill-sustained pulse and atrial beat are found in association with the murmur, the diagnosis is not seriously in doubt. If there is a history of appropriate symptoms – dyspnoea on effort, chest pain, palpitation or syncope – together with a family history of sudden death, the diagnosis becomes virtually certain, and further tests are merely confirmatory.

When there are no pressure gradients, the signs may be confined to the character of the pulse and to the atrial beat. But in some patients, there may be no definitely abnormal signs, and the diagnosis may be suggested by the electrocardiogram or echocardiogram. Mild cases with no symptoms and no physical signs and with borderline electrocardiographic appearances may be impossible to diagnose with certainty, especially when echocardiography, angiography and radionuclide studies are equivocal. This is particularly true in young athletic persons who have a high cardiac output, jerky pulse, physiological ejection systolic murmur and a high ejection fraction, and a suggestion of left ventricular hypertrophy.

The differentiation from hypertensive heart disease can be extremely difficult or even impossible. Clues that help are the characteristic late onset of the murmur found in hypertrophic cardiomyopathy, but not in systemic hypertension, and the left atrial pulsation and jerky ill-sustained arterial pulse. If the electrocardiogram shows severe left ventricular hypertrophy, left atrial enlargement with short PR interval and Q waves, the diagnosis of hypertrophic cardiomyopathy is supported. Mid-systolic closure of the aortic valve and systolic anterior movement of the mitral valve both occur in hypertrophic cardiomyopathy (usually associated with pressure gradients), but are rare in hypertension. However, the differentiation of hypertrophic cardiomyopathy associated with hypertension for hypertensive heart disease can be a matter for prolonged debate.

One of the most sensitive differential diagnoses lies between hypertrophic cardiomyopathy and 'angina with normal coronary arteries'. There may be no physical signs to suggest hypertrophic cardiomyopathy, and the history may be only that of angina of effort. The electrocardiogram may be normal or non-specific, though unexplained left ventricular hypertrophy may provide a clue to the diagnosis of hypertrophic cardiomyopathy. Special attention should be paid to the *size* of the coronary arteries on angiography; they are wide of lumen and of smooth bore. Also the morphology of the left ventricle is characteristic in hypertrophic cardiomyopathy and usually makes the diagnosis (*see below*, under Angiocardiography). Prior to angiography, if there are any clinical signs remotely suggestive of hypertrophic cardiomyopathy, or the electrocardiogram shows unexplained left ventricular hypertrophy, echocardiography should be performed. However, a negative echocardiographic result does not exclude the possibility of hypertrophic cardiomyopathy.

When atrial fibrillation has developed, the diagnosis becomes even more difficult because the characteristic left atrial beat disappears and the pulse becomes less typical.

When severe mitral regurgitation has occurred, the systolic murmur becomes pansystolic and is followed by a third heart sound and short decrescendo mid-diastolic murmur. The resemblance then to rheumatic mitral valve disease becomes overwhelming, and the true diagnosis can only be known by further investigation. The echocardiograph is suggestive and the angiocardiogram is usually diagnostic.

FURTHER INVESTIGATIONS

Electrocardiographic (Holter) monitoring

The frequency of serious arrhythmia and the relation between sudden death and arrhythmia[7] make regular electrocardiographic monitoring essential, especially as much arrhythmia is undetected by the patients[1,6-10].

Monitoring should be for a minimum of 24 hours – usually 48 hours is advisable.

The frequency with which Holter monitoring should be carried out has not been formally laid down. In patients with poor prognostic factors (young age, strong family history, symptoms and signs) it should be not less than at 3-monthly intervals; with others, at 6-monthly intervals, except those with minimal risk factors (see Chapters 2.2 and 2.3) who can be assessed at yearly intervals. Frequently multifocal multiform ectopic beats or runs of ventricular tachycardia are indications for antiarrhythmic therapy (see Chapters 2.2 and 2.3).

Angiocardiography

Angiocardiography is the definitive diagnostic test, revealing the characteristic morphology of the left ventricle and its contractile pattern. While angiography is not always needed in clear-cut cases, it is essential when any doubt as to diagnosis exists and when mitral regurgitation is in question.

The characteristic feature of the left ventricle is massive hypertrophy of the septum, free wall and papillary muscle area, with an angulated shape of the cavity which appears to be bent in its central portion. Entrapment of contrast media in the massive columnae carnae may impart a stellar appearance to the cavity of the ventricle. In systole, the apex and mid-portion are empty, or almost empty, of contrast media, the ventricular cavity being reduced to a triangular portion beneath the aortic valve. Sometimes a globule of contrast medium may be trapped at the apex of the cavity, apparently isolated and cut off from the proximal area of the ventricle. Contraction is rapid and powerful. In diastole, the ventricular volume appears to be normal and does not reveal the severe disorder of relaxation that exists (Figure 2.2.3).

The characteristic elimination of the cavity in systole is present in 90% of patients; the remainder show enlargement of papillary muscles, while less than 5% show dilatation of the cavity. Dilatation only occurs in the presence of additional problems such as massive myocardial infarction, extreme mitral regurgitation or advanced congestive heart failure.

Right ventricular angiography in some cases shows the massive septum bulging into the right ventricle. Simultaneous right and left ventricular injections have been used to outline the ventricular septum.

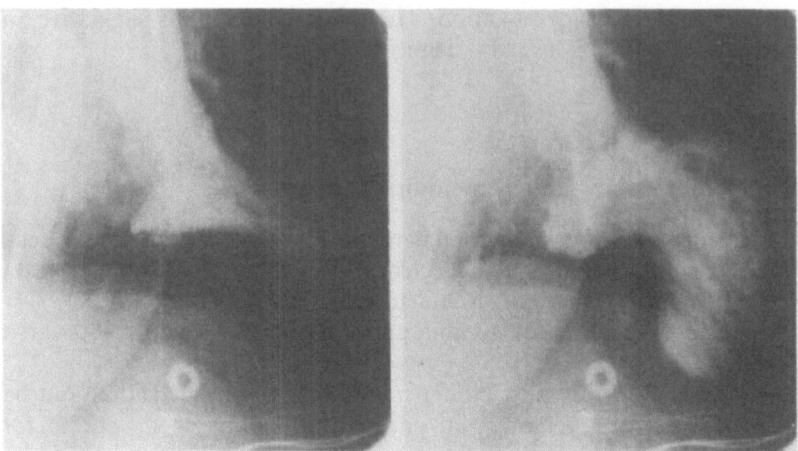

Figure 2.2.3 Anteroposterior cineangiogram of the left ventricle in hypertrophic cardiomyopathy showing (L) systolic frame with elimination of mid and apical portions of the left ventricle, and (R) diastolic frame emphasizing the angulation of the ventricle, with normal volume but slight mitral regurgitation

Care is needed in the interpretation of the appearances, for if the normal left ventricle is subjected to an increase in positive inotrophy or to hypovolaemia the cavity may be eliminated[11]. Thus it behoves the investigator also to assess both the shape of the ventricle and the degree of hypertrophy in making an angiographic diagnosis of hypertrophic cardiomyopathy. But in any event, the diagnosis should never be made on angiographic grounds alone, but always in the light of the clinical picture and results of other investigations.

VENTRICULAR FUNCTION

Systolic function

Powerful contraction of the left ventricle results in rapid expulsion of the contents in the first half or two thirds of systole. The hypertrophied chamber contracts with great force, and the muscle squeezes the body and the apex of the left ventricle, thus eliminating (rather than obliterating) the cavity except for a triangular proximal portion below the aortic valve. The anterior cusp and subvalvar apparatus of the mitral valve meet the hypertrophied septum sharply, creating eddies, vortices and pressure gradients. These gradients may be persistent but are often variable and tend to come and go with differing circumstances. They are provoked by positive inotropic stimulation such as excitement or exercise, and by circumstances which reduce the volume of the left ventricle, such as hypotension or hypovolaemia. Gradients are relieved by negative inotropic intervention, and by increases in ventricular volume and by adrenergic blocking agents or calcium blocking agents.

It has been suggested that a Venturi mechanism operates. The negative lateral pressure of the narrow jet of blood being expelled from the left ventricle draws the anterior mitral leaflet into the left ventricular outflow tract and causes the obstruction and the mitral regurgitation[12].

On the other hand, true obstruction has long been questioned[13], and more recently work by Murgo et al.[14] has suggested that gradients are likely to be due to rapid and complete emptying of the ventricle. Flow velocity in the aorta may be actually increased when a gradient develops on provocation by exercise or amyl nitrite.

Further evidence against true obstruction lies in the ephemeral nature of the gradients, the lack of correlation between gradients and prognosis or symptoms, and the high ejection fraction (70–90%) in many cases both with and without gradients.

Diastolic function

Left ventricular end-diastolic pressure is commonly raised, especially on effort. A reduced rate of filling of the left ventricle was postulated by Stewart et al.[15], due possibly to increased stiffness of the hypertrophied and fibrotic myocardium[16]. Myofibrillar disarray may add to the stiffness by creating a basket-weave arrangement.

More recently, prolongation of relaxation and of left ventricular filling rate with delay of mitral valve opening has been shown[17,18]. Peak filling rate is reduced, time to peak filling rate prolonged[19]. Both the timing and sequence of relaxation are abnormal, as is the rate of relaxation[20]. Abnormalities of relaxation and wall movement are regional as well as global. The rapid filling period is prolonged and abnormal as a result of both impaired relaxation and abnormal shape of the left ventricular cavity[2].

Newer techniques of investigation

Isotope radionuclide methods have been used to study ventricular function in hypertrophic cardiomyopathy.

Radionuclide angiography was used by Bonow et al.[19] to study left ventricular time-activity curves.

Hanrath et al.[21] used thallium 201 to study the left ventricle and showed localized defects of perfusion in the ventricular septum, probably due to ischaemia or fibrosis. Positron emission tomography (PET) has been used to study the blood flow and metabolic characteristics of the myocardium by our group. Regional uptake of rubidium 82 was found to be reduced in the septum as compared with the free wall of the left ventricle[9].

More recently our group studied the significance of gradients in hypertrophic cardiomyopathy using gated blood pool studies. The percentage of stroke volume ejected in the first third of systole, the initial 50% and the first 80% of systole was greater in hypertrophic cardiomyopathy than in normals, but there was no difference between the patients with, and those without gradients. These results favour the hypothesis that the presence of gradients is not a true indication of left ventricular obstruction[22]. Using similar techniques, the ejection fraction was shown to be 70–90% in many patients with hypertrophic cardiomyopathy.

THE RELATION OF SUDDEN DEATH TO VENTRICULAR FUNCTION

Apart from ventricular arrhythmia, the other probable cause for sudden death is haemodynamic. It is likely that resistance to filling of the left ventricle (which has abnormal relaxation) is increased by tachycardia and by positive inotropic influences. The elimination of the ventricular cavity in systole further augments the difficulty of filling of the left ventricle and thus can lead to cardiac arrest. We have reported one patient in whom this or a similar mechanism operated[23].

The future may see genetic probes to detect patients who are especially prone to die suddenly and to identify receptors for abnormal catecholamine function in the myocardium.

References

1. McKenna, W.J., Deanfield, J., Faruqui, A., England, D., Oakley, C.M. and Goodwin, J.F. (1981). Prognosis in hypertrophic cardiomyopathy: role of age and clinical electrocardiographic and haemodynamic features. *Am. J. Cardiol.*, **47**, 532–8
2. Goodwin, J.F. (1982). The frontiers of cardiomyopathy. *Br. Heart J.*, **48**, 1–18
3. Nagle, R.E., Boicourt, O.W., Gillam, P.M.S. and Mounsey, J.P.D. (1966). Cardiac impulse in hypertrophic cardiomyopathy. *Br. Heart J.*, **28**, 419–25
4. McKenna, W.J., Borgraffe, M., England, D., Deanfield, J., Oakley, C.M. and Goodwin, J.F. (1982). The natural history of left ventricular hypertrophy in hypertrophic cardiomyopathy: an electrocardiographic study. *Circulation*, **66**, 1233–40
5. Shapiro, L.M. and McKenna, W.J. (1983). Distribution of left ventricular hypertrophy in hypertrophic cardiomyopathy: a two-dimensional echocardiographic study. *J. Am. Coll. Cardiol.*, **2**, 437–44
6. Doi, Y.L., Deanfield, J., McKenna, W.J., Dargie, H.J., Oakley, C.M. and Goodwin, J.F. (1980). Echocardiographic differentiation of hypertensive heart disease and hypertrophic cardiomyopathy. *Br. Heart J.*, **44**, 395–400
7. McKenna, W.J., England, D., Doi, Y.L., Deanfield, J., Oakley, C.M. and Goodwin, J.F. (1981). Arrhythmias in hypertrophic cardiomyopathy; I Influence on prognosis. *Br. Heart J.*, **46**, 168–73
8. Goodwin, J.F. and Krikler, D.M. (1976). Arrhythmias as a cause of sudden death in hypertrophic cardiomyopathy. *Lancet*, **2**, 937–40
9. Krikler, D.M., Davies, J., Rowland, E., Goodwin, J.F., Evans, R.C. and Shaw, D.B. (1980). Sudden death in hypertrophic cardiomyopathy: associated accessory atrioventricular pathways. *Br. Heart J.*, **43**, 245–51
10. Maron, B.J., Roberts, W.C., Edwards, J.E., McAllister, H.A. Jr., Foley, D.D. and Epstein, S.E. (1978). Sudden death in patients with hypertrophic cardiomyopathy: characterisation of 26 patients without functional limitations. *Am. J. Cardiol.*, **41**, 803–10
11. Grose, R., Maskin, C., Spinola-Franco, H. and Yipintsoi, T. (1981). Production of left ventricular cavity obliteration in normal man. *Circulation*, **64**, 448–58
12. Wigle, E.D., Rakowski, H., Pollick, C., Henderson, M.A. and Ruddy T.D. (1981). Future trends in cardiomyopathy. *Prog. Cardiol.*, **10**, 175–203
13. Criley, J.M., Lewis, K.B., White, R.I. Jr. and Ross, R.S. (1965). Pressure gradients without obliteration: a new concept of hypertrophic subaortic stenosis. *Circulation*, **32**, 881–7

14. Murgo, J.P., Alter, B.Z., Dorethy, J.F., Altobelli, S.A. and McGranahan, G.M. (1980). Left ventricular ejection dynamics in hypertrophic cardiomyopathy. In Sekiguchi, M. and Olsen, E.C.J. (eds.) *Cardiomyopathy*. pp. 45–65. (Tokyo: University of Tokyo Press)
15. Stewart, S., Mason, D.R. and Braunwald, E. (1968). Impaired rate of left ventricular function in idiopathic hypertrophic subaortic stenosis and valvular aortic stenosis. *Circulation*, **37**, 8–14
16. Oakley, C.M. (1971). Hypertrophic obstructive cardiomyopathy: pattern of progression. In Wolstenholme, G. and O'Connor, M. (eds.) *Hypertrophic Obstructive Cardiomyopathy*. (Ciba Foundation Study Group No. 37). pp. 9–39. (London: Churchill)
17. Sanderson, J.E., Gibson, D.G., Brown, D.J. and Goodwin, J.F. (1977). Left ventricular filling in hypertrophic cardiomyopathy: an angiographic study. *Br. Heart J.*, **39**, 661–70
18. Sanderson, J.E., Traile, T.A., St. John Sutton, M.G., Brown, D.J., Gibson, D.G. and Goodwin, J.F. (1978). Left ventricular relaxation and filling in hypertrophic cardiomyopathy, an echocardiographic study. *Br. Heart J.*, **40**, 596–601
19. Bonow, R.O., Rosing, D.R., Bacharach, S.L. *et al.* (1980). Effects of verapamil on left ventricular systolic function and diastolic filling in patients with hypertrophic cardiomyopathy. *Circulation*, **64**, 707–96
20. Alvares, R.F., Shaver, J.A., Gamble, W.H. and Goodwin, J.F. (1984). Isovolumic relaxation period in hypertrophic cardiomyopathy. *J. Am. Coll. Cardiol.*, **3**, 71–81
21. Hanrath, P. *et al.* (1981). Myocardial thalium imaging in hypertrophic obstructive cardiomyopathy. *Eur. Heart J.*, **2**, 177
22. Sugrue, D., Dickie, S., Oakley, C.M. and Lavender, J.P. (1984). Haemodynamic significance of left ventricular gradient in hypertrophic cardiomyopathy. *Br. Heart J.*, **51**, 113
23. McKenna, W.J., Harris, L. and Deanfield, J. (1982). Syncope in hypertrophic cardiomyopathy. *Br. Heart J.*, **47**, 177–9

2.3
Treatment and prognosis

D.D. SUGRUE AND W.J. McKENNA

NATURAL HISTORY

Adults

The symptomatic course in hypertrophic cardiomyopathy (HCM) is extremely variable. The majority of adult patients live for many years with few or no symptoms and only a minority are severely symptomatic[1]. Furthermore, symptoms often remain stable or improve spontaneously, a fact which has important implications when trying to assess the response to therapy. Loogen et al.[2] reported that 28 of 47 (60%) patients remained stable on no treatment during a mean follow-up period of 6.7 years and Adelman et al.[3] noted that 56 of 60 (93%) patients developed symptoms an average of 10 years after diagnosis, while only 40 patients (60%) deteriorated to functional class IV an average of 5 years after the onset of symptoms. In our own series of 254 patients, the average age at onset of symptoms was 29 years and only 26% developed progressive symptoms (Figure 2.3.1)[4]. Spontaneous changes in the magnitude of left ventricular gradients, either an increase, reduction or loss, occur in a minority of patients. These changes are usually associated with deterioration in symptomatic status[5].

The natural history of the disease has been documented in several large series[1-4,6-9]. In reviewing these data, three pertinent facts must be kept in mind: (1) all of the available studies are based exclusively on hospital populations and are therefore biased in favour of severely symptomatic patients, (2) many patients included in these series were treated and do not therefore truly represent the natural history of the disease and (3) diagnostic criteria have changed with time. Thus patients included in the earlier years of these natural history studies might not be directly comparable to patients included at a later date. It is of interest that recent information from the Framingham data base has shown that unexplained left ventricular hypertrophy is present in 2% of a free living population over the age of 65 years[10]. Thus it is possible that hypertrophic cardiomyopathy is a relatively common disease with a more benign prognosis than has previously been appreciated.

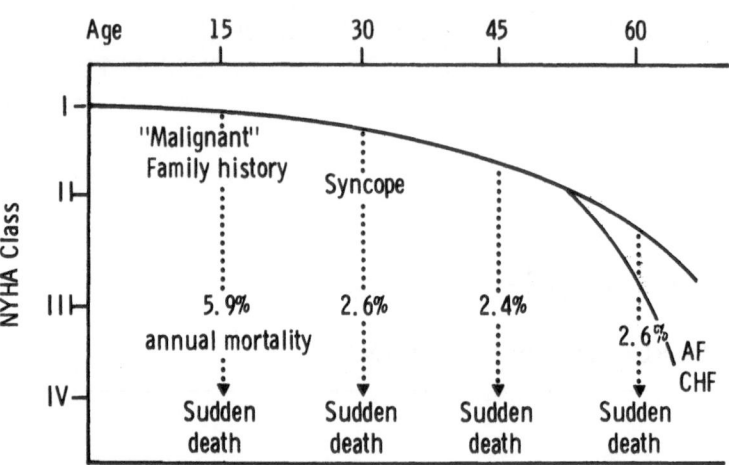

Figure 2.3.1 A suggested natural history of hypertrophic cardiomyopathy. AF = atrial fibrillation; CHF = congestive heart failure; NYHA = New York Heart Association. (From McKenna and Goodwin[47], with permission)

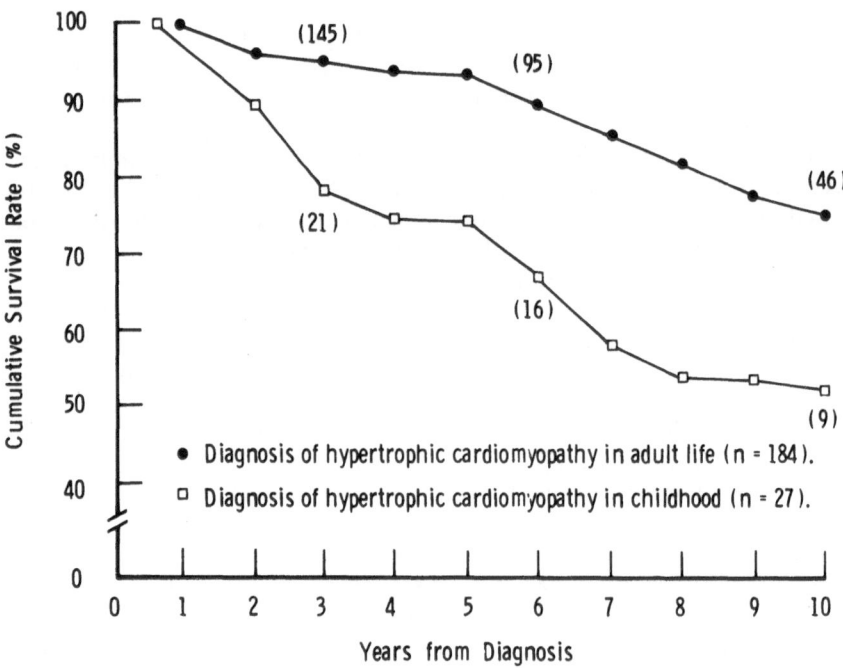

Figure 2.3.2 Cumulative survival curve from the year of diagnosis for 211 medically treated patients. (From McKenna *et al.*[4])

Among adult patients with hypertrophic cardiomyopathy, death is most frequently sudden and unexpected[4]. In a retrospective analysis of the natural history of the disease in 254 patients followed for up to 21 years (mean 6), there were 58 deaths of which 32 occurred suddenly[4]. Additional causes of death included: congestive cardiac failure ($n = 6$), postoperative death following myotomy/myectomy ($n = 9$), cerebral embolism ($n = 1$), endocarditis ($n = 2$) and non-cardiac causes ($n = 7$). One patient died during an electrophysiological study. In these patients, the annual mortality was approximately 2.5% per year (Figure 2.3.2).

Neonates and infants

There is a relative paucity of reported cases of hypertrophic cardiomyopathy in the neonatal period and in infancy but the available evidence suggests that the natural history of the disease in this age group may be somewhat different to that described for adults. In a recent multicentre study, 10 of 20 (50%) infants who were diagnosed during the first year of life died during a mean follow-up period of 5.5 years[11]. The causes of death included congestive cardiac failure ($n = 5$), postoperative death ($n = 2$), sudden death ($n = 2$), and unrelated ($n = 1$). Altogether, nine of 11 infants who were in congestive failure died. These data suggest that for children diagnosed during the first year of life, the prognosis is poor and is related to ventricular function.

Children

The prognosis in children appears to depend, to some extent, on the clinical presentation. In general, children who present between the ages of 5 and 15 have a poor prognosis with an annual mortality rate of approximately 4%. Children who are diagnosed through screening of families in whom a sibling has died suddenly also have a poor prognosis[12] although the precise annual mortality is uncertain. Children who are diagnosed because of the detection of an asymptomatic murmur or because of paroxysmal symptoms including syncope also have a surprisingly poor prognosis with an annual mortality rate from sudden death of approximately 4% per year[13]. Children who present with moderate or severe symptoms, with limitation of exercise tolerance, have a poor prognosis related to progressive symptoms; these children either die suddenly or secondary to congestive heart failure[14]. Much further information is required on the natural history of the disease in infancy and childhood in order to better understand the aetiology of this myocardial disease and to optimize treatment for these children.

Questions which are of critical importance in the management of patients with hypertrophic cardiomyopathy include: (1) What is the mechanism of sudden death?, (2) Can patients who are at risk for sudden death be preselected? and (3) Can sudden death be prevented?

MECHANISM OF SUDDEN DEATH

In the final analysis, all sudden cardiac deaths are arrhythmic in origin. Thus it is not the terminal arrhythmia *per se* which is of prime interest but the antecedent events. Although asystole has been documented in one patient with hypertrophic cardiomyopathy[15], it seems much more likely that ventricular fibrillation is the terminal event in the majority of patients who die suddenly. The evidence in support of this observation includes the following: (1) ventricular fibrillation has been documented in a small number of patients at the time of resuscitation[16] and (2) ventricular fibrillation was induced by programmed ventricular stimulation at the time of cardiac surgery in five of 17 patients with the disease[17]. Several other potential mechanisms of sudden death have been documented but none would appear to be common (Figure 2.3.3). There are isolated reports of complete heart block in patients with HCM[18,19], but symptomatic conduction disease and overt sinus node and atrioventricular nodal disease is uncommon[4]. An accessory atrioventricular connection has been a focus of considerable attention as a potential cause of sudden death in these patients[20] but rapid antegrade conduction of atrial fibrillation has only been documented at the time of electrophysiology study in one patient[21]. There are many other isolated reports of overt pre-excitation in patients with HCM[22,23] and James and Marshall[24] noted persistence of the fetal pattern of atrioventricular junctional histology in 13 of 22 young patients with hypertrophic cardiomyopathy who died suddenly. They have emphasized the potential for this tissue to provide accessory routes for atrioventricular conduction, although electrocardiographic evidence of pre-excitation was not reported in any of these patients. A number of facts, however, suggest that pre-excitation is unlikely to provide a common substrate for sudden death in these patients. First, overt pre-excitation is uncommon; we found that the distribution of PR interval duration in 254 patients was identical to the normal population and only four patients had overt pre-excitation[4]. Second, although it is possible that these patients could have an accessory pathway without evidence of pre-excitation on the surface electrocardiogram, such pathways are typically left-sided freewall pathways[25] and therefore the functional significance of the histological findings reported by James and Marshall must be questioned. Third, of 13 patients studied in the electrophysiology laboratory by Ingham *et al.*[26] none had enhanced AV nodal conduction nor evidence of accessory pathway conduction and, although seven had discontinuous AV nodal refractory curves, none had inducible supraventricular tachycardia. Finally, despite the large number of patients who have undergone ambulatory monitoring, neither antidromic tachycardia nor atrial fibrillation with pre-excited ventricular complexes has ever been reported.

The role of acute myocardial ischaemia or infarction as a cause of sudden death in HCM has received little attention but is potentially of importance. It is clear that hypertrophic cardiomyopathy and coronary artery disease may coexist[27-29], but of greater interest was the recent report by Maron *et*

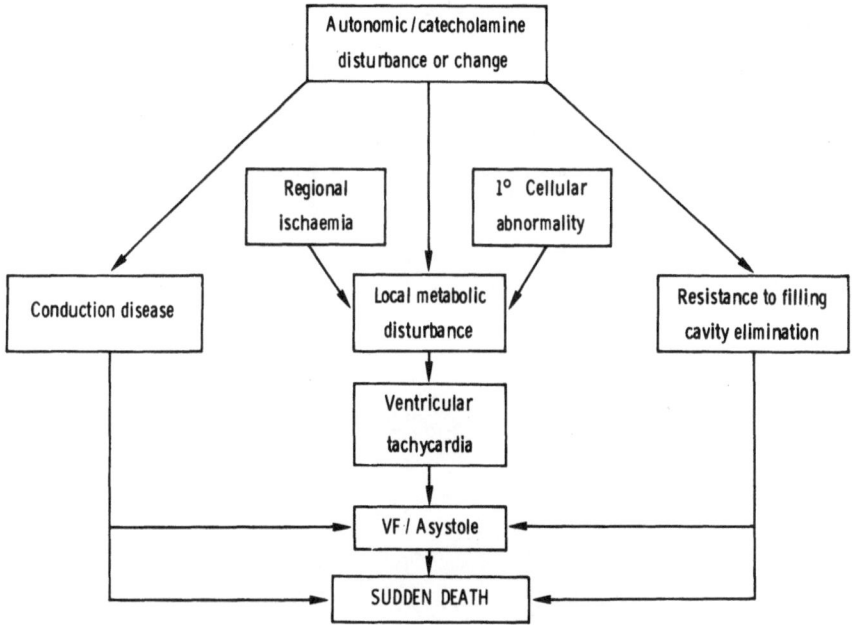

Figure 2.3.3 Potential mechanisms of sudden death in hypertrophic cardiomyopathy

al.[30] of seven patients with transmural myocardial infarction in the absence of significant large vessel coronary disease. Of these, six had narrowing of intramural coronary arteries, three had evidence of subepicardial scarring and all had areas of subendocardial fibrosis. In six of seven, myocardial infarction was clinically silent.

The role of haemodynamic abnormalities in the pathogenesis of sudden death is uncertain. Brock[31] suggested that patients might experience left ventricular outflow tract spasm or shutdown in a manner analogous to right ventricular outflow tract spasm in Fallot's tetralogy but, although conceptually appealing, this phenomenon has never been documented. The fact that an equal number of patients with and without outflow gradients die suddenly[4,12] and that surgery which abolishes gradients does not prevent sudden death (*see below*) suggests that other factors must also be important.

PREDICTION OF PATIENTS AT RISK FOR SUDDEN DEATH

Given the wide variation in symptomatic course and prognosis, the ability to distinguish those patients with a good prognosis from those at high risk is of importance in devising a rational treatment strategy. Considerable efforts have been directed at trying to define a clinical profile of the high risk patient. Using a stepwise discriminant analysis, we determined the prognostic importance of 24 clinical, haemodynamic and electrocardiographic variables in 254 patients[4]. The combination of the following four variables was best predictive of subsequent death: age less than 14 years at diagnosis,

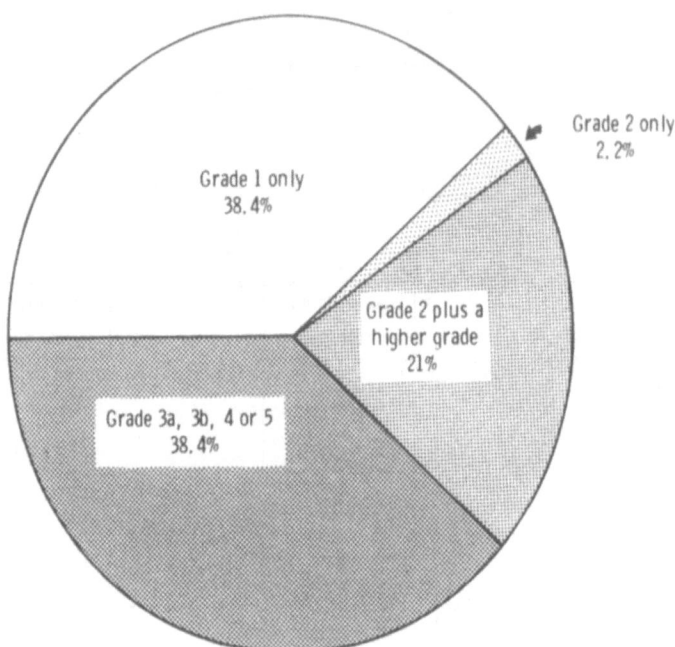

Figure 2.3.4 The incidence of ventricular arrhythmia grades 1–5 in 86 patients with hypertrophic cardiomyopathy during 3 days of ambulatory electrocardiographic monitoring

previous syncopal episodes, severe dyspnoea at last follow-up and a family history of hypertrophic cardiomyopathy and sudden death. In this analysis and in subsequent studies, the prognostic importance of two haemodynamic variables, left ventricular end-diastolic pressure and outflow gradients was evaluated. Left ventricular end-diastolic pressure showed a variable correlation with functional classification[7,9] and no correlation with sudden death[4,32], while the proportion of patients with left ventricular gradients was similar in survivors and those who died suddenly. The relationship between gradient and sudden death has also been evaluated in five studies in a total of 532 patients of whom 93 died suddenly[4,7,9,12,33]. A relationship could not be demonstrated in any of these series. Though helpful, the previously mentioned clinical profile of the high risk patient has a limited predictive value (false negative 30%, false positive 27%) and requires further refinement with assessment of variables which are more likely to be important determinants of sudden death.

The high incidence of arrhythmias in patients with hypertrophic cardiomyopathy was not fully recognized before the development of ambulatory monitoring[34–37]. In a recent series of 100 consecutive patients who underwent 72 hours of ambulatory monitoring, 29 had one or more episodes of ventricular tachycardia (Figure 2.3.4)[34]. The majority of these patients also had frequent and complex ventricular extrasystoles. The characteristics of the episodes of ventricular tachycardia (VT) are of interest and included the following: the episodes were all non-sustained (3–27 beats,

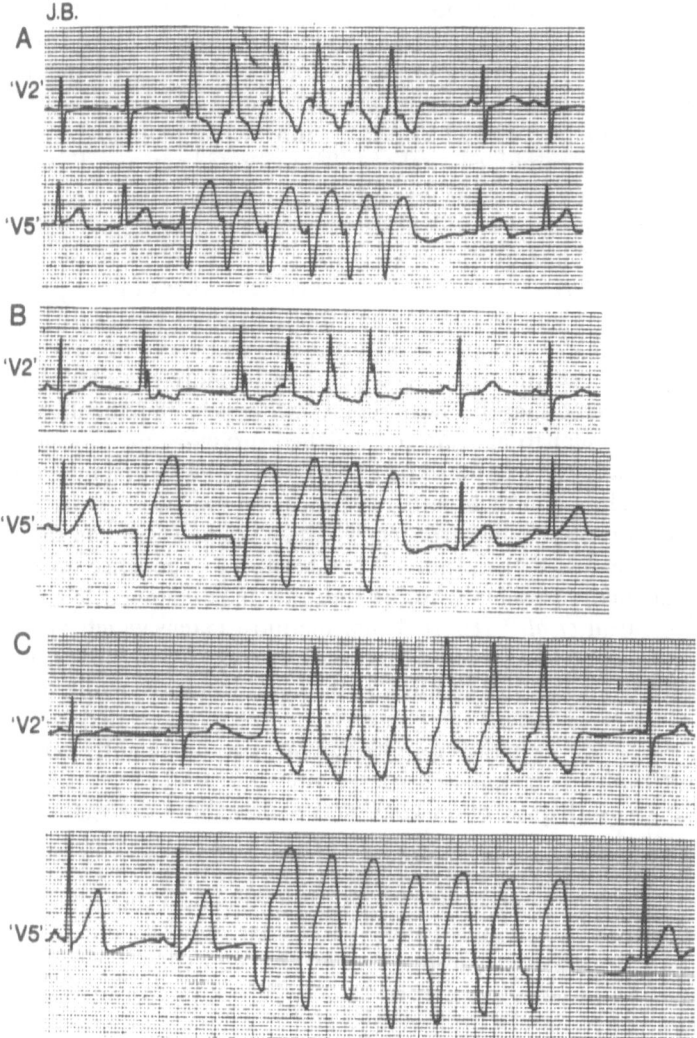

Figure 2.3.5 Typical episodes of ventricular tachycardia recorded during ambulatory e.c.g. monitoring in a patient with hypertrophic cardiomyopathy

mean 8), the morphology was usually multiform, rates were usually slow (mean 140 beats/minute), 40% of episodes occurred between midnight and 8.00 a.m. and all episodes were asymptomatic (Figure 2.3.5)[34].

Supraventricular arrhythmias are also common in hypertrophic cardiomyopathy[35,37] and may occasionally be associated with troublesome symptoms, systemic emboli[38] or haemodynamic deterioration. Seven per cent of patients are in established atrial fibrillation at the time of diagnosis[9] and during the next 5 years a further 7% can be expected to develop this arrhythmia. Established atrial fibrillation or paroxysmal supraventricular tachycardia are more common in patients with ventricular tachycardia[4].

Established atrial fibrillation is generally associated with a poor prognosis[4,7,8] although not specifically related to subsequent sudden death[4]. Ventricular tachycardia, however, documented by ambulatory monitoring, is an important clinical marker of poor prognosis. This relationship has been noted in two independent studies[35,37] in which ambulatory monitoring was performed in a combined total of 168 unoperated patients. Forty-one of 168 (25%) had ventricular tachycardia and of these, nine died suddenly during a mean follow-up period of 3 years, whereas four of 127 without VT died suddenly. Of interest however is the fact that 32 of those with VT survived. Thus VT is a sensitive but non-specific marker of poor prognosis.

A priori, one might anticipate that those patients who had the most hypertrophy would have the 'worst disease' and therefore the poorest prognosis. However, the situation appears to be more complex than this. Maron *et al.*[32] found that the mean septal thickness in 78 patients who died suddenly was similar to age and sex matched survivors and Savage *et al.*[36] could not find a linear relationship between ventricular septal thickness and frequency of VPCs although patients with septal thickness greater than or equal to 20 mm had a higher frequency of high grade VPCs than those with septal thickness less than 20 mm. It has been our experience and that of others[33] that many patients who die suddenly have minimal hypertrophy. However, Maron *et al.*[39] reported that the most extensive left ventricular wall cellular disorganization found at necropsy occurred in those patients in whom sudden unexpected death was the first definitive manifestation of cardiac disease. Electrical irritability is likely to be related to cellular disorganization and it is therefore likely that it is the 'quality' rather than the 'quantity' of hypertrophied myocardium which is of prognostic importance. At present, there is no *in vivo* marker of cellular disorganization. A systematic study of the relationship between myocardial mass and prognosis has not been performed.

The relationship between myocardial structure and ventricular arrhythmias is unclear. It is assumed that the cellular disarray and myocardial fibrosis provide an anatomical substrate for ventricular arrhythmias. *In vitro* studies of the electrical properties of hypertrophied myocardium have described a variety of electrical abnormalities including low resting potentials, reduced potassium ion conductance, lengthening of action potential duration, after potentials, triggered activity, split upstrokes and electrically silent areas[40-42]. Coltart and Meldrum[43] recorded the transmembrane action potential in a single cardiac myofibril excised from a patient with hypertrophic cardiomyopathy using a microelectrode technique and found a prolonged repolarization time and decreased rate of rise of the action potential. It was postulated that these abnormalities were due to an abnormal transmembrane permeability to sodium, potassium and magnesium ions. Thus cellular studies would tend to confirm that the hypertrophied heart is electrically unstable; additional experiments using a canine model have shown an increased incidence of sudden cardiac death in dogs with left ventricular hypertrophy subjected to coronary artery occlusion[44].

There has been much speculation about the potential importance of impaired left ventricular relaxation, filling and compliance. Goodwin[20] hypothesized that patients with hypertrophic cardiomyopathy would be at particular risk from the combination of increased heart rate and decreased filling which would lead to a marked decline in stroke output with concomitant cardiovascular collapse and sudden death. We have recently examined the possible prognostic significance of impaired left ventricular function in two separate studies[45,46]. In one study, left ventricular angiograms performed at diagnosis in 88 patients were digitized and the relation between haemodynamic indices of ejection and filling and the subsequent course was examined[45]. During a mean follow-up period of 8 years, 11 patients died suddenly. These patients had lower normalized peak rates of ejection and filling at diagnosis compared to survivors. In an independent cross-sectional study, the relation of previously determined prognostic indicators (ventricular tachycardia, syncope, family history of hypertrophic cardiomyopathy and sudden death) and gated equilibrium radionuclide indices of resting left ventricular ejection and filling was determined in 84 patients[46]. Ejection and/or filling were significantly impaired in those patients with one or more of these indicators of poor prognosis. Impairment of left ventricular filling could be an important determinant of whether ventricular tachycardia is well tolerated or is associated with acute haemodynamic deterioration and death. Additional longitudinal studies are required to determine if those patients with ventricular tachycardia who survive have normal left ventricular filling. This information is of great potential clinical importance because it might obviate the need for anti-arrhythmic treatment in such patients.

CAN SUDDEN DEATH BE PREVENTED?

Because of the lack of controlled trials, the impact of conventional medical therapy and surgery on prognosis is difficult to assess. We have previously reviewed the published experience of the effect of β-blocker therapy and surgical myotomy/myectomy on prognosis[47]. Five medical series were reviewed (159 patients) and the overall mortality was 7.5% (range 0–12.9%). Six surgical series were reviewed (282 patients) and the overall mortality was 17% (range 7.5–25.5%). Recently, Borggrefe et al.[48] have reported that the prevalence of ventricular arrhythmias was unchanged following myotomy/myectomy in 31 patients who underwent 48 h ambulatory electrocardiographic monitoring before and after surgery. In the multicentre study reported by Shah et al.[6], 18 of 101 (18%) patients on propranolol therapy died suddenly; in Maron's study 19 of 78 (24%) patients who died suddenly were taking propranolol in a dose which was $\geqslant$120 mg per day[32], and in another study ten of 77 patients (13%) who were treated with propranolol (120–240 mg daily) died during an average follow-up period of 4.7 years[2]. However, Frank et al.[49] reported no mortality in 22 patients followed for an average of 5 years and treated with 'complete' β-receptor blocking doses of propranolol (mean daily dose 462 mg, range 260–640). Several aspects of this unique study deserve

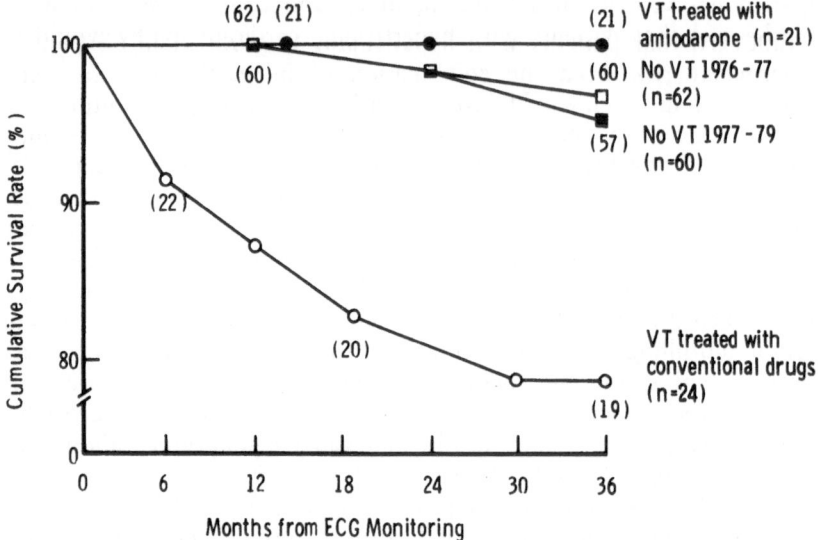

Figure 2.3.6 Cumulative survival for 24 patients with ventricular tachycardia (VT) treated with conventional antiarrhythmic agents (○), 21 patients with ventricular tachycardia treated with amiodarone (●), 62 patients with no ventricular tachycardia during e.c.g. monitoring between 1976 and 1977 (□) and 60 patients without ventricular tachycardia during e.c.g. monitoring performed between 1977 and 1979 (■). The probability of cardiac death equals the total number of deaths for the year divided by the adjusted number at risk minus the number of deaths due to other causes

further comment. Cardiac rhythm status off treatment was not documented in all patients; patients were not stratified according to prognostic indicators; seven patients had systemic hypertension and seven were given antiarrhythmic drugs in addition to propranolol.

Currently, there is only one study which deals with the impact of calcium channel blockers on prognosis. Haberer *et al.*[50] reported a significantly lower annual mortality (1.8%) in 14 patients treated with verapamil 360 mg daily for a mean of 3.7 years; this compared to an average mortality of 6.3% in 15 patients treated with propranolol and 6.3% in 20 patients on no treatment. Again, these data must be interpreted with caution because patients were not stratified according to risk.

Recently we have presented data which indicate that amiodarone improves survival in one subset of patients with hypertrophic cardiomyopathy who are at high risk, i.e. those with ventricular tachycardia (Figure 2.3.6)[51]. During the years 1976 and 1977, 86 patients with hypertrophic cardiomyopathy underwent 72 h ambulatory monitoring and ventricular tachycardia was documented in 24. Ventricular arrhythmias were treated in these patients with conventional antiarrhythmic drugs (mexiletine, disopyramide, quinidine). Seven of 84 patients died during a follow-up of 3 years and of these five had previously documented ventricular tachycardia. During the next 2 years (1978–79) the next 82 consecutive patients underwent 48 h ambulatory monitoring; of these 21 had ventricular tachycardia. These patients were treated with amiodarone, 150–400 mg daily (median 300 mg). Ventricular tachycardia was suppressed during repeat electrocardiographic monitoring. There were three sudden deaths during a mean follow-up of 3 years but none of these deaths occurred in the treatment group. Thus control of ventricular tachycardia with amiodarone was associated with improved 3-year survival ($p < 0.04$) compared to conventional agents in matched non-parallel treatment groups.

MANAGEMENT

Treatment of patients with hypertrophic cardiomyopathy has two distinct objectives, namely the amelioration of symptoms and the prevention of complications, particularly sudden death. A rational treatment programme should be based on an understanding of the pathophysiology of symptoms (something which is poorly understood) and on an understanding of the natural history of the disease (something which is now partially understood – see above). Valid interpretation of the published results of medical and surgical therapy is made difficult by a number of factors, including (1) a paucity of controlled trials of therapy (surgical treatment has never been subjected to a randomized control trial), (2) failure to stratify patients according to prognosis, (3) use of subjective and therefore imprecise criteria such as change in functional status to assess the response treatment, (4) relatively short duration of follow-up and (5) variations in both the dosage of prescribed medications and in surgical technique.

Before detailing our approach to treatment it is appropriate that the cumulative experience of the haemodynamic and symptomatic effects of medical and surgical therapy be reviewed (Figure 2.3.7).

	Dyspnea	Exercise Duration	Chest Pain	LVEDP	LVOT Gradient	Diastolic Function
Propranolol	↓	↑	↓↓	↑↓	↓	↑↓
Verapamil	↓↓	↑↑	↓↓	↑↓	↓↓	↑↑
Surgery	↓↓↓	↑↑	↓↓↓	↑↓	↓↓↓	ND

Figure 2.3.7 Assessment of the effects of treatment on symptoms and left ventricular function in hypertrophic cardiomyopathy based on our own experience and a review of the literature. LVEDP = left ventricular end-diastolic pressure; LVOT = left ventricular outflow tract; ND = not done

β-BLOCKERS

Use of β-blockers in this disease was prompted by the demonstration of an apparent excess of noradrenaline in tissue removed from the interventricular septum at the time of surgery[52] and by the observation that exercise and catecholamines led to an intensification of outflow tract gradients[53]. To date, only practolol[54,55], propranolol[54–59] and acebutolol[60] have been studied acutely; the results of one single-blind[61] and one double-blind[62] trial of chronic oral β-blocker therapy in this disease have been reported. When given intravenously, β-blockers reduce or abolish provoked gradients[54–57,63]; most – though not all – studies have shown that these drugs have little effect on resting gradients. Chronic oral therapy also has little effect on gradient[61,63,64] and it is unclear whether improvement is related to the abolition of outflow gradients, to improvement in diastolic relaxation and filling or to both. Haemodynamic studies have shown that β-blockers improve left ventricular compliance[57–60], but in a recent echocardiographic study it was noted that the effect of β-blockers on left ventricular filling was variable and unpredictable[65]. Much of the information on the beneficial effect of β-blockers on symptoms is anecdotal. Nevertheless, it is generally agreed that β-blockers ameliorate symptoms, particularly chest pain[61–63,66], in 50–70% of patients, although this effect is not always maintained during long term therapy. Hubner et al.[62] compared the effects of propranolol 320 mg daily, practolol 800 mg daily and placebo, each given in a double-blind manner for 4 weeks, on the symptomatic status of 16 patients with hypertrophic cardiomyopathy. Dyspnoea was improved by propranolol only in those patients with severe limitation (NYHA grades 3 and 4) and propranolol caused a significant reduction in the frequency of chest pain. There is no evidence that propranolol in clinical doses prevents progression of or induces regression in cardiac hypertrophy. In our hands, propranolol in moderate dose (280 mg daily) did not reduce the incidence of ventricular extrasystoles or ventricular tachycardia[67]. Large dose β-blockers may cause significant symptomatic side-effects, particularly lethargy. β-Blockers such as atenolol which do not cross the blood–brain barrier tend to cause less subjective side-effects and, although objective data on the efficacy of these newer compounds on the symptomatic status of patients with this disease are not available, it is reasonable to presume that there should be no difference between subgroups of β-blockers in this regard.

CALCIUM ANTAGONISTS

Use of calcium antagonists in hypertrophic cardiomyopathy was stimulated by (1) the observation that metabolic and anatomical abnormalities which are thought to be the result of increased transmembrane calcium flux in the Syrian hamster model of cardiomyopathy can be prevented by these drugs[68] (it must be emphasized that there is no conclusive evidence linking abnormalities of myocardial metabolism to human hypertrophic cardiomyopathy), (2) the suggestion that calcium antagonists might prevent ventricular arrhythmias[20] and (3) the proposed relationships between the positive inotropic action of catecholamines and increased concentrations of intracellular calcium[68]. Most clinical experience has been gained using verapamil[69-79]. When given intravenously, verapamil is negatively inotropic[70-72] but improves regional[71] and global[78,79] left ventricular relaxation and filling characteristics in most but not all patients[72,77]; gradients are also usually decreased or abolished. Data obtained both from detailed haemodynamic studies and from observations on the effect of verapamil on cultured monolayers of avian ventricular cells have shown that these alterations in left ventricular filling are a consequence of improved left ventricular compliance and not simply a manifestation of altered loading conditions[80]. The acute haemodynamic response to verapamil is not always favourable or predictable, however[72]. Epstein and Rosing[81] reported that following intravenous verapamil there was an increase in pulmonary capillary wedge pressure in four of 19 patients in whom this measurement was previously normal, while left ventricular end-diastolic pressure increased in five of ten patients in whom this measurement was previously normal. In those patients who show a pronounced fall in systemic blood pressure in response to intravenous verapamil, outflow tract gradients may actually increase. Of 120 patients treated with chronic oral verapamil over a 3-year period and reported by the NIH group[81], eight developed acute pulmonary oedema and three of these patients died. Significant electrophysiological complications also occurred in some patients, including sinus arrest (2%), sinus bradycardia with junctional escape rhythm (11%) and Mobitz type II block (1%). Sudden death, possibly related to an adverse haemodynamic response, has been reported[82]. The limited data which are currently available on the long term symptomatic response to chronic verapamil therapy show that symptoms are ameliorated in approximately 70%[69,74,75] of patients and there is an objective improvement in exercise capacity[74]. The efficacy and safety of verapamil in patients with more severe symptoms and haemodynamic impairment, however, are uncertain. A decrease in left ventricular hypertrophy and intraventricular septal thickness following chronic oral verapamil therapy has been reported[76] but, although of great interest, these data must be viewed with caution because of the limitations of the methodologies used to assess myocardial hypertrophy. The speculation that some ventricular arrhythmias are slow channel dependent and may therefore be prevented by drugs like verapamil has not proven to be the case in hypertrophic cardiomyopathy. In our hands, verapamil (240–480 mg daily) did not reduce the incidence of ventricular extrasystoles or ventricular tachycardia[83].

When given acutely, nifedipine also improves left ventricular relaxation and filling in these patients without depressing systolic function[84,85]. As with verapamil, profound hypotension and an increase in outflow tract gradient can occur. By comparing the effects of nifedipine and sodium nitroprusside on diastolic function in patients with hypertrophic cardiomyopathy, it has been demonstrated that the favourable effects of nifedipine on left ventricular diastolic function result both from systemic vasodilatation and from a direct myocardial relaxant effect[86]. Knowledge of the long term effects of nifedipine therapy are limited to observations in one patient in whom there was sustained symptomatic improvement after chronic oral therapy for 35 weeks[84]. In a recent acute study it has been demonstrated that the combination of nifedipine and propranolol appears to have more favourable haemodynamic effects than nifedipine alone[57]. It was postulated that the vasodilatory effects of nifedipine were counteracted by the adrenergic receptor blockade associated with propranolol. There are no long term data currently available on this drug combination.

SURGERY

Surgical proponents have advocated and used a variety of procedures since the late 1950s including septectomy, myotomy/myectomy, via a trans-aortic, transatrial or transventricular approach, and isolated mitral valve replacement[47,87]. Although it is generally agreed that only those patients who are refractory to medical therapy should be subjected to surgery, this definition will vary in different centres. Much of the published data relates to case reports or series of less than 20 patients. The long term results of surgery have been reported in six series each containing more than 30 patients. This experience in 282 patients was recently summarized[47]. Eighty per cent of these patients were NYHA functional class III or IV; the perioperative mortality ranged from 4% to 16.2% and the late mortality from 5% to 10% (mean follow-up 5.2–7 years). The largest individual experience to date has recently been reported from the National Institutes of Health where 217 patients have been operated on between January 1960 and April 1979[88]. The patients ranged in age from 9 to 76 years (median 44); duration of postoperative follow-up ranged from 1 to 19 years (mean 4.4 years). There were 18 perioperative deaths (8%), 25 (12%) late deaths of whom 14 died from cardiac causes. Eight of these patients died suddenly and unexpectedly. Of the 170 surviving patients, 147 (86%) reported improvement in symptomatic status by at least one functional class. Surgery is effective in abolishing left ventricular gradients in the majority of patients; left ventricular end-diastolic pressure usually declines and mitral regurgitation is usually improved or abolished. Objective improvement in exercise capacity following surgery has been demonstrated by Redwood et al.[89] in 25 of 28 (89%) patients and radionuclide ejection fraction has been normal or above normal following surgery in 19 of 21 patients studied by Borer et al.[90]. Thus, in the short term, myotomy/myectomy improves symptoms and does not appear to impair left ventricular systolic function although there is a higher incidence of late congestive cardiac failure in these patients compared to patients treated medically.

The mechanism whereby surgery abolishes symptoms is unknown. It is unlikely to be the result of a placebo effect alone. However it is equally unlikely to be a direct result of the abolition of left ventricular gradients because these gradients do not relate to symptoms. There is, however, some tenuous evidence that symptoms are related to impaired relaxation and diastolic filling[91-92]. Detailed studies of the effects of surgery on left ventricular diastolic filling and coronary blood flow, and on the natural history of left ventricular hypertrophy, have not been performed; such studies are urgently required.

APPROACH TO TREATMENT

At diagnosis, all patients should have at least 48 hours of ambulatory electrocardiographic monitoring and an assessment of left ventricular function. Ambulatory monitoring is more sensitive than treadmill exercise testing in the detection of arrhythmias in these patients[36,67]. Currently, two-dimensional echocardiography is the imaging modality of choice and in addition to assessing left ventricular function allows an assessment of the extent and distribution of left ventricular hypertrophy[93,94]; with the addition of Doppler echocardiography, left ventricular gradients and mitral regurgitation can be quantitated[95,96]. We also use high temporal resolution equilibrium radionuclide cineangiography to assess left ventricular systolic and diastolic function, as this is a non-invasive and highly reproducible technique which can be repeated serially. Routine diagnostic cardiac catheterization is not necessary. In general, we reserve catheterization to address the following specific questions: to assess haemodynamics in patients who are being considered for surgery; to quantitate the severity of mitral regurgitation; to assess coronary anatomy in patients over 40 years of age with angina; to evaluate a concomitant cardiac disease process; to confirm the diagnosis when it is in doubt.

Treatment must be individualized. General measures applicable to all patients include the use of antibiotic prophylaxis for patients undergoing potentially infective procedures, i.e. dental extractions. Patients with paroxysmal or established atrial fibrillation should be anticoagulated. Sympathomimetic drugs and strenuous exercise should be avoided and, as in any patient with a chronic cardiac disability, general psychological support is of great importance. Genetic counselling[97] and family screening by echocardiography and ambulatory monitoring[98] are mandatory provided that patients are agreeable.

β-Blockers are the mainstay of treatment for symptomatic patients, but there is no particular merit in treating asymptomatic patients without arrhythmia with 'prophylactic' β-blockers. These drugs are best for chest pain. Although the largest experience has been gained using propranolol, there is no *a priori* reason to believe that other β-blockers may not be equally effective. If β-blockers are not tolerated, are contraindicated or are unsuccessful in relieving symptoms, we use verapamil. Up to 720 mg per day can be used if it is tolerated and symptoms warrant this dose. Therapy with verapamil should be initiated in hospital and under close supervision, as some patients respond adversely. Verapamil should not be used in specific subgroups of patients. It has been recommended that patients with a raised pulmonary capillary wedge pressure, patients with a low systolic blood pressure and those with recurrent paroxysmal nocturnal dyspnoea or orthopnoea should not be treated with verapamil[81]. However, these are often the patients with refractory symptoms. For patients with chest pain not responding to medical therapy and with documented coronary artery disease, coronary artery bypass surgery can be performed without any special risk[99], although anaesthetists should be aware of the importance of a stable blood volume.

The only specific risk factor which has been identified for sudden death which can be treated is ventricular arrhythmia. Our current policy is to treat all patients with ventricular tachycardia, defined as greater than or equal to three consecutive ventricular extrasystoles at a rate greater than 120 beats/minute or frequent ventricular extrasystoles defined as peak hourly count of greater than 30 or a 24 h total of greater than 250, with amiodarone. Control of ventricular arrhythmia is usually achieved within 1 week with 600–800 mg daily and can be maintained with chronic daily administration of 200–400 mg. We also use amiodarone in the treatment of refractory established atrial fibrillation with a ventricular rate greater than 100 beats/minute despite digoxin and propranolol, and in patients with troublesome or sustained supraventricular tachycardia or paroxysmal atrial fibrillation. As amiodarone is associated with a high incidence of side-effects, many of which are dose and duration related, it is important to use the minimum effective maintenance dose. Patients on amiodarone should be re-evaluated with electrocardiographic monitoring at 3–6-month intervals. The daily dose of amiodarone can then be decreased or increased in 50–200 mg increments depending on the presence or absence of arrhythmias, side-effects and plasma drug levels. If amiodarone is unsuccessful in controlling ventricular arrhythmias, another antiarrhythmic drug such as quinidine or disopyramide may be added with careful surveillance of the Q–T interval. Doses of digoxin and anticoagulants need to be reduced by approximately 50% in patients starting amiodarone therapy. Serious side-effects seldom develop during therapy with a daily dose of 300 mg or less. We do not use programmed ventricular stimulation to assess the efficacy of amiodarone therapy nor do we favour this approach, as advocated by others[100], in patients with recurrent syncope without documented arrhythmia. Programmed ventricular stimulation may be dangerous in these patients because of difficulty in cardiopulmonary resuscitation[21]. Furthermore, there appears to be a high incidence of non-specific false positive responses to programmed stimulation, particularly when an aggressive stimulation protocol is used[17].

For patients with a left ventricular gradient who are in cardiac failure, vasodilator therapy is contraindicated and diuretics should be used with caution. The predominant haemodynamic fault underlying the failure should be ascertained, i.e. systolic pump failure or diastolic compliance failure; digoxin may be particularly helpful in the former while β-blockers may aid the latter. Only those patients who are refractory to medical therapy or who have severe mitral regurgitation should be operated on. Currently, transaortic myotomy/myectomy is the surgical procedure of choice. Mitral valve replacement should be reserved for the minority of patients (approximately 3%) who have severe mitral regurgitation. We do not favour surgery for asymptomatic patients with left ventricular gradients because of the significant operative mortality and because surgery does not eliminate the risk of late sudden death. It has been suggested that surgery may be helpful in patients who have had a previously documented cardiac arrest, but the evidence is anecdotal and difficult to interpret in the absence of controls[101]. Morrow et al.[101] reported the results of myotomy/myectomy in nine patients, all of whom had a left ventricular gradient with minimal functional limitation and who had a previous cardiac arrest. One patient died in the perioperative period, one died suddenly 9 months postoperatively and the remainder were alive from 9 months to 5.5 years following surgery.

Pregnancy is well tolerated in patients with hypertrophic cardiomyopathy without any specific risks; epidural anaesthesia and hypovolaemia should however be avoided[102].

The potentially deleterious haemodynamic effects of VVI pacing should be carefully looked for in patients requiring permanent pacemaker implantation; in a minority of these patients AV sequential pacing should offer significant haemodynamic benefits[103] because of their dependence on atrial systole to maintain stroke volume; such patients can be identified by non-invasive assessment of the atrial contribution to filling volume from a radionuclide activity time-curve.

Management of patients who are asymptomatic or minimally symptomatic but who have large left ventricular gradients, or of patients with adverse prognostic features such as a family history of sudden death or a young age at diagnosis, is controversial and there are no definite guidelines regarding optimal management at the present time.

Ventricular arrhythmias are relatively uncommon in children with the disease. Children with a high risk clinical profile but without documented arrhythmias pose a difficult management problem. Our current policy is to treat such patients with low dose amiodarone, based on the hypothesis that this agent will decrease ventricular irritability and prevent sudden death. The mortality and morbidity of a surgical procedure must be carefully balanced against any putative benefits in these patients who have nothing to gain from a symptomatic standpoint and in whom the risk of sudden death may not be diminished by myotomy/myectomy.

References

1. Braunwald, E., Lambrew, C.T. and Rockoff, S.D. (1964). Idiopathic hypertrophic subaortic stenosis: I. A description based upon an analysis of 64 patients. *Circulation*, 29–30 (Suppl. IV), 3
2. Loogen, F., Kuhn, H. and Krelhaus, W. (1978). Natural history of hypertrophic obstructive cardiomyopathy. In Kaltenbach, M. *et al.* (eds.) *Cardiomyopathy and Myocardial Biopsy.* pp. 268–99. (New York: Springer)
3. Adelman, A.G., Wigle, E.D., Ranganathan, N., Webb, G.D., Kidd, B.S.L., Bigelow, W.G. and Silver, M.D. (1972). The clinical course in muscular subaortic stenosis. *Ann. Intern. Med.*, 77, 515–25

4. McKenna, W.J., Deanfield, J., Faruqui, A., England, D., Oakley, C.M. and Goodwin, J.F. (1981). Prognosis in hypertrophic cardiomyopathy: role of age and clinical, electrocardiographic and hemodynamic features. *Am. J. Cardiol.*, 47, 532–8

5. Shah, P.M., Adelman, A.G., Wigle, E.D., Gobel, F.L., Burchell, H.B., Hardarson, T., Curiel, R., de la Calazada, C., Oakley, C.M. and Goodwin, J.F. (1974). The natural (and unnatural) history of hypertrophic obstructive cardiomyopathy. *Circ. Res.*, 34–5 (Suppl. II) 179–95

6. Swan, D.A., Bell, B., Oakley, C.M. and Goodwin, J.F. (1971). Analysis of symptomatic course and prognosis and treatment of hypertrophic cardiomyopathy. *Br. Heart J.*, 33, 671–85

7. Ciro, E., Maron, B.J., Bonow, R.O., Cannon, R.O. and Epstein, S.E. (1984). Relation between marked changes in left ventricular outflow tract gradient and disease progression in hypertrophic cardiomyopathy. *Am. J. Cardiol.*, 53, 1103–9

8. Hardarson, T., de la Calazada, C.S., Curiel, R. and Goodwin, J.F. (1973). Prognosis and mortality in hypertrophic obstructive cardiomyopathy. *Lancet*, 2, 1462–7

9. Frank, S. and Braunwald, E. (1968). Idiopathic hypertrophic subaortic stenosis. Clinical analysis of 126 patients with emphasis on the natural history. *Circulation*, 37, 759–88

10. Savage, D.D., Abbot, R.D., Padgett, S., Anderson, S.J. and Garrison, R.J. (1983). Epidemiologic features of left ventricular hypertrophy in normotensive and hypertensive patients. In ter Keuts Med, J. and Schipperheyn, J.J. (eds.) *Cardiac Left Ventricular Hypertrophy*. pp. 3–12. (Boston, The Hague: Martinus Nijhoff)

11. Maron, B.J., Tajik, A., Ruttenberg, H.G., Graham, J.P., Atwood, G.F., Victorica, B.E., Lie, J.J. and Roberts, W.C. (1982). Hypertrophic cardiomyopathy in infants: clinical features and natural history. *Circulation*, 65, 7–17

12. Maron, B.J., Lipson, L.C., Roberts, W.C., Savage, D.D. and Epstein, S.E. (1978). Malignant hypertrophic cardiomyopathy identification of a subgroup of families with unusually frequent premature death. *Am. J. Cardiol.*, 41, 1133–40

13. McKenna, W.J. and Deanfield, J.E. (1984). Hypertrophic cardiomyopathy: an important cause of sudden death. *Arch. Dis. Child.*, 59, 971–5

14. Maron, B.J., Henry, W.L., Clark, C.E., Redwood, D.R., Roberts, W.C. and Epstein, S.E. (1976). Asymmetric septal hypertrophy in childhood. *Circulation*, 53, 9–19

15. Joseph, S., Balcon, R. and McDonald, L. (1972). Syncope in hypertrophic obstructive cardiomyopathy. *Br. Heart, J.*, 26, 874–6

16. Ciro, E. and Maron, B.J. (1983). Unusual long-term survival following cardiac arrest in hypertrophic cardiomyopathy. *Am. Heart J.*, 105, 145–7

17. Anderson, K.P., Stinson, E.B., Derby, G.C., Dyer, P.E. and Mason, J.W. (1983). Vulnerability of patients with obstructive hypertrophic cardiomyopathy to ventricular arrhythmia induction in the operating room. *Am. J. Cardiol.*, 51, 811–6

18. Chmielewzki, C.A., Riley, R.S., Mahendran, A. and Most, A.S. (1971). Complete heart block as a cause of syncope in asymmetric septal hypertrophy. *Am. Heart J.*, 93, 91–3

19. Johnson, A.D. and Dailey, P.O. (1975). Hypertrophic subaortic stenosis complicated by high degree heart block: successful treatment with an atrial synchronous ventricular pacemaker. *Chest*, 67, 491

20. Goodwin, J.F. and Krikler, D.M. (1976). Hypothesis. Arrhythmia as a cause of sudden death in hypertrophic cardiomyopathy. *Lancet*, 2, 937–40

21. Krikler, D.M., Davies, M.J., Rowland, E., Goodwin, J.F., Evans, R.C. and Shaw, D.W. (1980). Sudden death in hypertrophic cardiomyopathy: associated accessory atrioventricular pathways. *Br. Heart J.*, 43, 245–51

22. Touboul, P., Kirkorian, G., Atallah, G., Cahen, P., de Zulossa, C. and Moleur P. (1984). Atrioventricular block and pre-excitation in hypertrophic cardiomyopathy. *Am. J. Cardiol.*, 53, 961–3

23. Hauser, A.M., Gordon, S. and Timmis, G.C. (1984). Familial hypertrophic cardiomyopathy and pre-excitation. *Am. Heart J.*, 107, 176–9

24. James, T.N. and Marshall, T.K. (1975). De subitaneis mortibus. XIII. Asymmetrical hypertrophy of the heart. *Circulation*, 51, 1149–66

25. Sung, R.J., Gelband, H., Castellanos, A., Aranda, J.M. and Myerburg, R.J. (1977). Clinical and electrophysiologic observations in patients with concealed accessory atrioventricular bypass tracts. *Am. J. Cardiol.*, **40**, 839–47

26. Ingham, R.E., Mason, J.W., Rossen, D.M., Goodman, D.J. and Harrison, D.C. (1978). Electrophysiologic findings in patients with idiopathic subaortic stenosis. *Am. J. Cardiol.*, **41**, 811–6

27. Gulotta, S.J., Hamby, R.I., Alsonsen, A.L. and Ewing, K. (1972). Co-existent idiopathic hypertrophic subaortic stenosis and coronary arterial disease. *Circulation*, **46**, 890–6

28. Lardani, H., Serrano, J.A. and Villamil, R.J. (1978). Hemodynamics and coronary angiography in idiopathic hypertrophic subaortic stenosis. *Am. J. Cardiol.*, **41**, 476–81

29. Walston, A. and Behar, V.S. (1976). Spectrum of coronary artery disease in idiopathic hypertrophic subaortic stenosis. *Am. J. Cardiol.*, **38**, 12–16

30. Maron, B.J., Epstein, S.E. and Roberts, W.C. (1979). Hypertrophic cardiomyopathy and transmural myocardial infarction without significant atherosclerosis of the extramural coronary arteries. *Am. J. Cardiol.*, **43**, 1086–1102

31. Brock, R. (1957). Functional obstruction of the left ventricle (acquired subvalvular aortic stenosis). *Guy's Hosp. Rep.*, **106**, 221–38

32. Maron, B.J., Roberts, W.C. and Epstein, S.E. (1982). Sudden death in hypertrophic cardiomyopathy: a profile of 78 patients. *Circulation*, **65**, 1388–94

33. Maron, B.J. Roberts, W.C., Edwards, J.E., McAllister, H.A., Foley, D.D. and Epstein, S.E. (1978). Sudden death in patients with hypertrophic cardiomyopathy: characterization of 26 patients without functional limitation. *Am. J. Cardiol.*, **41**, 803–10

34. McKenna, W.J. (1983). Arrhythmia and prognosis in hypertrophic cardiomyopathy. *Eur Heart J.*, **4** (Suppl. F), 225–34

35. McKenna, W.J., England, D., Doi, Y.I., Deanfield, J.E. Oakley, C. and Goodwin, J.F. (1981). Arrhythmia in hypertrophic cardiomyopathy. I: Influence on prognosis. *Br. Heart J.*, **46**, 168–72

36. Savage, D.D., Seides, S.F., Maron, B.J., Myers, D.J. and Epstein, S.E. (1979). Prevalence of arrhythmias during 24 hour electrocardiographic monitoring and exercise testing in patients with obstructive and non-obstructive hypertrophic cardiomyopathy. *Circulation*, **59**, 866–75

37. Maron, B.J., Savage, D.D., Wolfson, J.K. and Epstein, S.E. (1981). Prognostic significance of 24 hour ambulatory electrocardiographic monitoring in patients with hypertrophic cardiomyopathy: a prospective study. *Am. J. Cardiol.*, **48**, 252–7

38. Furlan, A.J., Craciun, A.R., RaJu, N.R. and Hart, N. (1984). Cerebrovascular complications associated with idiopathic hypertrophic subaortic stenosis. *Stroke*, **15**, 282–4

39. Maron, B.J., Anan, J.J. and Roberts, W.C. (1981). Quantitative analysis of the distribution of cardiac muscle cell disorganization in the left ventricular wall of patients with hypertrophic cardiomyopathy. *Circulation*, **63**, 882–94

40. Heller, L.J. (1979). Augmented after contractions in papillary muscles from rats with cardiac hypertrophy. *Am. J. Physiol.*, **6**, 649–54

41. Aronson, R.S. (1981). After potentials and triggered activity in hypertrophied myocardium from rats with renal hypertension. *Circ. Res.*, **48**, 720–7

42. Cameron, J.S., Myerburg, R.J. and Wong, S.S. (1983). Electrophysiologic consequences of chronic experimentally induced left ventricular pressure overload. *J. Am. Coll. Cardiol.*, **2**, 481–7

43. Coltart, D.J. and Meldrum, S.J. (1970). Hypertrophic cardiomyopathy: an electrophysiological study. *Br. Med. J.*, **4**, 217–8

44. Koyanagi, S., Eastham, C. and Marcus, M.L. (1982). Effects of chronic hypertension and left ventricular hypertrophy on the incidence of sudden cardiac death after coronary artery occlusion in conscious dogs. *Circulation*, **65**, 1192–7

45. Newman, H., McKenna, W.J., Oakley, C.M. and Goodwin, J.F. (1984). The relation of the left ventricular function and sudden death in hypertrophic cardiomyopathy. (Abstr.) *J. Am. Coll. Cardiol.*, **3**, 620

46. Sugrue, D., Dickie, S., Myers, M., Lavender, J.P. and McKenna, W.J. (1983). The relation of left ventricular function to prognostic features in hypertrophic cardiomyopathy. (Abstr), *Circulation*, **68** (Suppl.), 111–61

47. McKenna, W.J. and Goodwin, J.F. (1981). The natural history of hypertrophic car-diomyopathy. *Curr. Probl. Cardiol.*, **6**, 5–26
48. Borggrefe, M., Kuhn, H., Koninger, H.H., Stoter, H., Breithardt, G., Loogen, F., Schulte, H.D. and Bircks, W. (1983). Arrhythmias in hypertrophic obstructive and non-obstructive cardiomyopathy. *Eur. Heart J.*, **4** (Suppl. F.), 245–51
49. Frank, M.J., Abdulla, A.M., Canedo, M.J. and Saylors, R.E. (1978). Long-term medical management of hypertrophic obstructive cardiomyopathy. *Am. J. Cardiol.*, **42**, 993–1001
50. Haberer, T., Hess, O.H., Jenni, R. and Krayenbuhl, H.P. (1983). Hypertrophic obstruc-tive cardiomyopathy: spontaneous course in comparison to long-term therapy with propranolol and verapamil. *Z. Kardiol.*, **72**, 487–93
51. McKenna, W.J., Oakley, C.M. and Goodwin, J.F. (1983). The influence of amiodarone on survival in hypertrophic cardiomyopathy. *Circulation*, **68**, 111–61 (Abstr.)
52. Pearce, A.G.E. (1964). The histochemistry and electron microscopy of obstructive cardiomyopathy. In Wolstenholme, G.E.W. and O'Connor, M. (eds.) *Cardiomyopathy*. pp. 132–64. (London: Churchill)
53. Wigle, E.D. (1965). Cardiovascular drugs in muscular subaortic stenosis. *Fed. Proc.*, **24**, 1279–86
54. Harrison, D.C. Braunwald, E., Glick, G., Mason, D.T., Chidsey, C.A. and Ross, J. Jr. (1964). Effects of beta-adrenergic blockade on the circulation with particular reference to patients with hypertrophic cardiomyopathy. *Circulation*, **29**, 84–98
55. Cherian, G., Brockington, L.F., Shah, P.M., Oakley, C.M. and Goodwin, J.F. (1966). Beta-adrenergic blockade in hypertrophic obstructive cardiomyopathy. *Br. Med. J.*, **1**, 895–8
56. Matlof, H.J. and Harrison, D.C. (1973). Acute haemodynamic effects of practolol in patients with idiopathic hypertrophic subaortic stenosis. *Br. Heart J.*, **35**, 152–7
57. Landmark, K., Sire, S., Thaulow, E., Amlie, J.P. and Nitter-Hauge, S. (1982). Haemody-namic effects of nifedipine and propranolol in patients with hypertrophic obstructive cardiomyopathy. *Br. Heart J.*, **48**, 19–26
58. Webb-Peploe, M.M., Croxson, R.S., Oakley, C.M. and Goodwin, J.F. (1971). Car-dioselective beta-adrenergic blockade in hypertrophic obstructive cardiomyopathy. *Postgrad. Med. J.* (Suppl.), **47**, 93–7
59. Swanton, R.H., Brooksby, I.A.B., Jenkins, B.S. and Webb-Peploe, M.M. (1977). Haemodynamic studies of beta blockade in hypertrophic obstructive cardiomyopathy. *Eur. J. Cardiol.*, **5/4**, 327–41
60. Lewis, B.S. Mijha, A.S., Bakst, A., Purdon, K. and Gotsman, M.S. (1974). Haemodyna-mic effects of beta blockade in hypertrophic cardiomyopathy using Sectral (Acebutalol, M. and B 17803A). *Cardiovasc. Res.*, **8**, 249–62
61. Rookmaker, W.A., Nieveen, J., Kruizinga, K. and Blickman, J.R. (1971). Beta-adrenergic blockade in the treatment of left sided hypertrophic obstructive cardiomyopathy (HOCM). *Acta Med. Scand.*, **189**, 427–31
62. Hubner, P.J.B., Ziady, G.M., Lane, G.K. Hardarson, T., Scales, B., Oakley, C.M. and Goodwin, J.F. (1973). Double blind trial of propranolol and practolol in hypertrophic. cardiomyopathy. *Br. Heart J.*, **35**, 1116–23
63. Flamm, M.D., Harrison, D.C. and Hancock, E.W. (1968). Muscular subaortic stenosis: prevention of outflow obstruction with propranolol. *Circulation*, **38**, 846–58
64. Stenson, R.E., Flamm, M.D., Harrison, D.C. and Hancock, E.W. (1973). Hypertrophic subaortic stenosis. Clinical and hemodynamic effects of long-term propranolol therapy. *Am. J. Cardiol.*, **31**, 763–73
65. Adelman, A.F. Shah, P.M., Gramiak, R. and Wigle, E.D. (1970). Long-term propranolol therapy in muscular subaortic stenosis. *Br. Heart J.*, **32**, 804–11
66. Alvares, R.F. and Goodwin, J.F. (1982). Non-invasive assessment of diastolic function in hypertrophic cardiomyopathy on and off beta adrenergic blocking drugs. *Br. Heart J.*, **48**, 204–12
67. McKenna, W.J. Chetty, S., Oakley, C.M. and Goodwin, J.F. (1980). Arrhythmia in hypertrophic cardiomyopathy: exercise and 48 hour ambulatory electrocardiographic assessment with and without beta-adrenergic blocking therapy. *Am. J. Cardiol.*, **45**, 1–5

68. Chatterjee, K., Raff, G., Anderson, D. and Parmley, W.W. (1982). Hypertrophic cardiomyopathy therapy with slow channel inhibiting agents. *Prog. Cardiovasc. Dis.*, **25**, 193–208

69. Kaltenbach, M., Hopf, R., Kober, G., Bussman, W.D., Keller, M. and Petersen, Y. (1978). Verapamil treatment of hypertrophic cardiomyopathy. In Kaltenbach, M. *et al.* (eds.) *Cardiomyopathy and Myocardial Biopsy*. pp. 316–31. (New York: Springer)

70. Rosing, D.R., Kent, D.M., Borer, J.S., Seides, S.F. Maron, B.J. and Epstein, S.E. (1979). Verapamil therapy: a new approach to the pharmacologic treatment of hypertrophic cardiomyopathy I. Hemodynamic effects. *Circulation*, **60**, 1201–7

71. Hanrath, P., Mathey, D.G., Kremer, P., Sonntag, F. and Bleifeld, W. (1980). Effect of verapamil on left ventricular isovolumic relaxation time and regional left ventricular filling in hypertrophic cardiomyopathy. *Am. J. Cardiol.*, **45**, 1258–64

72. Ten Cate, F.J., Serruys, P.W., Mey, S. and Roelandt, J. (1983). Effects of short-term administration of verapamil on LV relaxation and filling dynamics measured by a combined hemodynamic ultrasonic technique in patients with hypertrophic cardiomyopathy. *Circulation*, **68**, 1274–9

73. Bonow, R.O., Ostrow, H.G., Rosing, D.R., Cannon, R.O., Lipson, L.C., Maron, B.J., Kent, K.M., Bacharach, S.L. and Green, M.V. (1983). Effects of verapamil on left ventricular systolic and diastolic function in patients with hypertrophic cardiomyopathy: pressure-volume analysis with a non-imaging scintillation probe. *Circulation*, **68**, 1062–73

74. Rosing, D.R., Kent, K.M., Maron, B.J. and Epstein, S.E. (1979). Verapamil therapy: a new approach to the pharmacologic treatment of hypertrophic cardiomyopathy II. Effects on exercise capacity and symptomatic status. *Circulation*, **60**, 1208–13

75. Hasin, Y., Lewis, B.S., Weiss, A.T. and Gotsman, M.S. (1981). Long-term effects of verapamil in hypertrophic cardiomyopathy. *Int. J. Cardiol.*, **1**, 243–51

76. Troesch, M., Hirzel, H.O., Jenni, R. and Krayenbuhl, H.P. (1979). Reduction of septal thickness following verapamil in patients with asymmetric septal hypertrophy. (Abstr.) *Circulation*, **60**, 111–55

77. Thompson, D.S., Wilmhurst, P., Juul, S.M., Waldron, C.B., Jenkins, B.S., Coltart, D.J. and Webb-Peploe, M.M. (1983). Pressure-derived indices of left ventricular isovolumic relaxation in patients with hypertrophic cardiomyopathy. *Br. Heart J.*, **49**, 259–67

78. Bonow, R.O., Frederick, T.M., Bacharach, S.L., Green, M.V., Goose, P.W., Maron, B.J. and Rosing, D.R. (1983). Atrial systole and left ventricular filling in hypertrophic cardiomyopathy: effects of verapamil. *Am. J. Cardiol.*, **51**, 1386–91

79. Bonow, R.O., Rosing, D.R., Bacharach, S.L., Green, M.V., Kent, K.M., Lipson, L.C., Maron, B.J., Leon, M.B., Epstein, S.E. (1981). Effects of verapamil on left ventricular systolic function and diastolic filling in patients with hypertrophic cardiomyopathy. *Circulation*, **64**, 787–96

80. Lorell, B.H. and Barry, W.H. (1984). Effects of verapamil on contraction and relaxation of cultured chick embryo ventricular cells during calcium overload. *J. Am. Coll. Cardiol.*, **3**, 341–8

81. Epstein, S.E. and Rosing, D.R. (1981). Verapamil: its potential for causing serious complications in patients with hypertrophic cardiomyopathy. *Circulation*, **64**, 437–44

82. Perrot, B., Danchin, N. and Terrier de la Chaise, A. (1984). Verapamil: a cause of sudden death in a patients with hypertrophic cardiomyopathy. *Br. Heart J.*, **51**, 532–4

83. McKenna, W.J., Harris, L., Perez, G., Krikler, D.M., Oakley, C. and Goodwin, J.F. (1981). Arrhythmia in hypertrophic cardiomyopathy. II. Comparison of amiodarone and verapamil in treatment. *Br. Heart J.*, **46**, 173–8

84. Lorell, B.H., Paulus, W.J., Grossman, W., Wynne, J., Cohn, P.F. and Braunwald, E. (1980). Improved diastolic function and systolic performance in hypertrophic cardiomyopathy after nifedipine. *N. Engl. J. Med.*, **303**, 801–3

85. Lorell, B.H., Paulus, W.J., Grossman, W. Wynne, J. and Cohn, P.F. (1982). Modification of abnormal left ventricular diastolic properties by nifedipine in patients with hypertrophic cardiomyopathy. *Circulation*, **65**, 499–507

86. Paulus, W.J., Lorell, B.H., Craig, W.E., Wynne, J., Murgo, J.P. and Grossman, W. (1983). Comparison of the effects of nitroprusside and nifedipine on diastolic properties

in patients with hypertrophic cardiomyopathy: altered left ventricular loading or improved muscle inactivation? *J. Am. Coll. Cardiol.*, **2**, 879–86

87. Morrow, A.G. (1978). Hypertrophic subaortic stenosis: operative methods utilized to relieve left ventricular outflow obstruction. *J. Thorac. Cardiovasc. Surg.*, **76**, 423–30

88. Maron, B.J., Koch, J.P., Kent, K.M., Epstein, S.E. and Morrow, A.G. (1980). Results of surgery for idiopathic hypertrophic subaortic stenosis. *Cardiovasc. Med.*, **5**, 145–54

89. Redwood, D.R., Goldstein, R.E., Hirshfeld, J., Borer, J.F., Morganroth, J., Morrow, A.G. and Epstein, S.E. (1979). Exercise performance after septal myotomy and myectomy in patients with obstructive hypertrophic cardiomyopathy. *Am. J. Cardiol.*, **44**, 215–20

90. Borer, J.S., Bacharach, S.L., Green, M.V., Kent, K.M., Rosing, D.R., Seides, S.F., Morrow, A.G. and Epstein, S.E. (1979). Effect of septal myotomy and myectomy on left ventricular systolic function at rest and during exercise in patients with IHSS. *Circulation*, **60** (Suppl. I), 82–7

91. Sanderson, J.E., Traill, T.A., St. John Sutton, M.G., Brown, D.J., Gibson, D.G. and Goodwin, J.F. (1978). Left ventricular relaxation and filling in hypertrophic cardiomyopathy. *Br. Heart J.*, **40**, 596–601

92. St. John Sutton, M.G., Tajik, A.J., Smith, H.C. and Ritman, E.L. (1980). Angina in idiopathic hypertrophic subaortic stenosis. *Circulation*, **61**, 561–8

93. Maron, B.J., Gottdiener, J.S. and Epstein, S.E. (1981). Patterns and significance of distribution of left ventricular hypertrophy in hypertrophic cardiomyopathy. *Am. J. Cardiol.*, **48**, 418–28

94. Shapiro, L.M. and McKenna, W.J. (1983). Distribution of left ventricular hypertrophy in hypertrophic cardiomyopathy: a two-dimensional echocardiographic study. *J. Am. Coll. Cardiol.*, **2**, 437–44

95. Lima, C.O., Sahn, D.J., Valdes-Cruz, L.M., Allen, H.D. Goldberg, S.J., Grenadier, E. and Barron, J.V. (1983). Prediction of the severity of left ventricular outflow tract obstruction by quantitative two-dimensional echocardiographic doppler studies. *Circulation*, **68**, 348–54

96. Kinoshita, N., Nirura, Y., Okamoto, M., Miyatake, K., Nagata, S. and Sakakibara, H. (1983). Mitral regurgitation in hypertrophic cardiomyopathy. Non-invasive study by two-dimensional Doppler echocardiography. *Br. Heart J.* **49**, 574–83

97. Emanuel, R. and Withers, R. (1983). Genetics of the cardiomyopathies. In *Prog. Cardiol.*, **12**, 211–23

98. Bjarnasson, I., Hardarson, T. and Jonsson, S. (1982). Cardiac arrhythmias in hypertrophic cardiomyopathy. *Br. Heart J.*, **48**, 198–203

99. Gill, C.C., Duda, A.M., Kitazume, H., Kramer, J.R. and Loop, F.D. (1982). Idiopathic hypertrophic subaortic stenosis and coronary atherosclerosis. Results of coronary artery bypass alone and myectomy combined with coronary artery bypass. *J. Thorac. Cardiovasc. Surg.*, **84**, 856–60

100. Kowey, P.R., Eisenberg, R. and Engel, T.R. (1984). Sustained arrhythmias in hypertrophic obstructive cardiomyopathy. *N. Engl. J. Med.*, **310**, 1566–9

101. Morrow, A.G., Koch, J. Maron, B.J., Kent, K.M. and Epstein, S.E. (1980). Left ventricular myotomy and myectomy in patients with obstructive hypertrophic cardiomyopathy and previous cardiac arrest. *Am. J. Cardiol.*, **46**, 313–6

102. Oakley, G.D.C., McGarry, K., Limb, D.G. and Oakley, C.M. (1979). Management of pregnancy in patients with hypertrophic cardiomyopathy. *Br. Med. J.*, **1**, 1749–50

103. Shemin, R.G., Scott, W.E., Kastl, D.G. and Morrow, A.G. (1979). Hemodynamic effects of various modes of cardiac pacing after operation for idiopathic hypertrophic subaortic stenosis. *Ann. Thorac. Surg.*, **27**, 137–40

3.1
Pathology, causes and relation to myocarditis

E.G.J. OLSEN

INTRODUCTION

This condition of the heart muscle, of worldwide distribution[1], manifests itself pathologically by hypertrophy of the myocardium and dilatation.

This type of cardiomyopathy in particular has masqueraded under a variety of synonyms which included idiopathic cardiomegaly[2], idiopathic hypertrophy of the heart[3], obscure cardiomyopathy[4], acute reversible heart failure[5], cryptogenic heart disease[6], Nigerian (African) heart muscle disease[7], cardiac disorders of unknown aetiology[8], non-familial idiopathic cardiomyopathy[9] and Jamaican cardiomyopathy[10].

In Chapter 1 reference to the term 'dilated cardiomyopathy' has already been made. As congestive heart failure may not supervene prior to the patient's demise, this term is preferred following the World Health Organization/International Society and Federation of Cardiology Task Force recommendation[11], based on Goodwin's original concepts.

PATHOLOGY

When patients die they have usually reached the end stage of the disease. Macroscopically, the heart is dilated, often to an extreme degree, involving all cardiac chambers. Heart weights are usually double the normal but occasionally weights exceeding 1000 g are found[1,12]. The heart muscle is often pale and 'flabby'. The appearances of the epicardium are usually unremarkable. On opening the cardiac chambers, the walls are often of normal dimensions (for the left ventricle up to 15 mm and for the right ventricle 3 mm at the conus) despite the hypertrophy which is invariably present[13]. This is due to dilatation masking the often severe degree of hypertrophy (Figure 3.1.1). The endocardium is frequently thicker than normal, non-specific in distribution. Thrombus is superimposed in approximately 60% of patients – most frequently in the apical region, but it can occur elsewhere[14]. Cross-sectioning the ventricles may show foci of fibrous tissue particularly prominent towards the inner layers of the myocardial

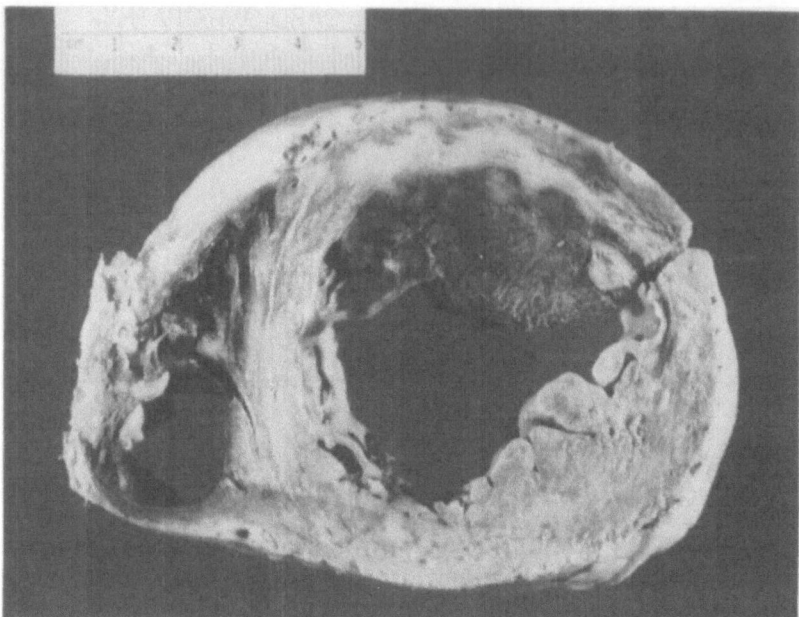

Figure 3.1.1 Cross-section of the ventricles from a patient with dilated cardiomyopathy. Despite the severe degree of hypertrophy, the myocardial wall thicknesses fall within the normal range. Note the superimposed thrombus

walls[15]. The coronary arteries are usually normal but very occasionally some atherosclerosis may be present, which is however insignificant compared to the global involvement of the myocardium[16]. By definition no other intracardiac abnormalities are present.

Death can, however, occur at any stage and therefore hypertrophy alone or with mild dilatation may only be found particularly in those patients in whom heart failure had not supervened prior to death[12].

HISTOLOGY

The myocardial fibres are in normal and in regular alignment, and show nuclear changes of hypertrophy in the form of vesicular changes or pyknosis. Despite obvious nuclear changes of hypertrophy, the myocardial fibre diameters may be normal (up to 12 μm) (Figure 3.1.2). This dissociation of nuclear appearance to cell size is due to stretching or attenuation of the fibres[1,12,15,17]. Occasionally attenuation of muscle fibres is not present and the changes of hypertrophy, including an increase in fibre width, is all that can be recognized. Rarely hypertrophy may be so severe that despite dilatation, attenuation is not recognizable in the myocardial tissue.

The foci of fibrous replacement noted macroscopically represent replacement of myocardial fibres due to necrosis. These changes are interpreted as being consequent to dilatation. In addition focal areas of increase of interstitial collagen tissue may also be found (Figure 3.1.2).

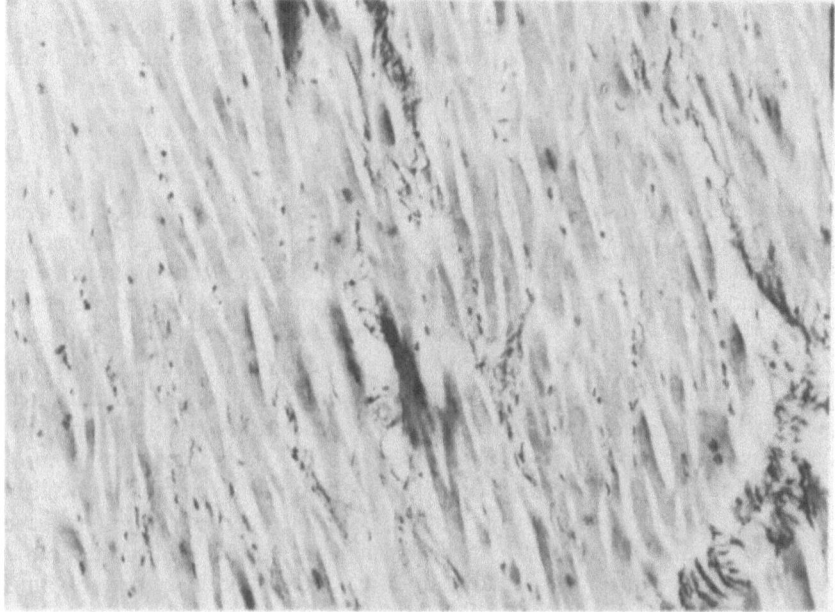

Figure 3.1.2 Photomicrograph showing myocardial fibres in regular alignment and normal myocardial cell fibre diameter. Nuclear changes in the form of pyknosis or vesicular change denoting hypertrophy are evident. This discrepancy is due to attenuation. Foci of fibrous replacement can also be seen. Elastic Van Gieson × 130

The intramyocardial vessels are usually absolutely normal[18]; occasionally, however, some intimal thickening may be present, frequently situated in sites of fibrous replacement but without significantly compromising the lumina. It is believed that these changes are also secondary to dilatation rather than being aetiologically related.

The endocardium is often focally thickened to a mild or moderately severe degree. The prominence of the smooth muscle component can be striking, which denotes that dilatation has been present for at least several months[17].

Focal accumulations of lymphocytes are a frequent finding; these are non-specific and must not necessarily be interpreted as representing myocarditis. Not infrequently, however, changes identical to myocarditis are found[20]; this aspect will be discussed in detail below.

The histological changes are therefore non-specific – consisting of a hypertrophied, dilated myocardium, together with varying severity of a chronic inflammatory infiltrate, indistinguishable from myocarditis.

HISTOCHEMISTRY

Extensive studies, including investigation on glycogen, succinic dehydrogenase, non-specific esterases and phosphatases, have been undertaken. An increase, decrease or normal distribution of these substances has been found. They are usually non-specific, and merely reflect the degree of hypertrophy and the severity and, to some extent, the duration of heart failure that had been present[21] (Figure 3.1.3).

ELECTRON MICROSCOPY

At this level of investigation changes of hypertrophy are found[22,23]. These consist of the myocardial fibrils being in regular alignment but occasionally small foci of irregular alignment can be found together with an increase in inter- and intrafibrillar connections. Mitochondria are usually increased above the normal (one mitochondrion per two sarcomeres). They are usually normal in size and shape but cristolysis can occasionally be observed (Figure 3.1.4). The nuclear membranes are convoluted and pores can often be clearly observed, believed to facilitate the RNA mediated protein synthesis[24]. The tubular system is dilated and the Golgi apparatus prominent. The intercellular spaces are often widened and collagen fibrils as well as occasional lymphocytes may be found. Varying degrees of degenerative changes can also be observed, including myelin figures, membrane-bound vesicles and dissolution of actin and myosin. Oedema of the capillary wall is also sometimes observed. This is interpreted as a non-specific feature, being frequently present in tissue obtained by bioptome[12] (Figure 3.1.5).

MORPHOLOGICAL DIAGNOSIS

Though clinically, together with modern investigatory procedures, any possible cause of cardiomegaly can be excluded, only if a full postmortem is carried out can the diagnosis be established with absolute certainty. As far as the heart is concerned, apart from hypertrophy and dilatation, no other observable abnormalities are present. In many specific heart muscle diseases, cardiac involvement also results in a hypertrophied, dilated heart. Necropsy is therefore essential to exclude any possible cause which may not have resulted in any clinical manifestations. Histological examination is also essential to exclude possible myocarditis, haemachromatosis or leukaemic infiltration, not readily discernible with the naked eye[25].

The technique of biopsy, recovering endomyocardial tissue by bioptome[25], has permitted additional morphological studies to be undertaken in the hope of defining possible diagnostic criteria with negative results. Morphometric studies have also not yielded any positive results[19,26]. When the histological changes described above are present, and provided that clinically other conditions resulting in heart failure have been excluded, diagnosis is possible. Experience has however shown that hypertrophy alone with or without evidence of dilatation in the endocardium may only be present and occasionally no morphological abnormalities are found. These patients usually present to the physician with vague chest pain or show minor electrocardiographic changes, such as left bundle branch block[27]. These two groups of patients are of particular interest as they may well represent the earliest manifestations of this disease.

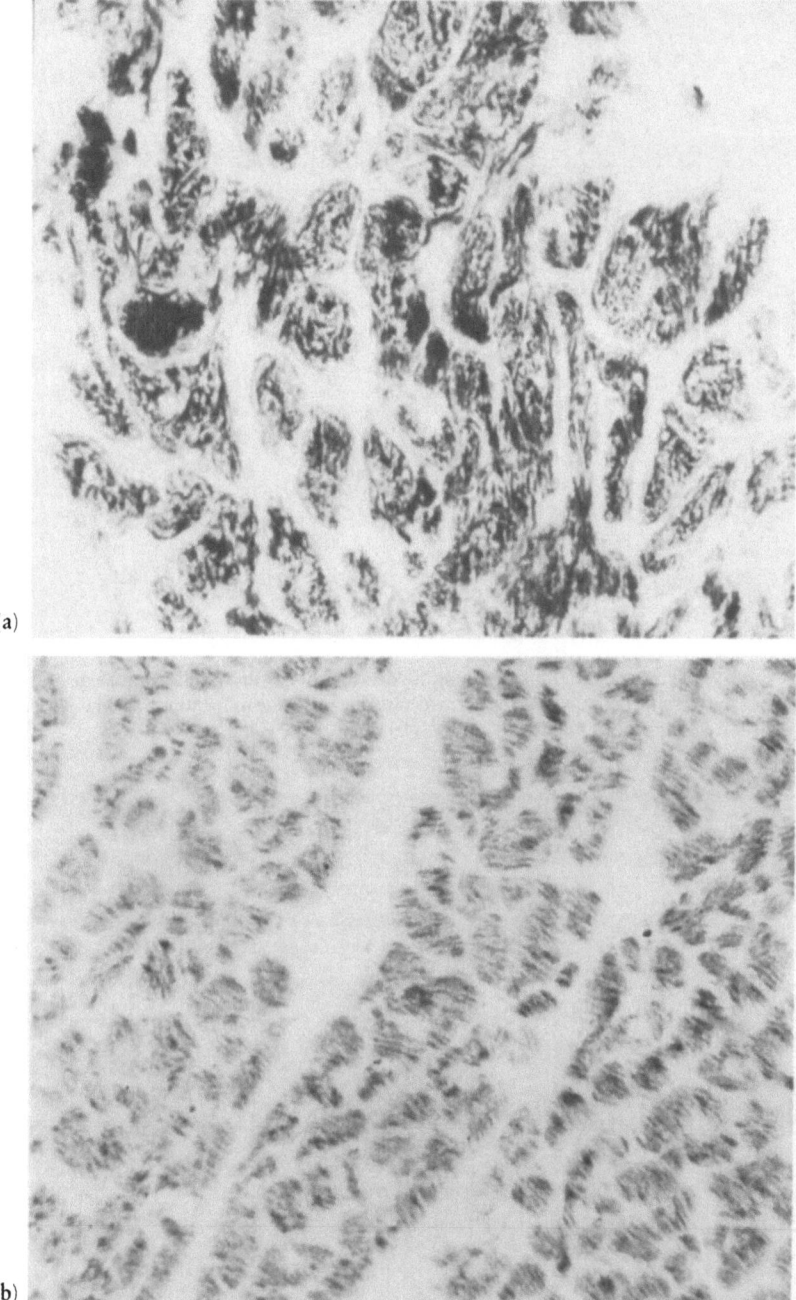

Figure 3.1.3 (a) The section has been stained to show a patchy increase of succinic dehydrogenase from a patient with a short history of non-specific symptoms. MTT × 250. (b) Photomicrograph of a similarly treated sample from a patient with a longstanding history of dilated cardiomyopathy and congestive heart failure showing widespread depletion. MTT × 250

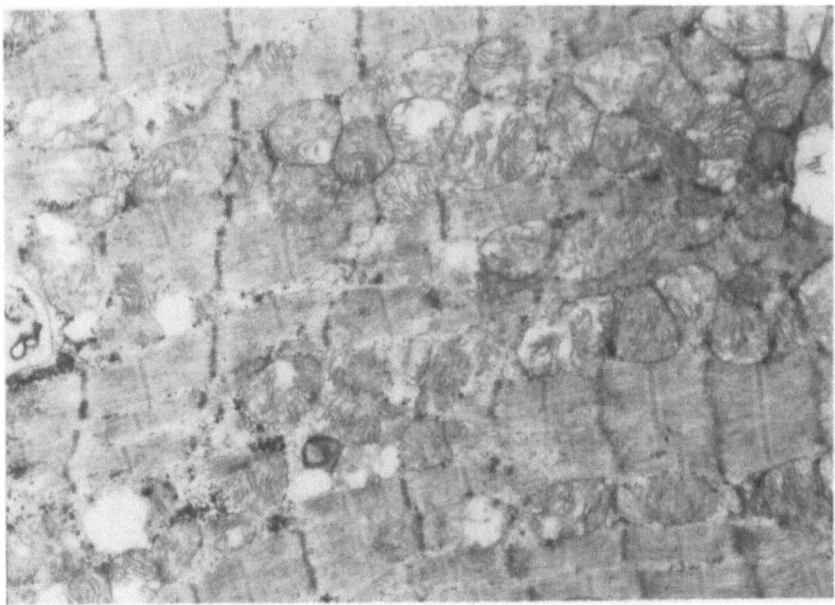

Figure 3.1.4 Electron micrograph showing myocardial fibrils in parallel alignment and an increase of mitochondria of up to three per two sarcomeres. Some mitochondria show evidence of cristolysis. Uranyl acetate and lead citrate × 11 600

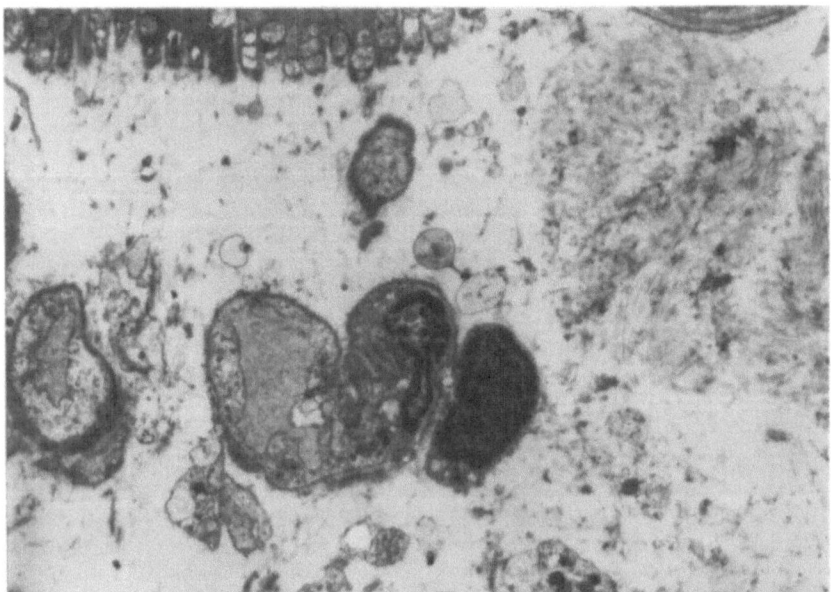

Figure 3.1.5 Electron micrograph of an intercellular space showing capillaries with oedema in their walls. This finding is non-specific. In addition collagen fibrils abound. Uranyl acetate and lead citrate × 4300

Electronmicroscopic examination has also not yielded any diagnostic criteria. Degenerative changes are found in hypertrophy due to known causes. Foci of irregular fibrillar alignment are also found in hypertrophy due to known causes as well as in other conditions such as hypertrophic cardiomyopathy. In that condition disarray of myocardial fibrils is, however, widespread, whereas in dilated cardiomyopathy and hypertrophy due to known causes, foci of irregular arrangement are very few and far between[28].

DIFFERENTIAL DIAGNOSIS

Two conditions are morphologically identical to dilated cardiomyopathy. The first is heart failure due to alcoholic abuse, and no differences between the two conditions have been established[29] (Figure 3.1.6). Recourse to

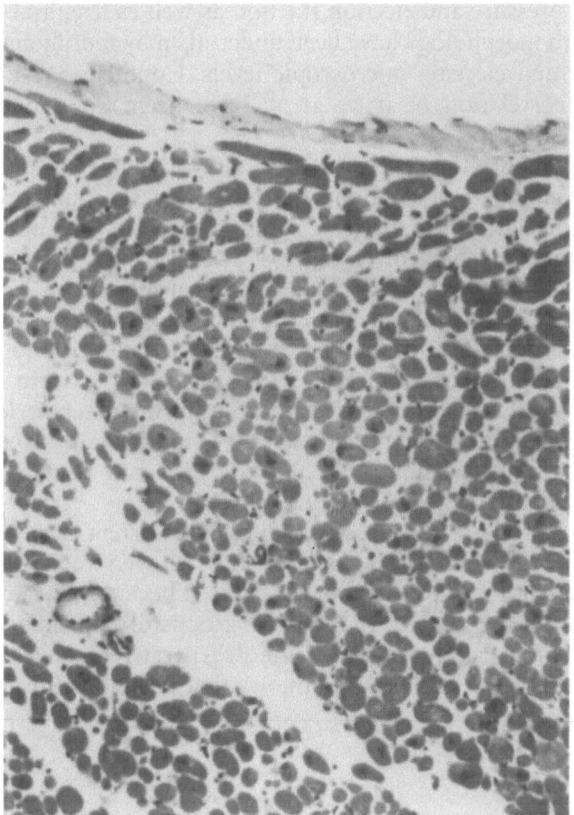

Figure 3.1.6 Cross-section of an endomyocardial biopsy, showing predominantly normal diameter of myocardial fibres and nuclear changes of hypertrophy. The endocardium is mildly thickened, containing some prominent smooth muscle fibres. A normal arteriole has been included in the section. The appearances are non-specific and are morphologically indistinguishable from dilated cardiomyopathy. H & E × 140

enzymatic examination has to be undertaken. It has been shown that creatinine phosphokinase, lactic dehydrogenase, malic dehydrogenase, α-hydroxybutyric dehydrogenase and glutamic oxaloacetic transaminase are significantly greater in patients with alcohol abuse than in patients with dilated cardiomyopathy[30]. A higher percentage of H-subunits has been found in patients with heart failure due to excess alcoholic intake compared to patients with cardiomyopathy of similar haemodynamic state[31].

The other condition which is identical, morphologically, to dilated cardiomyopathy is heart failure occurring towards the end of pregnancy or in the puerperium[29]. The relation to pregnancy makes identification of these patients easy. The causes of the condition are unknown but possible aetiological suggestions have included malnutrition, infection, auto-immunity and local customs.

Correlative studies of haemodynamic parameters such as left ventricular end diastolic pressure and ejection fraction as well as length of history and prognosis with morphology have been undertaken by morphometric techniques at light and electron microscopic levels. Conflicting results showing either good correlation or none at all have been reported by different groups[32,33].

An extensive morphometric study, relating volume per cent of interstitial collagen to haemodynamic parameters, length of history and prognosis has shown no correlation whatever[19,26,34]. These results are not surprising. Calculating the coefficient of variance showed a value to 80·5% between two biopsies from the same ventricle. It has been shown that if five or more biopsies are taken the coefficient of variance is sufficiently low reflecting fairly accurately the state of the rest of the myocardium[35].

The reasons for the discrepancy in results by this group from some others may be due to the investigators concentrating on different features, for example the interstitium or volume fraction of interstitial collagen tissue, or due to lack of sufficient number of biopsies, or it may be that correlations may be coincidental.

As far as prognosis is concerned, a points system has been devised evaluating the degenerative changes[36]. It has been found that for an individual patient prognosis cannot be assessed because death can occur at any stage during the disease. A trend for groups of patients was however established in that the more severe the degenerative changes, the poorer the prognosis became. It therefore follows that prognosis for an individual patient cannot be given[34].

CAUSES

By definition the causes of dilated cardiomyopathy are unknown. As it is often the case, if an aetiology is not known innumerable suggestions have been made.

Deficiency of succinic dehydrogenase[37]

As has already been noted in the section on Histochemistry, varying degrees of this substance are found. Deficiency occurs in most patients with a longstanding history or in those with severe heart failure. It is now believed that a decrease in succinic dehydrogenase is secondary to heart failure rather than causally related to dilated cardiomyopathy[21].

Abnormalities of the small vessels[38]

Morphological abnormalities are only rarely found and even when they occur the vessels affected are usually insufficient in severity or number, which could explain the widespread myocardial changes. Oedema of the capillary walls is also considered non-specific[12] (*see above*). Reaction of vessels to substances such as prostaglandins may well occur but these do not result in morphologically recognizable changes.

A possible infective agent[39]

Suggestions that a protozoan may be involved have not been conclusively substantiated. The possibility of misinterpretation has been entertained[40].

Systemic hypertension

The possibility that dilated cardiomyopathy is systemic hypertension in disguise[41] has also not been confirmed morphologically by examining renal and other tissues. Hypertension occurring in some patients with dilated cardiomyopathy is well known but this may be a coincidental association.

Possible multifactorial aetiology

It may be that a multifactorial aetiology is the likely explanation, probably influenced by a factor or factors as yet, however, not established[42].

RELATION TO MYOCARDITIS

Viral infection and immunological abnormalities

There is now persuasive evidence that an infectious-immune mechanism may be operative in a significant number of patients with dilated cardiomyopathy[20]. It is relevant to review briefly the clinical and pathological features pointing to such a possible mechanism. In previously healthy individuals cardiac symptoms often develop some time after an upper respiratory infection. Periodic heart failure follows for no obvious cause. Many patients respond well to corticosteroid therapy, particularly in the early phase of the disease. Heart reactive antibodies, immunoglobulins, antinuclear antibodies and serological positive findings to rheumatoid

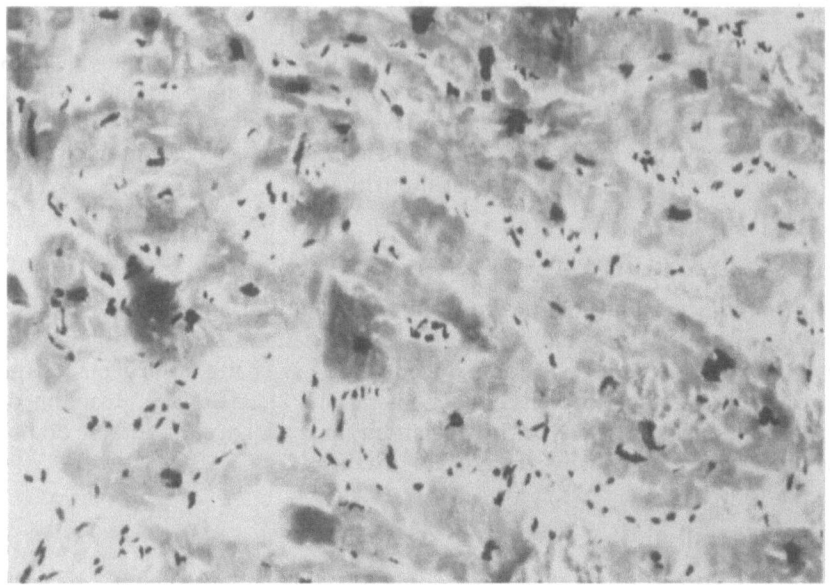

Figure 3.1.7 Endomyocardial biopsy from a patient clinically suspected to suffer from dilated cardiomyopathy. Widening of the interstitium is present in which a mild increase in chronic inflammatory cells can be seen. Fraying of myocardial fibres in close proximity to inflammatory cells can be seen. H & E × 235

disease as well as syphilis have been demonstrated in some patients. γ-Globulins have been demonstrated in heart tissue obtained by biopsy. Changes in the myocardium including an increase in interstitial fibrous tissue and an inflammatory infiltrate consisting of lymphocytes and other mononuclear cells have not infrequently been found[43].

Let us first consider the morphological features. Reference to lymphocytes in the myocardium has already been made[19]. Frequently, the changes of myocarditis now defined as 'the presence of inflammatory cells in the myocardium with evidence of fraying of adjacent myocardial fibres but without concomitant sequential fibre necrosis' are evident[20,44] (Figure 3.1.7).

In almost 15% of over 600 patients with a suspected clinical diagnosis of dilated cardiomyopathy in whom endomyocardial biopsy examination had been undertaken, typical changes of myocarditis, satisfying the above criteria of definition, have been found (Olsen, E.J.G., personal observation, 1983).

In a subsequent study investigating 74 patients with a similar suspected diagnosis, biopsy tissue was reported as active, healing or healed myocarditis. In addition microneutralization antibody tests for Coxsackie B virus were undertaken. In 45% of 22 patients morphologically grouped as having active myocarditis, titres in dilutions of 1:320 or more were obtained[45]. In

Table 3.1.1 Patients investigated at King's College Hospital (January 1980 to May 1982)

	Total	Peak Coxsackie B Neutralization titre				
		<80	160	320	640	>1280
Acute myocarditis	22	9	3	4	3	3
Healing/healed myocarditis	16	9	4	2	—	1
COCM	36	23	6	6	1	—

the other groups of patients, healing or healed myocarditis was evident often without neutralization titres in relevant dilutions (Table 3.1.1).

Another study also yielded similar results. In this investigation, however, patients were principally suspected to have had a viral myocarditis. In 45% of these patients correlation between myocarditis morphologically and rising neutralization antibody titres existed (Bolte, H.-D. and Olsen, E.J.G., personal observations, 1981) (Figure 3.1.8).

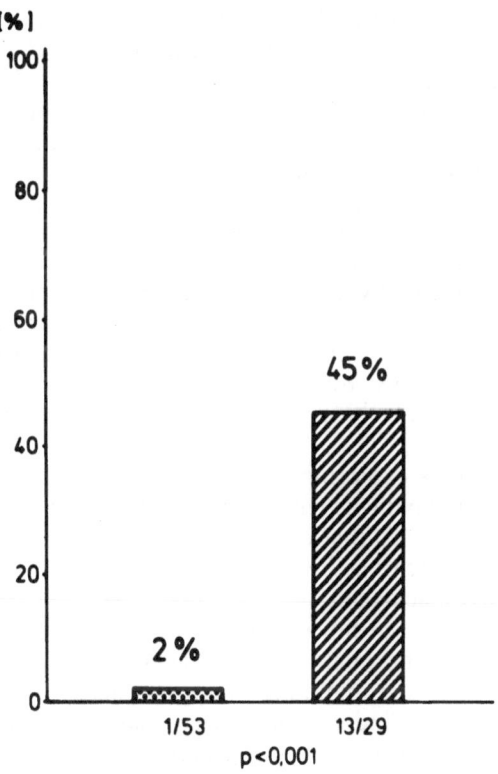

Figure 3.1.8 Myocardial biopsy. Morphological evidence of inflammation in COCM (left column) and viral carditis (right column). From Bolte, H.D., Olsen, E.G.J. et al. (unpublished)

Alternatively, titres in high dilutions may be present without morphological evidence of myocarditis. This was demonstrated in an investigation of 50 patients diagnosed as having dilated cardiomyopathy. Microneutralization antibody tests for Coxsackie B virus showed titres in dilutions of 1024 or more in 15 of these patients but only in one of 50 of age and sex matched control individuals[46]. Endomyocardial tissue had been obtained by bioptome in 11 of these 15 patients, showing non-specific features of dilated cardiomyopathy only, with no evidence of active myocarditis or myocarditis in the past.

These studies have demonstrated the close relation in a significant number of patients between myocarditis and clinically diagnosed dilated cardiomyopathy. The fact that immunological disturbances result in an inflammatory infiltrate is well established, and when these disturbances affect the heart, myocarditis may result. Although all the criteria of myocarditis are present the changes are usually mild.

What then is the evidence that immunological mechanisms consequent to a virus infection are operative?

Heart reactive antibodies have been found in various cardiovascular diseases among which cardiomyopathy is included. Dependent upon the method of assay used, prevalences of 17–40% have been established[47]. Although some workers have shown that these antibodies correlate with the severity and duration of cardiomyopathy[48], others have not[49]. It has been suggested that heart reactive antibodies are unlikely to be pathogenetically linked[47]. Further evidence was provided by the observation that in severely disabled patients undergoing transplantation, heart reactive antibodies were not present in the circulation prior to operation. Examination of cardiac tissue from the recipients showed extensive deposit of bound γ-globulin and complement. The likelihood that the heart severely affected by cardiomyopathy may preferentially fix heart reactive immunoglobulins to specific sarcolemmal and subsarcolemmal antigens, and thus prevent detection of heart reactive antibodies in the serum, has been entertained[50]. In endomyocardial tissue obtained by bioptome from patients with dilated cardiomyopathy preferential binding of IgG and IgA has been demonstrated[48].

A series of investigations exploring immunological disturbances consequent to a viral infection in patients with dilated cardiomyopathy has taken place in more recent years[43]. To that end, cell mediated immunity has been explored. One such approach has been the study of *in vitro* lymphocytic transformation to phytohaemagglutinin[51]. Patients with dilated cardiomyopathy as well as other cardiovascular diseases including ischaemic, rheumatic and congenital abnormalities, as well as control individuals have shown abnormal cell mediated immunity in approximately 40% of cases with cardiomyopathy. This finding emphasized that cases with dilated cardiomyopathy represent a heterogeneous group.

Sensitization to heart muscle was also demonstrated in some patients with cardiomyopathy using heart extract[51]. Reduced lymphocytic stimulation to phytohaemagglutinin has been confirmed by other workers[52], who also demonstrated an absolute reduction in the percentage of circulating T-lymphocytes.

Cell mediated immunity has also been investigated by leukocyte migration inhibition, using concanavalin A (mitogen) and human heart muscle extract (antigen) in patients with dilated cardiomyopathy and ischaemic heart disease together with controls[43]. Though no significant differences were noted in mean leukocyte migration inhibition, a distinct bimodal response above and below the 90% confidence limit of the control migration index was observed in cardiomyopathic patients. Five of the 12 patients with cardiomyopathy showed responses to concanavalin A above the 90% confidence limit of control. The findings were significant.

The role of cell mediated immunity has also been investigated by studying cell mediated cytotoxicity in several heart diseases including dilated cardiomyopathy[53]. Results showed lymphocytes were cytotoxic to cultured human heart cells in 30% of 73 patients with dilated cardiomyopathy and in 24% in other cardiac conditions, mainly rheumatic heart disease, and 4% of 49 control individuals. Thus lymphocytic toxicity was not specific to patients with cardiomyopathy but could occur as a result of myocardial damage due to a variety of causes.

The possibility that sensitized lymphocytes could be responsible for chronic myocardial damage has been entertained, based on experimental evidence. T-lymphocytes from infected mice with Coxsackie B-3 virus have been shown to be cytotoxic to infected syngeneic myocardial cells *in vitro*. The effect was abolished by antithymocytic serum[54].

T-suppressor-cell function which normally prevents excessive lymphoid proliferation has shown to be defective in man with dilated cardiomyopathy but not in coronary heart disease[55,56]. It may be that antibodies to viral infection act on the T-cell receptors, interfering with normal B-cell activity resulting in auto-immune antibodies. T-suppressor-cell dysfunction may also affect cell mediated immunity[43].

The defective T-cell function, and by inference, its normal function, is demonstrated by the study of 37 patients with cardiomyopathy undergoing cardiac transplantation for dilated cardiomyopathy. Six patients developed lymphoma. This did not occur in 54 patients with coronary heart disease[57]. These studies corroborate the role of T-cell lymphocytes.

All these studies have provided some insight into a possible mechanism of dilated cardiomyopathy operative in a substantial number of cases. Otherwise healthy individuals may be unusually susceptible to common virus infection triggering abnormal immunological responses which result in myocarditis and heart failure. Evidence for such a concept may be found experimentally. Active myocarditis followed infection with Coxsackie B virus in mice. Recovery of virus from myocardium in the early stages was possible. The active stage was succeeded by chronic myocarditis (when virus could no longer be recovered), showing foci of myocardial necrosis and a cellular infiltrate. It was suggested that these features resulted from an immune response initiated by persistent but non-infectious antigens or due to new antigens formed from necrotic myocardial fibres[58].

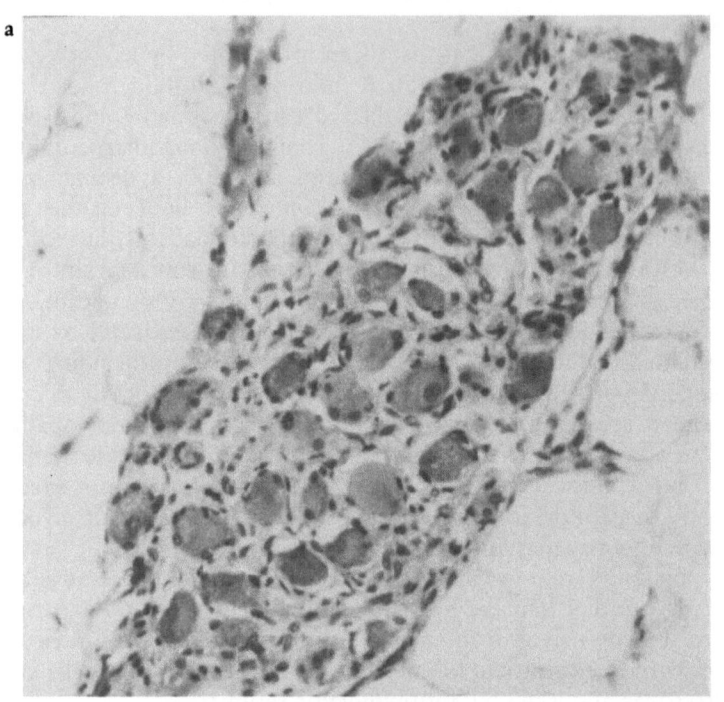

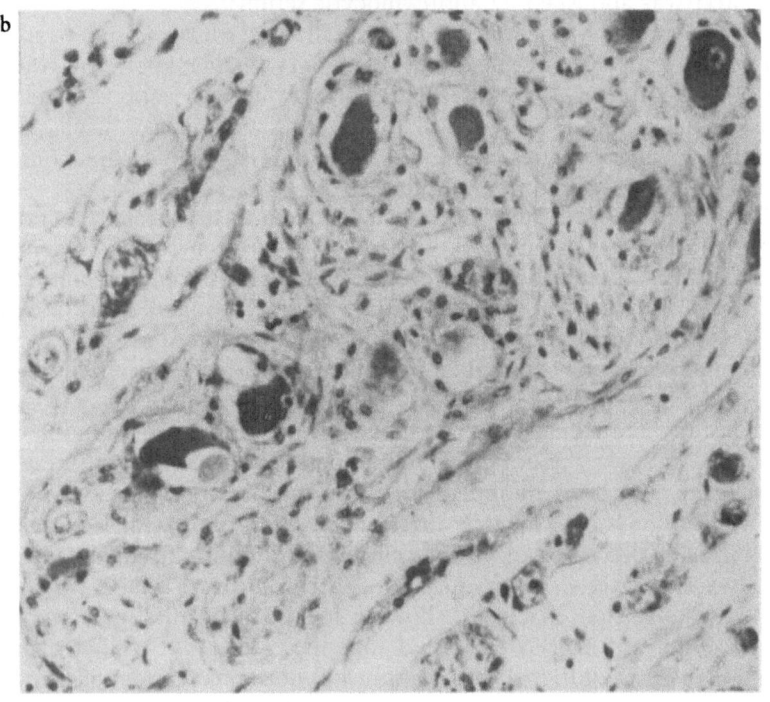

It is tempting to extrapolate from these experimental studies to man where similar changes are observed.

An additional morphological study has provided a further possible clue to the pathogenetic mechanism in dilated cardiomyopathy. Assessment of the number of neurons in the right atrium between the *venae cavae* has shown a significant reduction in the hearts of patients with dilated cardiomyopathy compared to normal controls (Figure 3.1.9). The strip of right atrial muscle was serially sectioned at 50 μm intervals (to avoid counting neuronal cells twice). In normal individuals the neuronal count averaged 6412 ± 377 (SE), whilst in patients with cardiomyopathy values of 4565 ± 471 (SE) were counted $(p < 0.002)$[59].

It may be that the final morphological expression of immunological abnormalities following virus infection in susceptible patients results in neuronal depopulation in some patients with dilated cardiomyopathy.

Considering these various aspects, there is therefore good evidence that myocarditis is closely linked to some patients with dilated cardiomyopathy. This does not, however, imply that when patients are infected with a virus heart failure due to viral myocarditis no longer occurs and all patients develop dilated cardiomyopathy. Subtle morphological differences exist. In heart failure, occurring in myocarditis, either due to bacterial, viral, fungal or rickettsial infection or indeed in the isolated form, the inflammatory infiltrate is usually severe and necrosis of adjacent myocardial fibres extensive. In the chronic phase, areas of fibrous replacement are scattered throughout the entire thickness of the ventricular walls. The pericardium is also frequently involved. In dilated cardiomyopathy in which virus may play a pathogenetic role, the inflammation occurring as a result of immunological abnormalities is mild, cellular necrosis is minimal and the pericardium is rarely involved. In cases of long standing the areas of fibrous replacement are limited to the inner layers of the myocardium[60].

Conclusion

Although the evidence of an infectious-immune pathogenesis in some patients with dilated cardiomyopathy is compelling, much work needs to be done to establish clearly the role of virus and myocarditis in these patients.

References

1. Olsen, E.G.J. (1972). Cardiomyopathies. *Cardiovasc. Clin.*, 4, 240
2. Levy, R.L. (1955). Idiopathic cardiomegaly. *J. Chron. Dis.*, 1, 292
3. Altman, H. and Stein, H (1956). Idiopathic hypertrophy of the heart in African children. *Br. Med. J.*, 1, 1207
4. Evans, B. (1957). Obscure cardiomyopathy. *Br. Heart J.*, 19, 164

Figure 3.1.9   (a) Neuronal cells closely packed of a right atrial intercaval strip from a normal individual. H & E × 160. Compare with (b) from a similar site from a patient with dilated cardiomyopathy. A severe reduction of neuronal cells, widely separated by collagen tissue can clearly be seen. H & E × 224

5. Grusin, H. (1957). Acute reversible heart failure. *Circulation*, **16**, 27
6. Higginson, J., Isaacson, C. and Simson, I. (1960). Pathology of cryptogenic heart disease. *Arch. Pathol.*, **70**, 497
7. Edington, G.M. and Jackson, J.G. (1963). Pathology of heart muscle disease and endomyocardial fibrosis in Nigeria. *J. Pathol. Bacteriol.*, **86**, 333
8. Stuart, K.L. and Hayes, J.A. (1963). A cardiac disorder of unknown aetiology in Jamaica. *Q. J. Med.*, **32**, 99
9. Hudson, R.E.B. (1970). The cardiomyopathies. Order from chaos. *Am. J. Cardiol.*, **25**, 70
10. Hill, K.R., Still, W.J.S. and McKinney, B. (1967). Jamaican cardiomyopathy. *Br. Heart J.*, **29**, 594
11. Report of the WHO/ISFC Task Force on the definition and classification of cardiomyopathies (1980) *Br. Heart J.*, **44**, 672
12. Olsen, E.G.J. (1981). Pathology of congestive cardiomyopathy. In Goodwin, J.F., Hjalmarson, A. and Olsen, E.G.J. (eds.) *Congestive Cardiomyopathy, Kiruna, Sweden, 1980.* pp. 66–74. (Mölndal, Sweden: AB Hässle)
13. Olsen, E.G.J. (1972). Pathology of primary cardiomyopathies. *Postgrad. Med. J.*, **48**, 732
14. Olsen, E.G.J. (1976). Pathologie der 'primären' Kardiomyopathien. *Munch. Med. Wochenschr.*, **118**, 735
15. Olsen, E.G.J. (1979). The pathology of cardiomyopathies. A critical analysis. *Am. Heart J.*, **98**(3), 385
16. Gau, G.T., Goodwin, J.F., Oakley, C.M., Olsen, E.G.J., Rahimtoola, S.H., Raphael, M.J. and Steiner, R.E. (1972). Q waves and coronary arteriography in cardiomyopathy. *Br. Heart J.*, **34**, 1034
17. Olsen, E.G.J. (1975). Pathological recognition of cardiomyopathy. *Postgrad. Med. J.*, **51**, 277
18. Olsen, E.G.J. (1978). Endomyocardial biopsy. *Invest. Cell Pathol.*, **1**, 139
19. Baandrup, U. and Olsen, E.G.J. (1981). Critical analysis of endomyocardial biopsies from patients suspected of having cardiomyopathy. I: Morphological and morphometric aspects. *Br. Heart J.*, **45**, 475
20. Olsen, E.G.J. (1983). Myocarditis, a case of mistaken identity. *Br. Heart J.*, **50**, 303
21. Olsen, E.G.J. (1978). Postmortem findings and histologic, histochemical, and electron microscopic findings of myocardial biopsies. In Kaltenbach, M., Loogen, F. and Olsen, F.G.J. (eds.) *Cardiomyopathy and Myocardial Biopsy.* pp. 52–61 (Berlin, Heidelberg, New York: Springer)
22. Olsen, E.G.J. (1974). Hypertrophy, hyperplasia and dilatation. In Olsen, E.G.J. (ed.) *The Pathology of The Heart.* pp. 26–30. (Stuttgart: Thieme)
23. Maron, B.J., Ferrans, V.J. and Roberts, W.C. (1975). Ultrastructural features of degenerated cardiac muscle cells in patients with cardiac hypertrophy. *Am. J. Pathol.*, **79**, 387
24. Legato, M.J. (1974). Nuclear pores in the human myofiber. *J. Mol. Cell Cardiol.*, **6**, 283
25. Olsen, E.G.J. (1977). Myocardial biopsy. In Hamer, J. (ed.) *Recent Advances in Cardiology.* No. 7. pp. 349–67. (Edinburgh, London and New York: Churchill Livingstone)
26. Baandrup, U., Florio, R.A., Rehahn, M., Richardson, P.J. and Olsen, E.G.J. (1981). Critical analysis of endomyocardial biopsies from patients suspected of having cardiomyopathy. II: Comparison of histology and clinical/haemodynamic information. *Br. Heart J.*, **45**, 487
27. Kuhn, H., Breithardt, G., Knieriem, H.J., Köhler, E., Lösse, B., Seipel, L. and Loogen, F. (1978). Prognosis and possible presymptomatic manifestations of congestive cardiomyopathy (COCM). *Postgrad. Med. J.*, **54**, 451
28. Olsen, E.G.J. (1982). Myocardial disarray revisited. (Leader.) *Br. Med. J.*, **285**, 991
29. Olsen, E.G.J. (1980). *The Pathology of the Heart.* 2nd Edn. p. 327. (London: Macmillan)
30. Richardson, P.J. and Atkinson, L. (1980). Enzyme activities in endomyocardial biopsy samples from patients with cardiomyopathy. In Bolte, H.-D. (ed.) *Myocardial Biopsy.* pp. 97–101. (Berlin, Heidelberg, New York: Springer)
31. Bolte, H.-D., Schultheiss, P., Cyran, J. and Goss, F. (1980). Binding of immunoglobulins in the myocardial (biopsies) in cardiomyopathies. In Bolte, H.-D. (ed.) *Myocardial Biopsy.* pp. 85–93. (Berlin, Heidelberg, New York: Springer)

32. Kunkel, B., Lapp, H., Kober, G. and Kaltenbach, M. (1978). Light microscopic evaluation of myocardial biopsies. In Kaltenbach, M., Loogen, F. and Olsen, E.G.J. (eds.) *Cardiomyopathy and Myocardial Biopsy*. pp. 62–70. (Berlin, Heidelberg, New York: Springer)

33. Davies, M.J., Brooksby, I.A.B., Jenkins, B.S., Cankovic-Darracott, S., Swanton, R.H., Coltart, J. and Webb-Peploe, M.M. (1977). Left ventricular endomyocardial biopsy II: The value of light microscopy. *Catheter. Cardiovasc. Diagn.*, 3, 123

34. Baandrup, U., Florio, R.A., Roters, F. and Olsen, E.G.J. (1981). Electron microscopic investigation of endomyocardial biopsy samples in hypertrophy and cardiomyopathy. A semiquantitative study in 48 patients. *Circulation*, 63, 1289

35. Baandrup, U., Florio, R.A. and Olsen, E.G.J. (1982). Do endomyocardial biopsies represent the morphology of the rest of the myocardium? A quantitative light microscopic study of single v. multiple biopsies with the King's bioptome. *Eur. Heart J.*, 3, 171

36. Kuhn, H., Breithardt, G., Knieriem, H.J., Loogen, F., Both, A., Schmidt, W.A.K., Stroobandt, R. and Gleichmann, U. (1975). Die Bedeutung der endomyokardialen Katheterbiopsie für die Diagnostik und die Beurteilung der Prognose der kongestiven Kardiomyopathie. *Dtsch. Med. Wochenschr.*, 100, 717

37. Kobernick, S.D., Mandell, G.H., Zirkin, R.M. and Hashimoto, Y. (1963). Succinic dehydrogenase deficiency in idiopathic cardiomyopathy. *Am. J. Pathol.*, 43, 661

38. James, T.N. (1964). An etiologic concept concerning the obscure myocardiopathies. *Prog. Cardiovasc. Dis.*, 7, 43

39. Braimbridge, M.V., Darracott, S., Chayen, J., Bitensky, L. and Poulter, L.W. (1967). Possibility of a new infective aetiological agent in congestive cardiomyopathy. *Lancet*, 1, 171

40. Van Noorden, S., Olsen, E.G.J. and Pearse, A.G.E. (1971). Hypertrophic obstructive cardiomyopathy, a histological, histochemical and ultrastructural study of biopsy material. *Cardiovasc. Res.*, 5, 118

41. Oakley, C.M. (1972). Clinical definitions and classification of cardiomyopathies. *Postgrad. Med. J.*, 48, 703

42. Goodwin, J.F. (1978). Introduction, problems and aims of the Multicentre Research Project. *Postgrad. Med. J.*, 54, 431–2

43. Das, S.K., Stein, L.D., Reynolds, R.T., Thebert, P. and Cassidy, J.T. (1981). Immunologic studies in cardiomyopathy and pathophysiologic implications. In Goodwin, J.F., Hjalmarson, A. and Olsen, E.G.J. (eds.) *Congestive Cardiomyopathy, Kiruna, Sweden, 1980*. pp. 87–93. (Mölndal, Sweden: AB Hässle)

44. Olsen, E.G.J. In Goodwin, J.F., Hjalmarson, A. and Olsen, E.G.J. (eds.) *Congestive Cardiomyopathy, Kiruna, Sweden, 1980*. Discussion, p. 122. (Mölndal, Sweden: AB Hässle)

45. Richardson, P.J., Daly, K. and Gishen P. (1984). Haemodynamic findings in biopsy-proven acute myocarditis. In Bolte, H.-D. (ed.) *Viral Heart Disease*. p. 265 (Berlin, Heidelberg, New York, Tokyo: Springer–Verlag)

46. Cambridge, G., MacArthur, C.G.C., Waterson, A.P., Goodwin, J.F. and Oakley, C.M. (1979). Antibodies to Coxsackie B viruses in congestive cardiomyopathy. *Br. Heart J.*, 41, 692

47. Das, S.K. and Cassidy, J.T. (1973). Antiheart antibodies in patients with systemic lupus erythematosus. *Am. J. Med. Sci.*, 265, 275

48. Bolte, H.-D. and Schultheiss, P. (1978). Immunological results in myocardial diseases. *Postgrad. Med. J.*, 54, 500

49. Kirsner, A.B., Hess, E.V. and Fowler, N.O. (1973). Immunologic findings in idiopathic cardiomyopathy: a prospective serial study. *Am. Heart J.*, 86, 625

50. Das, S.K., Callen, J.P., Dodson, N.V. and Cassidy, J.T. (1971). Immunoglobulin binding in cardiomyopathic hearts. *Circulation*, 44, 612

51. Das, S.K., Petty, R.E., Meengs, W.L. and Tubergen, D.G. (1976). Cell mediated immunity in cardiomyopathy. *Circulation*, 53/54 (Suppl. 2), II–22

52. Sachs, R.N. and Lanfranchi, J. (1978). Cardiomyopathies primitives et anomalies immunitaires. *Coeur Med. Intern.*, 17, 193

53. Jacobs, B., Matsuda, Y., Deodhar, S. and Shirey, E. (1979). Cell-mediated cytotoxicity to cardiac cells of lymphocytes from patients with primary myocardial disease. *Am. J. Clin. Pathol.*, **72**, 1

54. Wong, C.Y., Woodruff, J.J. and Woodruff, J.F. (1977). Generation of cytotoxic T lymphocytes during Coxsackie virus B-3 infection. II. Characterization of effector cells and demonstration of cytotoxicity against viral-infected myofibers. *J. Immunol.*, **118**, 1165

55. Fowles, R.E., Bieber, C.P. and Stinson, E.B. (1979). Defective in vitro suppressor cell function in idiopathic congestive cardiomyopathy. *Circulation*, **59**, 483

56. Eckstein, R., Mempel, W. and Bolte, H.-D. (1982). Congestive cardiomyopathy and myocarditis. *Circulation*, **65**, 1224

57. Anderson, J.L., Bieber, C.P., Fowles, R.E. and Stinson, E.B. (1978). Idiopathic cardiomyopathy, age, and suppressor-cell dysfunction as risk determinants of lymphoma after cardiac transplantation. *Lancet*, **2**, 1174

58. Wilson, F.M., Miranda, Q.R., Chason, J.L. and Lerner, A.M. (1969). Residual pathologic changes following murine Coxsackie A and B myocarditis. *Am. J. Pathol.*, **55**, 253

59. Amorim, D.S. and Olsen, E.G.J. (1982). Assessment of heart neurons in dilated (congestive) cardiomyopathy. *Br. Heart J.*, **47**, 11

60. Olsen, E.G.J. (1983). Histomorphological relations between myocarditis and dilated cardiomyopathy. In Bolte, H.-D. (ed). *Viral Heart Disease.* p. 5 (Berlin, Heidelberg, New York, Tokyo: Springer-Verlag)

3.2
Clinical aspects, treatment and prognosis

R.O. BRANDENBURG

INTRODUCTION

Dilated (congestive) cardiomyopathy is defined as 'a form of cardio-myopathy in which there is impaired function of the heart as a pump with dilatation of the ventricles and reduced systolic function'[1]. In addition, the muscle dysfunction is of unknown cause[2].

The incidence of the disease appears to vary widely, but it is more common in less industrialized countries. In a Uganda hospital, the incidence was 19%[3]. In Ceylon (now Sri Lanka), it accounted for 26% of 150 patients with congestive heart failure[4]. In South Africa, it constituted 14% of cardiac deaths at autopsy in blacks[5]. In a defined population in Sweden, however, Torp noted an incidence of only 5.3 cases per 100 000 population using clinical criteria and 7.5 cases per 100 000 at postmortem study[6]. It seems clear the incidence is much higher than previously suspected. A recent estimate is that dilated cardiomyopathy is between a tenth and a quarter as common as 'ischaemic cardiomyopathy'[7]. The disease is more common in blacks and males, and is recognized most often in the middle decades.

CLINICAL ASPECTS

Clinically, it is necessary to exclude the common causes (coronary, hyper-tension, valvular, and congenital heart disease) and also heart muscle disease of known cause or associated with disorders of other systems[2]. In addition, there must be dilatation of the ventricles and impairment of systolic function.

The recognition of dilated cardiomyopathy may be early, an asymptomatic stage in which physical signs are subtle and minimal, or late, when the patient is in advanced congestive heart failure. For purposes of discussion of the clinical aspects of the disease, we will divide the course into three stages.

Stage I: asymptomatic stage

In the asymptomatic stage, slight cardiomegaly on a chest X-ray made during a routine clinical examination or an examination for insurance may be the first clue to the diagnoses. Another asymptomatic patient may have a normal cardiac silhouette, but a routine examination discloses non-specific electrocardiographic abnormalities or an arrhythmia not apparent to the patient. Physical examination at this time may be entirely normal or may disclose a fourth heart sound. The abnormal chest X-ray and/or electrocardiogram will usually lead to an echocardiogram being ordered. This will disclose some enlargement of the left ventricle with the left ventricular end-diastolic dimensions being between 5.5 and 6.5 cm and with a depressed ejection fraction between 0.40 and 0.50. It is this group of asymptomatic patients that causes difficulty in attempting to determine the incidence and natural history of dilated cardiomyopathy since few patients are diagnosed correctly at this stage.

Stage II: moderately severe disease

Patients in this category may continue to deny symptoms and be able to perform reasonably well. The majority, however, will have begun to notice effort fatigue and dyspnoea. In some patients, palpitations are the most troublesome symptom. The chest X-ray will almost always disclose some degree of cardiomegaly (Figure 3.2.1). The electrocardiogram will have a high likelihood of disclosing an abnormality, most often that of a left ventricular conduction delay or left ventricular hypertrophy. The echocardiogram in these patients will disclose a more severe degree of abnormality, with the left ventricular end-diastolic dimension being 6.5–7.5 cm and the ejection fraction being reduced to 0.20–0.40[8]. The left ventricle at this time has become resistant to filling due to wall stiffness and increased residual volume. Consequently, atrial contraction becomes a most important mechanism to maintain diastolic inflow. Therefore, a fourth heart sound is invariably present in the presence of normal sinus rhythm. A soft third sound and murmur of mitral regurgitation may also be present.

Stage III: severe

Most patients with dilated cardiomyopathy have first been detected at this level of ventricular dysfunction. They will have noted dyspnoea and fatigue with mild exertion; they usually have a heart murmur due to atrioventricular valve incompetence; or an episode of atrial or ventricular arrhythmia may have brought them to the attention of the physician. Occasionally, a systemic embolus is the event bringing the patient to the physician, though it becomes apparent later that the patient was having symptoms of functional impairment before the embolus occurred. The increase in atrial contraction is now no longer able to create an adequate stroke volume, cardiac output becomes inadequate and signs of backward failure also begin to appear.

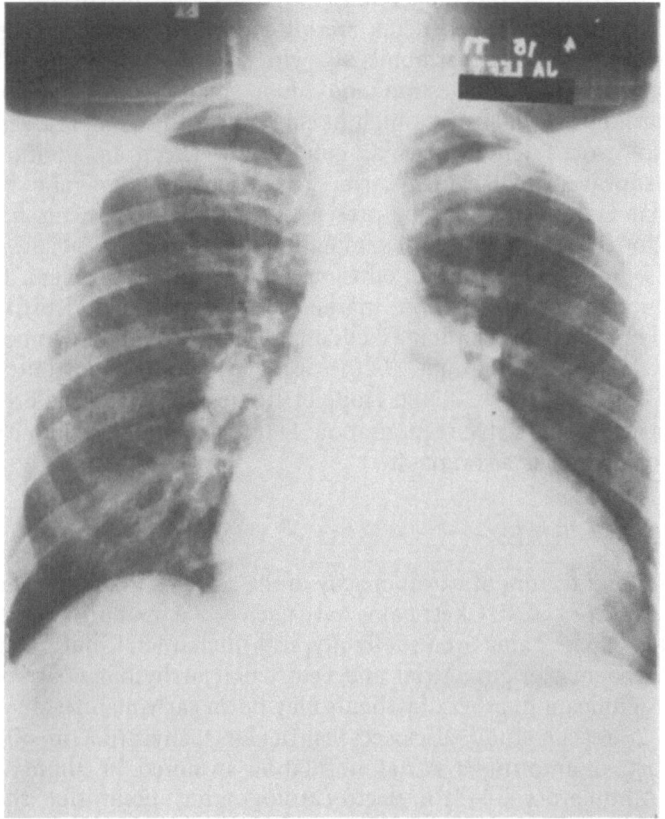

Figure 3.2.1 A 29-year-old male who 2 years earlier noted the onset of dyspnoea and congestive heart failure. Examination disclosed atrial and ventricular gallops and evidence of mitral and tricuspid valve incompetence. Chest X-ray disclosed marked cardiomegaly with dilatation of all cardiac chambers and pulmonary vascular congestion.

Dilatation of the right side of the heart is similar to that of the left side. Consequently, right-sided dilatation with tricuspid incompetence occurs simultaneously with evidence of left ventricular dysfunction and mitral valve incompetence. The patient seen for the first time at this point will have a narrow pulse pressure with cold blue extremities, small volume carotid pulsations, and an elevated jugular venous pressure with a prominent V wave due to tricuspid valve incompetence. The apical impulse is of poor quality, displaced to the left and often at the midaxillary line. A right ventricular lift is due to enlargement and overload of the right ventricle. Both atrial and ventricular gallop sounds are present, but may fuse into a single 'summation' gallop if tachycardia is present. The pansystolic murmur of mitral valve incompetence is present at the apex and at the lower sternal area the pansystolic murmur of tricuspid valve incompetence is also noted. With inspiration, atrial and ventricular gallop sounds may be identified over the right ventricle. At this time, pulmonary congestion, hepatomegaly due to vascular congestion, and oedema are all commonly present. Chest X-ray will disclose significant cardiomegaly with a globular cardiac silhouette, pulmonary vascular congestion and often small pleural effusions. The electrocardiogram will have a high likelihood of disclosing left ventricular hypertrophy or a left ventricular conduction defect. In addition, atrial ectopy, supraventricular tachycardias, ventricular ectopy and bursts of ventricular tachycardia may be present. Occasionally, patients have been referred for echocardiographic examination because the physician suspected the possibility of a pericardial effusion as the primary problem. Echocardiographic studies will disclose marked left ventricular and usually right ventricular dilatation with marked impairment of systolic function, an ejection fraction less than 0.20, displacement of the mitral valve towards the posterior wall, and Doppler studies will verify the presence of tricuspid and mitral valve regurgitation. Left atrial dilatation in the range of 5–6 cm or greater is also noted.

SPECIFIC FEATURES

The presenting feature of cardiomegaly in the asymptomatic stage has been noted in 16% of cases[9]. Chest pains have been noted in approximately 10% of patients[10]. The pains are usually atypical in character, but occasionally suggest ischaemic origin. Atrial and ventricular arrhythmias are common and in a significant number of patients may be an early manifestation of the disease[9]. A recent study disclosed ventricular tachycardia in 60% with ambulatory monitoring[11]. Atrial fibrillation is noted in about 20% of cases[12]. Ambulatory 24–48 h electrocardiographic monitoring should be routinely done because of the high incidence of atrial and ventricular arrhythmias[11]. Other features of the electrocardiogram are Q waves due to patchy fibrosis which may lead to suspicion of myocardial infarction[13,14]. Left axis deviation is common. Interventricular conduction defects, especially left bundle branch block, are common[15–17]. Sudden cardiac death, presumably related to the arrhythmias, usually occurs late in the course of the disease, but in some instances is early.

Systolic time intervals will disclose decreased left ventricular ejection time and a prolonged pre-ejection period[18]. M-mode and two-dimensional echocardiography are valuable adjuncts in the diagnosis and management of dilated cardiomyopathy[19]. Findings are those of increased ventricular dimensions together with a global decrease in systolic function. Septal and free wall thickness are usually normal, but there may be paradoxical movement of the septum. Mitral valve leaflet separation may be decreased due to decreased forward flow, intracardiac thrombi may be noted[20], and there may be an associated pericardial effusion (Figure 3.2.2).

Radionuclide imaging will disclose biventricular dilatation and a global decrease in contractility, particularly of the left ventricle. Reversible perfusion defects may be noted, suggesting ischaemic disease, but additional features will usually suggest the correct diagnosis[21]. An additional advan-

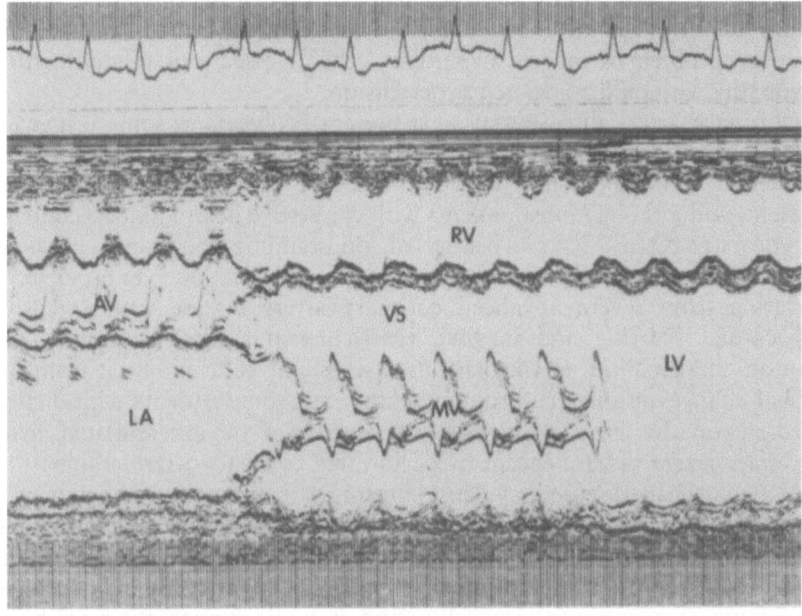

Figure 3.2.2 Echocardiogram in the 29-year-old male with the chest X-ray in Figure 3.2.1. Both ventricles and left atrium are dilated and ventricular contractility is reduced

tage of these studies is being able to obtain the results of treatment, both at rest and with exercise.

Cardiac catheterization will disclose angiographic and haemodynamic evidence of dilatation of the left ventricle with a global reduction in contraction, elevated end-diastolic pressures, and moderate elevations of pressures in the pulmonary artery and right heart[9,22,23]. Occasionally, right-sided involvement will predominate[24]. Left ventricular hypertrophy is present, but inappropriate to the degree of dilatation[24]. Mitral and tricuspid regurgitation are commonly present. The atria are often enlarged and mural thrombi may be seen. The coronary arteries are usually normal – occasionally, mild to modest coronary obstructive disease is present, but is discordant with the impairment in ventricular function.

DIFFERENTIAL DIAGNOSIS

Depending on the stage when the patient is seen, dilated cardiomyopathy may mimic or suggest hypertensive heart disease, coronary heart disease, valvular heart disease and chronic pericardial effusion.

Hypertension associated with cardiac failure is usually associated with a long history of hypertension, hypertensive changes in the retinal arteries and evidence of renal impairment. However, some patients with dilated cardiomyopathy have been noted to have mild hypertension before the onset of congestive heart failure. The hypertension disappears during the stage of congestive failure and then reappears when the congestive failure improves. In some instances, it is impossible to be certain whether the primary problem is that of hypertensive heart disease or dilated cardio-myopathy with mild associated hypertension.

Coronary artery disease may also present problems in some instances. The chest pain in dilated cardiomyopathy is usually atypical, but may mimic ischaemic pain. Risk factors for coronary artery disease, in addition, may be present, and although most patients with congestive heart failure secondary to coronary disease have a history of longstanding angina and previous infarctions, occasional patients do not give this history, and yet prove to be suffering from severe advanced coronary artery disease with extensive myocardial scarring and massive ventricular dilatation. Regional wall motion abnormalities in coronary disease usually differentiate it from the global changes in dilated cardiomyopathy, but some patients with dilated cardiomyopathy have dyskinesis, which cannot be differentiated from coronary artery disease except by performing coronary arteriography.

Valvular heart disease may cause difficulties in diagnosis if the patient is seen for the first time with advanced congestive heart failure with mitral and tricuspid valve incompetence and no prior information regarding the patient's difficulty. If the murmurs lessen or disappear following treatment with improvement in ventricular function, it would support the probability of a dilated cardiomyopathy. If the murmurs persist, and especially if they become louder, it suggests primary valvular disease. An occasional patient will present with advanced heart failure due to severe aortic stenosis, but the low output will obscure the usual signs of the disease. In this situation, serial examination, identification of valve calcification by echocardiographic examination and gradient determination by Doppler may resolve the problem.

If the patient has a short history preceded by a febrile illness suggesting a viral infection, the possibility of acute myocarditis must be considered. My personal experience has been that in patients with a short history and a preceding febrile illness, the diagnosis, in most instances, has proven to be dilated cardiomyopathy, rather than myocarditis.

A history of alcohol abuse in a patient presenting with features of dilated cardiomyopathy may pose a difficult problem. If the evidence of heart disease entirely disappears with cessation of alcohol, it can be concluded the cardiac dysfunction was secondary to alcohol. In most instances, alcohol has seemed only a possible accelerating factor in the disease process.

TREATMENT

The management of patients with dilated cardiomyopathy must take into account the stage of the disease, previous therapy if this has occurred, the patient's response and complicating features. The management programme can be divided into general measures, diet, toxin exposure and pharmaco-logical intervention.

General measures include weight reduction when indicated, avoidance of unusual stresses, activity level gauged to the degree of disease present, extra periods of rest, and proper treatment of any complicating medical problems such as anaemia or diabetes. Bed rest or modified bed rest with oxygen inhalation may be necessary and appropriate during periods of decompensation. Diet changes include sodium restriction, and when appropriate, caloric reduction. Avoidance of toxins includes primarily abstinence from alcohol.

Pharmacological intervention includes the use of diuretics, cardiotonic agents, vasodilators, anticoagulants, antiarrhythmic drugs, and perhaps in selected patients, β-blockers. Fluid retention with oedema can in most patients be well controlled with sodium restriction and the proper use of diuretic therapy with proper care to avoid hypovolaemia, hypokalaemia and hyponatraemia. Digitalis glycosides are important in controlling atrial fibrillation when present. There has been some controversy regarding use of digitalis with normal sinus rhythm, recognizing the relatively mild inotropic effect and the potential for digitalis toxicity[25]. It seems appropriate in most patients with congestive failure due to dilated cardiomyopathy to add the effects of this medication with careful monitoring, especially if diuretics are also necessary[26,27]. In those patients with moderate to severe disease with elevated peripheral arterial resistance, the use of vasodilators has been helpful. Nitroprusside alone, or in combination with dobutamine, has been used intravenously with haemodynamic monitoring[28]. Nitrates, both orally and percutaneously, have also been employed. Hydralazine has been used primarily for afterload reduction, while prazosin is effective for both preload and afterload reduction[29,30]. Captopril has impressed us with its therapeutic effect in the 'congestive stage'. It prevents the formation of angiotensin II, a powerful vasoconstrictor, prevents degradation of bradykinesis, a vasodilator peptide, and contributes to the accumulation of vasodilator prostaglandins. The haemodynamic effects are increased cardiac output, decreased systemic resistance, arterial pressure, and systemic and pulmonary venous pressure.

Salbutamol has been reported to improve both systolic and diastolic function in patients with dilated cardiomyopathy[31]. A new promising innovation in treatment has been the infusion of dobutamine twice weekly by a small portable infusion pump[32]. Despite the symptomatic improvement with the use of these agents, no reduction in morbidity or mortality has been noted[30]. Since thrombosis and systemic embolism are common, being noted in 18% of one series not receiving anticoagulants, anticoagulation is recommended, particularly in patients with congestive failure or atrial fibrillation, unless contraindications exist[17]. The use of β-adrenergic blocking agents in a disease with marked impairment of systolic function seems theoretically inappropriate. Objective evidence of improvement with prolonged survival has been claimed in some patients treated with β-blockers[33] – in addition, however, to worsening of their condition when the drug was withdrawn[34]. Other investigators have not found a benefit from β-blockers, however, and their current use must be considered controversial[35,36]. Quinidine, procainamide, and more recently amiodarone have been most frequently used for control of cardiac arrhythmias. Prophylactic therapy consists of influenza and pneumonia immunizations, prompt treatment of acute infectious disease, and abstinence from alcohol.

In a small number of carefully selected patients, cardiac transplantation may be appropriate since it is the only treatment yet shown to prolong life[37]. Mechanical circulatory assist devices may be necessary to sustain such patients for cardiac transplantation[29].

PROGNOSIS

The natural history and prognosis of dilated cardiomyopathy is quite variable related particularly to the stage in which the diagnosis is first made[9,38]. Patients seen in the asymptomatic stage with only a left bundle branch block or mild cardiomegaly on chest X-ray may remain this way for years[9,38]. In patients with symptoms and especially if congestive heart failure develops, the prognosis significantly worsens[17]. Even in the latter instance, however, there may be significant differences in survival periods[17]. Survival was 7–8 years with congestive heart failure in one study[39]. In another series, the 5-year mortality was 57%[10]. A long term study of symptomatic patients with dilated cardiomyopathy having cardiac catheterization at the Mayo Clinic between 1960 and 1973 disclosed that three quarters of the patients had an accelerated course to death with two thirds of the deaths occurring in the first 2 years[17]. The remaining quarter of patients had a normal survival with the majority noting improvement and a reduction in heart size (Figure 3.2.3). Factors noted to be independently predictive of a poor prognosis were (1) age 55 years or greater; (2) a cardiothoracic ratio of 0.55 or greater, (3) a cardiac index of less than $3 \, l/min/m^2$ and (4) left ventricular end-diastolic pressure $\geq 20 \, mmHg$[17]. Systemic embolization occurred in 18% of patients who did not receive anticoagulant therapy and in none of those receiving it[17]. The risk of systemic emboli in this study of dilated cardiomyopathy was ten times higher than in a series of patients with left ventricular aneurysm associated with myocardial infarction[40].

Prognosis has been noted for some time to be influenced by the degree of left ventricular hypertrophy present[22]. This may be reflected in the electrocardiogram[41], left ventricular posterior wall thickening by echocardiography[42], and/or by angiocardiography[24]. A necropsy study disclosed that long term survivors had thicker left ventricular walls, a greater left ventricular wall thickness to left internal diameter and greater heart weights[43].

Endomyocardial biopsy of both right and left ventricles has been studied relative to its prognostic value[44]. A morphological score to quantitate changes has been developed[45–47]. Results have not been consistent or reproducible[48], however, and the role of transvenous endomyocardial biopsy in determining prognosis in patients with dilated cardiomyopathy continues to be investigated[49–56]. Lack of uniform diagnostic criteria is an important feature in the lack of reproducible data.

The most common cause of death is severe left ventricular failure, but

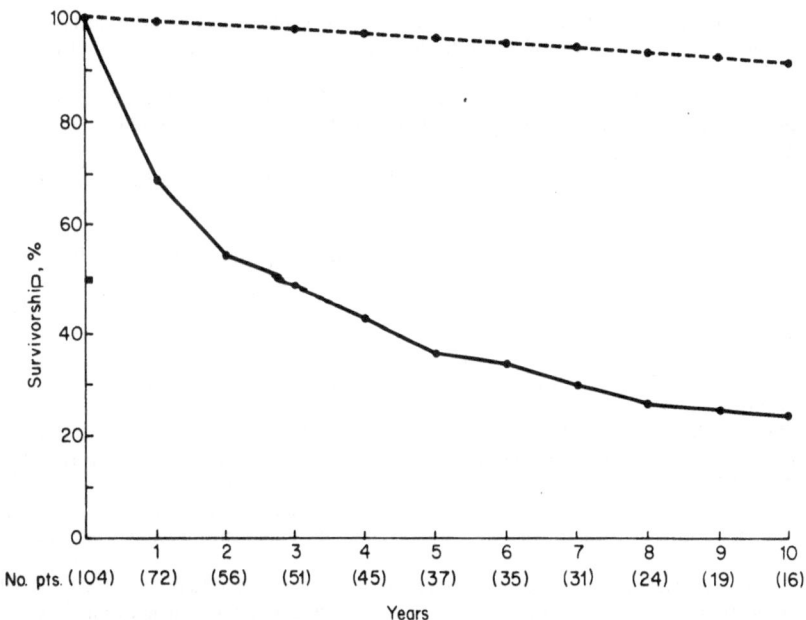

Figure 3.2.3 Observed survival plotted against time in years in 104 patients with diagnosis of idiopathic dilated cardiomyopathy (solid line). Dashed line is the control expected survival on the basis of age and sex distribution according to the death rates of the Minnesota 1970 White Population Life Table. The number of alive patients under observation at each follow-up interval is indicated in parentheses

arrhythmias have been noted in 14%[10] to 60% of cases[7,11,57]. Survival was reduced in patients with atrial fibrillation, multifocal ventricular premature contractions, and ventricular tachycardia on the routine electro- cardiogram[58,59]. With ambulatory monitoring a high incidence of ventricu- lar tachycardia has been described and half of the patients with a diagnosis of congestive cardiomyopathy died suddenly[60]. The effect of antiarrhythmic treatment on mortality is unknown, however, and the significance of finding ventricular tachycardia in dilated cardiomyopathy is also uncertain[11].

Ambulatory monitoring, echocardiography, and endomyocardial biopsy are procedures applied extensively in recent years. They have increased our knowledge and understanding of the disease, but aetiology continues to elude us and so, consequently, does definitive treatment. Investigational protocols for the development of treatment programmes to improve ven- tricular function and control ventricular arrhythmias appear appropriate despite lack of knowledge regarding aetiology.

References

1. Goodwin, J.F. (1981). Definition and identification of congestive cardiomyopathy. In Goodwin, J.F., Hjalmarson, A. and Olsen, E.G.J. (eds.) *Congestive Cardiomyopathy*. p. 10. (Mölndal, Sweden: AB Hässle)
2. Report of the WHO/ISCF Task Force on definition and classification of cardiomyopathies (1981). *Circulation*, 64, 437–8A

3. Somers, K. and D'Arbela, P.G. (1964). National topic on the epidemiology of cardiovascular disease: heart disease in Uganda. In *Proceedings of the Third Asian–Pacific Congress of Cardiology*. pp. 162–4. (Kyoto)
4. Obeyesehave, I. (1968). Idiopathic cardiomegaly in Ceylon. *Br. Heart J.*, 30, 226–35
5. Isaacson, C. (1977). The changing pattern of heart disease in South African blacks. *S. Afr. Med. J.*, 952, 793–8
6. Torp, A. (1981). Incidence of congestive cardiomyopathy. In Goodwin, J.F., Hjalmarson, A. and Olsen, E.G.J. (eds.) *Congestive Cardiomyopathy*. pp. 18–26. (Mölndal, Sweden: AB Hässle)
7. Johnson, R.A. and Palacios, I. (1982). Dilated cardiomyopathies of the adult. Part I. *N. Engl. J. Med.*, 1051, 1058
8. Wallentin, I. (1981). Non-invasive investigations in congestive cardiomyopathy. In Goodwin, J.F., Hjalmarson, A. and Olsen, E.G.J. (eds.) *Congestive Cardiomyopathy*, pp. 47–59. (Mölndal, Sweden: AB Hässle)
9. Hamby, R. (1970). Primary myocardial disease – a prospective clinical and hemodynamic evaluation in 100 patients. *Medicine*, 49, 55–78
10. Shirey, E.K., Proudfit, W.L. and Hawk, W.A. (1980). Primary myocardial disease: correlation with clinical findings, angiographic, and biopsy diagnosis. *Am. Heart J.*, 99, 198–207
11. Huang, S.K., Messer, J.F. and Denes, P. (1983). Significance of ventricular tachycardia in idiopathic dilated cardiomyopathy: observations in 35 patients. *Am. J. Cardiol.*, 51, 507–12
12. Mann, B., Ray, R., Goldberger, A.L., Shabetai, R., Green, C. and Kelly, M. (1981). Atrial fibrillation in congestive cardiomyopathy: echocardiographic and hemodynamic correlates. *Catheter. Cardiovasc. Diagn.*, 7, 387–95
13. Gau, G.T., Goodwin, J.F., Oakley, C.M., Olsen, E.G.J., Rahimtoola, S.H., Raphael, M.J. and Steiner, R.E. (1972). Q waves in coronary arteriography and cardiomyopathy. *Br. Heart J.*, 34, 1034–41
14. Pruitt, R.D., Curd, G.W. Jr. and Leachman, R. (1962). Simulation of electrocardiogram of apicolateral myocardial infarction by myocardial destructive lesions of obscure etiology (myocardiopathy). *Circulation*, 25, 506
15. Bettersby, E.J. and Glenner, G.G. (1961). Familial cardiomyopathy. *Am. J. Med.*, 30, 382
16. Evans, W. (1949). Familial cardiomyopathy. *Br. Heart J.*, 11, 68
17. Fuster, V., Gersh, B.J., Giuliani, E.R., Tajik, A.J., Brandenburg, R.O. and Frye, R.L. (1981). The natural history of idiopathic dilated cardiomyopathy. *Am. J. Cardiol.*, 47, 525–31
18. Weissler, A.M. (1977). Current concepts in cardiology. Systolic-time intervals. *N. Engl. J. Med.*, 296, 321
19. Engler, R., Ray, R., Higgins, C.B., McNally, C., Buxton, W.H., Bhargava, V. and Shabetai, R. (1982). Clinical assessment and follow-up of functional capacity in patients with chronic congestive cardiomyopathy. *Am. J. Cardiol.*, 49, 1832–7
20. DeMaria, A.N., Bommer, W., Lee, G. and Macon, D.T. (1980). Value and limitations of two-dimensional echocardiography in assessment of cardiomyopathy. *Am. J. Cardiol.*, 46, 1224–31
21. Saltissi, S., Hockings, B., Croft, D.N. and Webb-Pebloe, M.M. (1981). Thallium-201 myocardial imaging in patients with dilated and ischaemic cardiomyopathy. *Br. Heart J.*, 46, 290–5
22. Goodwin, J.F. (1970). Congestive and hypertrophic cardiomyopathies. A decade of study. *Lancet*, 1, 731
23. Pierpont, G.L., Cohn, J.N. and Franciosa, J.A. (1978). Congestive pathophysiology and response to therapy. *Arch. Intern. Med.*, 138, 1847–50
24. Feild, B.J., Baxley, W.A., Russell, R.O. Jr., Hood, W.P., Holt, J.H., Dowling, J.T. and Rackley, C.E. (1973). Left ventricular function and hypertrophy in cardiomyopathy with depressed ejection fraction. *Circulation*, 42, 1022–31
25. Johnston, G.D. and McDevitt, D.G. (1979). Is maintenance digoxin necessary in patients with sinus rhythm? *Lancet*, 1, 567–70
26. Arnold, S.B. (1980). Long-term digitalis therapy improves left ventricular function in heart failure. *N. Engl. J. Med.*, 303, 1443–8

27. Lee, D.C. (1982). Heart failure in outpatients: a randomized trial of digoxin versus placebo. *N. Engl. J. Med.*, 306, 699–701

28. Loeb, H.S., Bredakis, J. and Gunnar, R.M. (1977). Superiority of dobutamine over dopamine for augmentation of cardiac output in patients with chronic low output cardiac failure. *Circulation*, 55, 375–81

29. Pierpont, G.L. and Francis, G.S. (1982). Medical management of terminal cardiomyopathy. *Heart Transplant.*, 2, 18–27

30. Franciosa, J.A. (1982). Effectiveness of long-term vasodilator administration in the treatment of chronic left ventricular failure. *Prog. Cardiovasc. Dis.*, 24, 219–330

31. Sharma, B. and Goodwin, J.F. (1978). Beneficial effect of Salbutamol on cardiac function in severe congestive cardiomyopathy. Effect on systolic and diastolic function of the left ventricle. *Circulation*, 58, 449–60

32. Applefeld, M.M., Newman, K.A., Grove, W.R. *et al.* (1983). Intermittent continuous outpatient dobutamine infusion in the management of congestive heart failure. *Am. J. Cardiol.*, 51, 455–8

33. Swedberg, K., Hjalmarson, A., Waggstein, F. and Wallentin, I. (1980). Beneficial effects of long-term beta blockade in congestive cardiomyopathy. *Br. Heart J.*, 44, 117–33

34. Swedberg, K., Hjalmarson, A., Waggstein, F. and Wallentin, I. (1980). Adverse effects of beta blockade withdrawal in patients with congestive cardiomyopathy. *Br. Heart J.*, 44, 134

35. Skram, H. and Fitzpatrick, D. (1981). Double-blind trial of chronic oral beta blockers in congestive cardiomyopathy. *Lancet*, 2, 490

36. Skram, H. and Fitzpatrick, D. (1983). Beta blockade for dilated cardiomyopathy: the evidence against therapeutic benefit. *Eur. Heart J.*, 4 (Suppl. A), 179

37. Jamieson, S.W., Oyer, P.E., Bieber, C.P., Stinson, E.B. and Shumway, N.E. (1982). Transplantation for cardiomyopathy: a review of the results. *Heart Transplant.*, 2, 28

38. Oakley, C. (1978). Diagnosis and natural history of congested (dilated) cardiomyopathies. *Postgrad. Med. J.*, 54, 440–7

39. Koide, T., Kato, A., Takabatake, Y., Iizecka, M., Uchida, Y., Ozeki, K., Morooka, S., Kakihana, M., Scrizawa, T., Tanaka, S., Ohya, T., Momomura, S. and Murao, S. (1980). Variable prognosis in congestive cardiomyopathy. Role of left ventricular function, alcoholism, and pulmonary tuberculosis. *Jap. Heart J.*, 21, 451–63

40. Lapere, A.C. III, Steele, P.M., Kazmier, F.J., Chesebro, J.H., Vlietstra, R.E. and Fuster, V. (1983). Low incidence of systemic embolism in left ventricular aneurysm. A comparison with idiopathic dilated cardiomyopathy. *J. Am. Coll. Cardiol.*, 1(2), 704 (abstract)

41. Croxson, R.S. and Raphael, R.M. (1969). Angiographic assessment of congestive cardiomyopathy. *Br. Heart J.*, 31, 390–1

42. Kececioglu-Draelos, Z., Goldberg, S.J., Zalder-Crus, L.M., Allen, H.D. and Sahn, D.J. (1982). The importance of left ventricular wall thickening in severe dilated cardiomyopathy. *Am. J. Cardiol.*, 49, 1040 (Abstr.)

43. Benjamin, V.J., Schuster, E.H. and Bulkley, B.H. (1981). Cardiac hypertrophy in idiopathic dilated cardiomyopathy: a clinical pathological study. *Circulation*, 64, 412–47

44. Kawai, C., Fujiwara, H., Kawamura, K., Tsutsumi, J. and Noda, S. (1981). Value of cardiac biopsy in evaluating the prognosis in congestive cardiomyopathy. In Goodwin, J.F., Hjalmarson, A. and Olsen, E.G.J. (eds.) *Congestive Cardiomyopathy*. pp. 256–62. (Mölndal, Sweden: AB Hässle)

45. Kuhn, H., Briethardt, G., Kniesiem, H.J., Köhler, E., Lösse, B., Seipel, L. and Loogen, F. (1978). Prognosis and possible presymptomatic manifestations of congestive cardiomyopathy. *Postgrad. Med. J.*, 54, 451–9

46. Briethardt, G., Kuhn, H. and Knieriem, H.J. (1978). Prognostic significance of endomyocardial biopsy in patients with congestive cardiomyopathy. In Kaltenbach, E.M., Loogen, F. and Olsen, E.G.J. (eds.) *Cardiomyopathy and Myocardial Biopsy*. pp. 258–70. (Berlin, Heidelberg, New York: Springer)

47. Kuhn, H., Losse, B., Boch, H., Becker, R. and Hort, W. (1981). Prognosis of patients with cardiomyopathy – therapeutic, haemodynamic, morphologic, and metabolic aspects. In Goodwin, J.F., Hjalmarson, A. and Olsen, E.G.J. (eds.) *Congestive Cardiomyopathy*. pp. 213–20. (Mölndal, Sweden: AB Hässle)

48. Das, S., Kirlin, P., Zijen, P., Domenicercci, S., Wyns, W., Vletter, W. and Raelandt, J. (1983). Prospective determinants of survival in idiopathic dilated cardiomyopathy. *Circulation*, **68** (Suppl. III) 337 (Abstr.)
49. Shabetai, R. (1983). Cardiomyopathy. How far have we come in 25 years, how far yet to go. *J. Am. Coll. Cardiol.*, **1**, 252–63
50. Ferrans, V.J. and Roberts, W.C. (1978). Myocardial biopsy. A useful diagnostic procedure or only a research tool. (Editorial) *Am. J. Cardiol.*, **41**, 965–7
51. Fowles, R.E. and Mason, J.W. (1982). Myocardial biopsy. *Mayo Clin. Proc.*, **57**, 459–61
52. Olsen, E.G.J. (1981). Endomyocardial biopsy. *Br. Heart J.*, **40**, 95–8
53. O'Connell, J.B., Subramanian, R., Robinson, J.A. and Scanlon, P.J. (1984). Endomyocardial biopsy: techniques and applications in heart disease of unknown cause. *Heart Transplant.*, **3**, 132–44
54. Zee-Cheng, C.S., Tsai, C.C., Palmer, D.C., Codd, J.E., Pennington, D.G. and Williams, G.A. (1984). High incidence of myocarditis by endomyocardial biopsy in patients with idiopathic cardiomyopathy. *J. Am. Coll. Cardiol.*, **3**, 63–70
55. Baandrup, V., Floria, R.A., Rehahn, M., Richardson, P.J. and Olsen, E.G.J. (1981). Critical analysis of endomyocardial biopsies from patients suspected of having cardiomyopathy II. Comparison of histology and clinical/haemodynamic information. *Br. Heart J.*, **45**, 487–93
56. Baandrup, V., Floria, R.A., Roters, F. and Olsen, E.G.J. (1981). Electron microscopic investigation of endomyocardial biopsy samples in hypertrophy and cardiomyopathy. A semiquantitative study of 48 patients. *Circulation*, **63**, 1289–98
57. Franciosa, F.A., Wilen, M., Ziesche, S. and Cohn, J.N. (1983). Survival in men with severe chronic left ventricular failure due to either coronary heart disease or idiopathic dilated cardiomyopathy. *Am. J. Cardiol.*, **51**, 831–6
58. Hatle, L., Örjavik, O. and Storstein, O. (1976). Chronic myocardial disease. I. Clinical picture related to long-term prognosis. *Acta Med. Scand.*, **199**, 399–405
59. Segal, J.P., Stapleton, J.F., McClellan, J.R., Waller, B.F. and Harvey, W.P. (1978). Idiopathic cardiomyopathy: clinical features, prognosis, and therapy. *Current Probl. Cardiol.*, **3**(6), 947
60. Follansbee, W.P., Mickelson, E.L. and Morganrath, J.A. (1980). Non-sustained ventricular tachycardia in ambulatory patients: characteristics and associations with sudden cardiac death. *Ann. Intern. Med.*, **92**, 742–7

4
Restrictive cardiomyopathy

J. DAVIES

Restrictive cardiomyopathy is characterized by a restriction to diastolic filling and ventricular distensibility that can be produced by endocardial and/or myocardial lesions. The signs of 'heart failure' which result are not related to abnormal myocardial function, but are the result of back pressure due to impaired diastolic filling. Systolic function is usually well preserved. When this process becomes extensive, often as a result of superadded thrombus on top of endocardial scarring, the already small ventricular cavity may become 'obliterated'.

In the Western world amyloid infiltration is probably the commonest cause of restrictive cardiomyopathy, but throughout the world the most common cause is endomyocardial fibrosis with or without eosinophilia. In the temperate regions endomyocardial fibrosis is almost invariably associated with a marked eosinophilia. There are important haemodynamic differences between amyloid and endomyocardial fibrosis. In any part of the world the main important differential diagnosis in a patient suspected of suffering from restrictive cardiomyopathy is, of course, constrictive pericarditis.

DIFFERENTIAL DIAGNOSIS

The presence of pericardial calcium, often best appreciated on a lateral chest X-ray, is strongly suggestive of constrictive pericarditis. The presence of systolic murmurs indicating valvular dysfunction is much more suggestive of endocardial disease. Loud third heart sounds can occur in either condition, but these may be biventricular and asynchronous in endomyocardial fibrosis. Raised pulmonary artery pressure is uncommon in constrictive pericarditis and in this condition end-diastolic filling pressures in both ventricles are similar. Ventricular angiography frequently reveals cavity obliteration and valvular regurgitation in endomyocardial fibrosis (Figure 4.1). Endomyocardial biopsy may be needed to histologically confirm endocardial thickening.

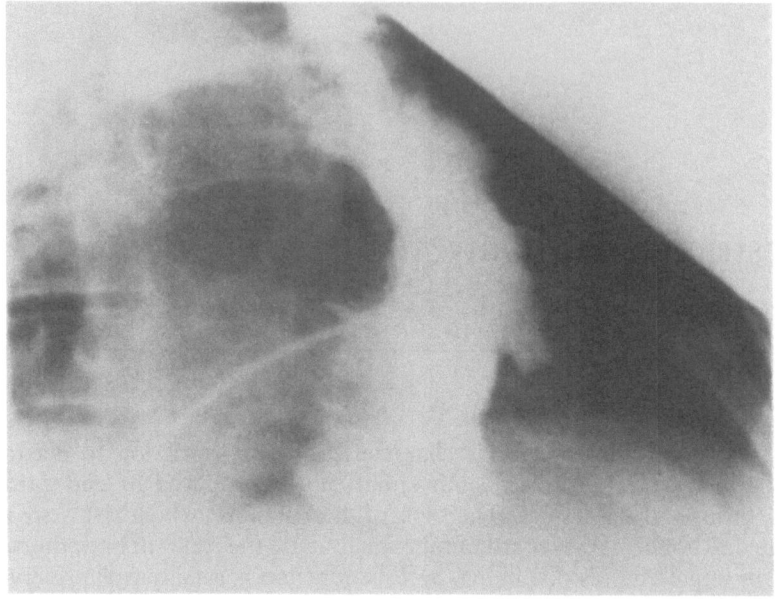

Figure 4.1 Right ventricular angiogram showing cavity obliteration and mild tricuspid incompetence

AMYLOID HEART DISEASE

Patients suffering amyloid heart disease (*see* Chapter 6), most commonly in association with systemic amyloidosis, may have impairment of systolic function and elevated filling pressures. Although abnormal signs may be confined to the heart, amyloid lesions may be seen on the tongue and mucous membranes. Nerve infiltration may result in peripheral neuropathies or autonomic dysfunction. The 'stiff' amyloid heart fills slowly throughout most of diastole and is therefore not assoicated with a third heart sound which, on the other hand, is common in endomyocardial fibrosis. This single physical sign may be very useful in clinically differentiating the two conditions. Rectal biopsy may be helpful but endomyocardial biopsy is very frequently positive in amyloid heart disease. There is no medical treatment for this condition and the prognosis is poor. Cardiac transplantation should be considered in young patients.

ENDOMYOCARDIAL FIBROSIS

The striking pathological similarities between endomyocardial fibrosis as it occurs in Europe, Africa and India have now been well established[1]. Although massive eosinophilia is the rule in Europe, eosinophilia is not a striking feature of this disease when it occurs in the tropics[2]. However, the fact that endomyocardial fibrosis occurs worldwide in the equatorial belt where parasitic infestation and eosinophilia are rife, begs the question whether the pathogenesis of these two conditions might be the same[3]. Clinically both conditions are similar except that in the tropics the severe right-sided form of the disease is more common and peripheral emboli are rare[4].

ENDOMYOCARDIAL FIBROSIS OCCURRING WITH EOSINOPHILIA

Endocardial scarring may occur as part of a generalized systemic condition with multisystem involvement, associated with marked eosinophilia. 'The hypereosinophilic syndrome' is defined as a cryptogenic hypereosinophilia, with persisting eosinophil counts of over $1.5 \times 10^9/l$, and evidence of tissue injury[5]. A wide range of organs may be affected but the main mortality and morbidity are due to cardiac involvement[5]. A careful search should be made for any possible cause of the eosinophilia such as parasites, hypersensitivity states and drugs and, if present, the underlying stimulus treated. The term 'hypereosinophilic syndrome' should be used when no cause can be found. Although tumours, particularly carcinoma of the bronchus and T-cell lymphomas, may produce hypereosinophilia, the hypereosinophilic syndrome itself appears not to be a leukaemia as the marrow is invariably full of mature and maturing eosinophils rather than blast cells. Eosinophil morphology however has been shown to be strikingly abnormal in this syndrome with a high incidence of vacuolated and degranulated forms (Figure 4.2). It has been postulated that the strongly positively charged major basic proteins within the eosinophil granules, when released into the circulation or locally into the tissues, actually induce tissue injury[6].

Medical treatment of hypereosinophilic syndrome

This follows several principles. The first is based on the recognition that associated malignancy is rare. The second is that the outlook depends mainly on the presence and the severity of the complications of the disease (e.g. thromboembolic, cardiovascular and neurological) rather than the overproduction of eosinophils themselves. Based on a retrospective study it appears that the use of steroids and cytotoxic drugs has greatly improved the prognosis of these patients[7]. When a patient with the hypereosinophilic syndrome complains of symptoms suggestive of cardiac damage, then treatment to lower the eosinophil count should be instituted as soon as possible. Direct histological evidence of tissue damage can be obtained by endomyocardial biopsy.

Recently the value of prednisolone was clearly shown in a study of 16 patients with progressive disease. Six responded to treatment with prednisolone and eight improved on prednisolone and hydroxyurea[8]. Patients with pulmonary eosinophilia, purpura, congestive cardiac failure and raised serum IgE levels appear to respond particularly well to steroids[9]. Some patients with mild disease require only short courses of treatment for

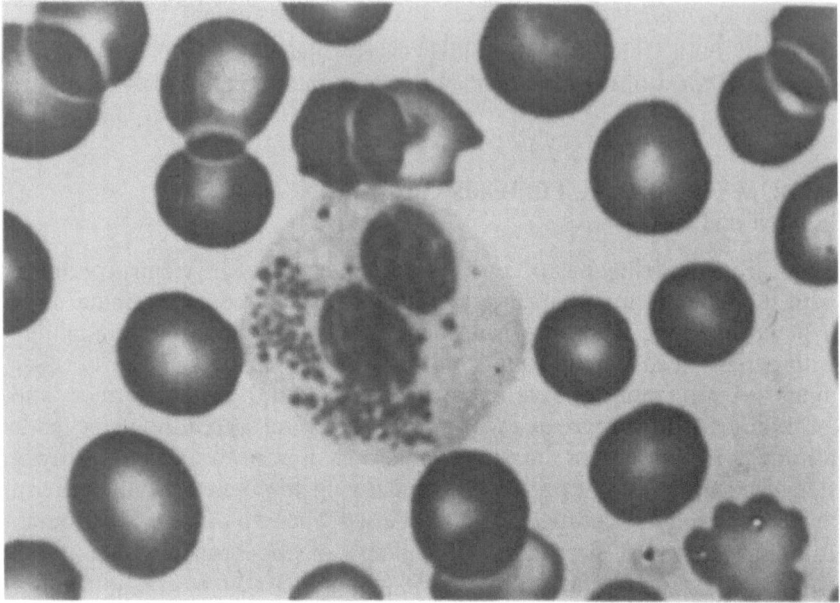

Figure 4.2 Morphologically abnormal eosinophils showing vacuolation and degranulation

episodes of increased disease activity[10]. The mechanism by which steroids affect tissue injury in the hypereosinophilic syndrome is not known. The main effect of steroids may be to inhibit the mechanisms which cause eosinophil activation and/or degranulation in tissues. It has been shown that when acute necrotic lesions are demonstrated on endomyocardial biopsy, steroid therapy can be useful in treating episodes of heart failure and also in preventing progression to the late fibrotic stage of the disease[11].

Hydroxyurea has been shown to be very useful in lowering eosinophil production and can also be beneficial in allowing reduction of steroid dosage in patients requiring maintenance treatment. In refractory patients vincristine almost invariably results in dramatic reduction of the eosinophil count. Patients notice a definite increase in well-being following intravenous injections of vincristine which can be repeated on a fortnightly basis for many months. The high incidence of thromboembolic problems in these patients, probably arising from superadded ventricular thrombus or endo-cardial scars, makes anticoagulation with warfarin and drugs that alter platelet function mandatory. Leukapharesis and plasma exchange can result in dramatic falls in eosinophil count over short periods and both procedures have been advocated in the acute management of aggressive disease associated with very high eosinophil counts.[12,13].

The medical and surgical treatment of the cardiac complications of the hypereosinophilic syndrome are the same as for endomyocardial fibrosis, occurring without eosinophilia (*see* following sections).

ENDOMYOCARDIAL FIBROSIS OCCURRING WITHOUT EOSINOPHILIA

Although also a rare disease in the tropics, endomyocardial fibrosis in certain areas accounts for up to 10% of paediatric cardiological admissions[14]. In a recent study designed to compare the clinical and cardiological features of endomyocardial disease in temperate and tropical regions, it was discovered that patients in the UK were older, had a male predominance, and they had a systemic illness: the 'hypereosinophilic syndrome'. On the other hand, patients in the tropical countries were younger, with an equal sex incidence, and were from poor, malnourished communities with heavy parasite loads, especially filariasis in India[4]. Interestingly, neither profound circulating blood eosinophilia nor abnormal degranulated eosinophil morphology was seen in tropical regions. However, the clinical effects of heart involvement, the echocardiographic features[15] and pathological specimens studied by endomyocardial biopsy and at postmortem were identical. It was observed that half of the UK patients presented in the early necrotic stage of the disease compared with tropical patients who presented with late fibrotic disease. In order to account for differences between patients in temperate and tropical regions, it was proposed that the nature of the underlying disease and the rate at which endomyocardial lesions develop determine the clinical nature of the disease. In temperate climates eosinophil granule products may produce a rapidly progressive form of the disease in patients with the 'hypereosinophilic syndrome', whereas the disease may take longer to develop in patients in tropical climates who have a less marked eosinophilia due to parasitic infections.

Medical treatment

Patients with late fibrotic lesions can be improved symptomatically with diuretics. Spironolactone is particularly useful as many have secondary hyperaldosteronism. Great care has to be taken, however, not to dehydrate these patients as this may further reduce volume and cardiac output. Arrhythmia, particularly atrial fibrillation, is common and may require digoxin therapy. After load reducing agents and calcium antagonists are not beneficial. As this group does not seem to suffer from thromboembolic problems to the same extent as those with hypereosinophilia, anticoagulation is less important.

Surgical treatment

An important advance in the treatment of endomyocardial fibrosis with or without eosinophilia has come from the introduction of surgical treatment. In the advanced stages, medical therapy is often ineffective and, in such patients, surgical decortication and/or valve replacement is safe and very

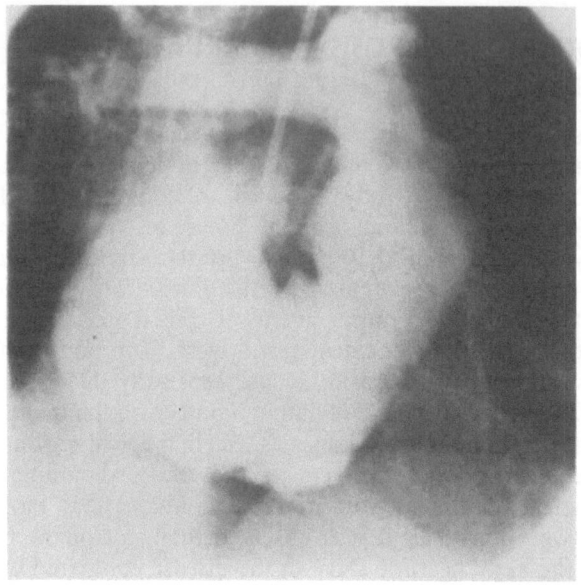

(a)

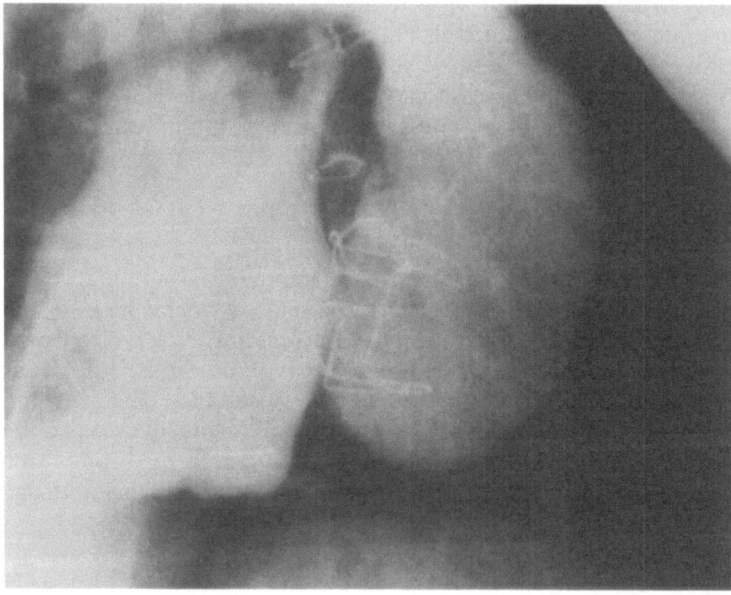

(b)

Figure 4.3 Pre (a) and post (b) right atrial angiograms in a young man with severe right ventricular endomyocardial fibrosis before and after decortication and xenograft tricuspid valve replacement

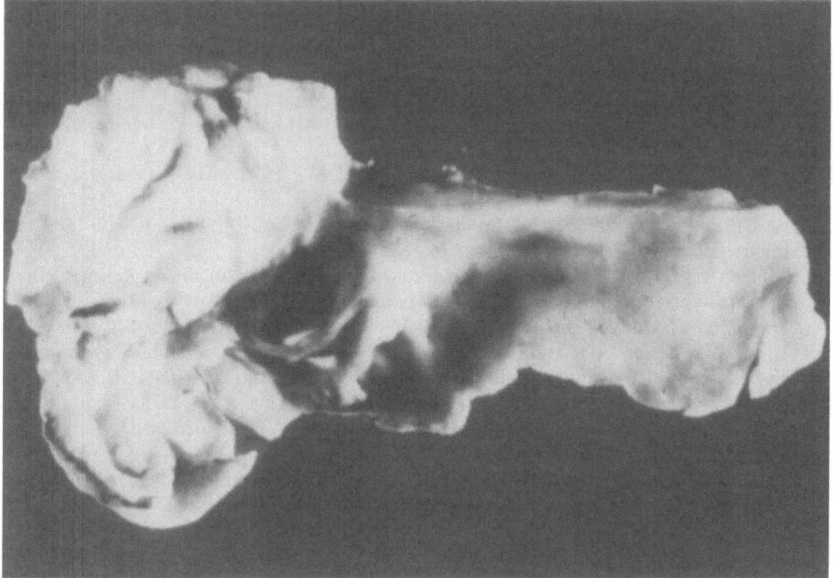

Figure 4.4   Ventricular endocardial fibrous tissue removed from the same patient as Figure 4.3

effective. These procedures have been shown to produce good long term results[16]. Even in the group with hypereosinophilia at operation, there has been no report of recurrence or progression of heart damage requiring further surgery in follow-up periods of up to 7 years[17,18] (Figures 4.3 and 4.4).

Each patient should be assessed on an individual basis depending on the site and extent of fibrosis and, while most patients require biventricular endocardectomy, some will greatly benefit from mitral valve replacement alone.

CONCLUSIONS

Restrictive cardiomyopathy should be carefully differentiated from constrictive pericarditis. When endomyocardial fibrosis occurs in the presence of hypereosinophilia, particularly in the presence of biopsy-proven necrotic cardiac damage, this should be treated with steroids and cytotoxic drugs. These patients should be anticoagulated. Medical treatment of endomyocardial fibrosis, with or without eosinophilia, is disappointing while surgical therapy is very encouraging.

References

1. Brockington, I.F. and Olsen, E.G.J. (1973). Loffler's endocarditis and Davies' endomyocardial fibrosis. *Am. Heart J.*, 85, 308–22

2. Patel, A.K., D'Arbela, P.G. and Somers, K. (1977). Endomyocardial fibrosis and eosinophilia. *Br. Heart J.*, **39**, 238–41
3. Olsen, E.G.J. and Spry, C.J.F. (1979). The pathogenesis of Loffler's endomyocardial disease and its relationship to endomyocardial fibrosis. *Prog. Cardiol.*, **8**, 281–303
4. Davies, J. and Spry, C.J.F., Vijayaraghavan, G. and de Souza, J.A. (1983). A comparison of the clinical and cardiological features of endomyocardial disease in temperate and tropical regions. *Postgrad. Med. J.*, **59**, 51–5
5. Chusid, M.J., Dale, D.C., West, B.C. and Wolff, S.M. (1975). The hypereosinophilic syndrome. *Medicine*, **54**, 1–27
6. Spry, C.J.F. and Tai, P.C. (1976). Studies on blood eosinophils. II. Patients with Lofflers cardiomyopathy. *Clin. Exp. Immunol.*, **24**, 423–34
7. Schooley, R.T., Parrillo, J.E., Wolff, S.M. and Fauci, A.S. (1980). Management of the idiopathic hypereosinophilic syndrome. In Mahmoud, A.A.F. and Austen, K.F. (eds.) *The Eosinophil in Health and Disease*. pp. 323–39. (New York: Grune and Stratton)
8. Parrillo, J.E., Fauci, A.S. and Wolff, S.M. (1977). The hypereosinophilic syndrome: dramatic response to therapeutic intervention. *Trans. Assoc. Am. Physicians*, **90**, 135–44
9. Bush, R.K., Geller, M., Busse, W.W., Flaherty, D.K. and Dickie, H.A. (1978). Response to corticosteroids in the hypereosinophilic syndrome: association with increased serum of IgE levels. *Arch. Intern. Med.*, **138**, 1244–6
10. Spry, C.J.F., Davies, J., Tai, P.C., Olsen, E.G.J., Oakley, C.M., and Goodwin, J.F. (1983). Clinical features of fifteen patients with the hypereosinophilic syndrome. *Q. J. Med.*, **52**, 1–22
11. Davies, J., Spry, C.J.F., Sapsford, R., Olsen, E.G.J., DuPerez, G., Oakley, C.M. and Goodwin, J.F. (1983). Cardiovascular features of eleven patients with eosinophilic endomyocardial disease. *Q. J. Med.*, **52**, 23–39
12. Blacklock, H.A., Cleland, J.F., Tan, P. and Pillai, V.M. (1979). The hypereosinophilic syndrome and leukapheresis. *Ann. Intern. Med.*, **91**, 650–1
13. Davies, J. and Spry, C.J.F. (1982). Plasma exchange or leukapheresis in the hypereosinophilic syndrome. *Ann. Intern. Med.*, **96–6**, 791
14. Nair, D.V. (1980). Endomyocardial fibrosis in Kerala State. *Indian Heart J.*, Teaching Series, No. 6, pp. 249–57
15. Vijayaraghavan, G., Davies, J., Sadanandan, S., Spry, C.J.F., Gibson, D.G. and Goodwin, J.F. (1983). Echocardiographic features of tropical endomyocardial disease in South India. *Br. Heart J.*, **50**, 450–9
16. Dubost, C., Maurice, P. and Gerbaux, A. (1976). The surgical treatment of constrictive fibrous endocarditis. *Ann. Surg.*, **184**, 303–7
17. Bell, J.A., Jenkins, B.S. and Webb-Peploe, M.M. (1976). Clinical, haemodynamic and angiographic findings in Lofflers eosinophilic endocarditis. *Br. Heart J.*, **38**, 541–8
18. Davies, J., Sapsford, R., Brooksby, I., Olsen, E.G.J., Spry, C.J.F., Oakley, C.M. and Goodwin, J.F. (1981). Successful surgical treatment of two patients with eosinophilic endomyocardial disease. *Br. Heart J.*, **46**, 73–81

5
Specific heart muscle diseases

N.K. WENGER

INTRODUCTION

Myocardial involvement in a variety of systemic diseases[1-3] may be manifest symptomatically – by congestive heart failure, arrhythmias, embolic phenomena, and even sudden death; by laboratory test abnormalities, particularly alterations of the electrocardiogram and the chest roentgenogram; or the diagnosis may be based on incidental findings at autopsy examination.

Because the myocardial involvement may be diffuse or localized, a wide variety of both structural and functional abnormalities are encountered. Additionally, there may be associated endocardial (valvular) and/or pericardial disease. Typically, the specific aetiological diagnosis depends considerably on the extracardiac manifestations of the disease, which predominate in the clinical presentation; less frequently, cardiovascular abnormalities dominate the clinical presentation of the illness. Clinical syndromes and myocardial morphological alterations may be comparable for many different aetiological categories.

This chapter will address the myocardial involvement in sarcoidosis; in infectious diseases of the myocardium; neurological and neuromuscular disorders; collagen vascular diseases; cardiac neoplasms; a variety of metabolic, haematological, and endocrine disorders; nutritional problems; chemical and drug effects; physical agent toxicities; and a number of miscellaneous systemic syndromes.

Amyloid heart disease is discussed as a restrictive cardiomyopathy in Chapter 6.

These disorders are important to identify because accurate diagnosis often enables specific treatment to be instituted.

SARCOIDOSIS[4,5]

Clinical manifestations

Systemic sarcoidosis is a granulomatous disorder with frequent cardiac manifestations and is characterized by relapses and spontaneous remissions;

it occurs most frequently in black women. Myocardial sarcoidosis occurs late in the course of the disease and has neither racial nor sex predilection.

Most patients with significant cardiac sarcoidosis have prominent manifestations of cardiovascular dysfunction. Dyspnoea and palpitations are frequent presentations, Stokes–Adams syncope may occur, and two thirds of patients with myocardial sarcoid die suddenly. Symptomatic evidence of cardiac involvement is a grave prognostic feature, with the majority of patients dying within 2 years of the onset of cardiac symptoms.

The predominant physical findings include tachycardia, arrhythmias, murmurs, particularly mitral regurgitation, and cardiac enlargement with and without congestive heart failure. Atrioventricular conduction disturbances, particularly complete heart block with Stokes–Adams syncope, are frequent; a significant number of patients who die of sarcoid heart disease have had complete heart block during the course of their disease. Myocardial sarcoid is an important cause of otherwise unexplained complete heart block in a young adult. Of equally grave prognosis are ventricular arrhythmias, which are often difficult to control and which also often result in sudden cardiac death. Congestive heart failure is more often secondary to chronic cor pulmonale than to myocardial sarcoidosis. Pericardial and valvular involvement are unusual, except for mitral annular calcification.

Laboratory data

The electrocardiogram (e.c.g.) is abnormal in about half of all patients with systemic sarcoidosis. The major abnormalities include supraventricular and ventricular arrhythmias and conduction abnormalities, particularly complete heart block. The electrocardiogram may mimic that of myocardial infarction. Hilar lymphadenopathy is the predominant abnormality on chest X-ray, with the radiological cardiac findings varying with the degree of pulmonary and myocardial involvement and the occurrence of pericardial effusion.

Exercise testing and ambulatory e.c.g. recording may help identify ventricular arrhythmias. Myocardial radionuclide imaging may identify areas of probable sarcoid infiltration. Endomyocardial biopsy may provide a definitive diagnosis and aid in decisions about therapy.

Pathology and pathophysiology

The most frequent morphological myocardial manifestation of systemic sarcoidosis is cor pulmonale, secondary to pulmonary sarcoidosis; myocardial sarcoidosis occurs in about 20% of patients studied at necropsy. Sarcoid granulomas may replace portions of the ventricular free wall and the papillary muscles, the ventricular septum, particularly its superior portion, the heart valves, pericardium, and aorta. These are non-caseating granulomas with multinucleate giant cells. There is often extensive myocardial damage, at times with aneurysm formation.

Treatment

Corticosteroid hormone therapy is recommended when myocardial involvement is identified, as it has been described to improve ventricular performance, although electrocardiographic abnormalities, including serious arrhythmias, have resolved both with and without corticosteroid therapy. Treatment with β-adrenergic blockade has been described to decrease the severity of arrhythmias and the incidence of sudden death; quinidine has also been effective. Conventional management of congestive heart failure is recommended. Pacemaker implantation may be life-saving.

INFECTIOUS DISEASES[6]

Clinical manifestations

Infectious myocarditis is an inflammatory process which can be caused by almost any infectious agent; it is most common in young adults. There is considerable aetiological variation dependent on the geographical location and the characteristics of the host. The cardiovascular manifestations vary widely, from patients who are essentially asymptomatic to those having severe heart failure, arrhythmias, conduction disturbances or even sudden cardiac death.

The predominant symptoms include dyspnoea, fatigue, palpitations and occasionally pleuropericardial pain. Arrhythmias may result in dizziness or syncope. Clinical evidence of the myocarditis characteristically becomes manifest during convalescence, concomitant with subsidence of the signs and symptoms of the systemic infection – muscle tenderness, upper respiratory symptoms, cutaneous eruptions, arthralgias, lymphadenopathy, nausea, vomiting, diarrhoea and malaise.

Tachycardia is frequent and is typically excessive for the degree of fever. Heart failure, manifest by dyspnoea and pulmonary congestion, is the most common of the severe presentations; cardiac enlargement, faint heart sounds, distension of the neck veins, atrial and ventricular gallop sounds, pulsus alternans, relative hypotension, hepatomegaly and peripheral oedema are encountered. A pericardial rub may be heard, and arrhythmias are frequent, as are pulmonary and systemic embolization.

Most adults with infectious myocarditis recover spontaneously. The number who progress to idiopathic congestive cardiomyopathy is not known; indeed the relationship between acute infectious myocarditis and congestive cardiomyopathy remains obscure. A minority of patients have recurrent or chronic myocarditis or die of an acute fulminant myocarditis.

Laboratory data

Cardiac enlargement as detected radiographically may be due to ventricular dilatation, pericardial effusion, or both. The characteristic electrocardiographic abnormalities, in addition to the arrhythmias and conduction defects, are sinus tachycardia and non-specific repolarization (ST–T) changes. Echocardiography and radionuclide ventriculography can be used to assess ventricular function and wall motion, and ambulatory electro-cardiography may document the arrhythmias. Recently, right ventricular endomyocardial biopsy has been advocated to differentiate infectious myocarditis from other causes of congestive cardiomyopathy, with evidence of an inflammatory process constituting an indication for corticosteroid hormone or other immunosuppressive therapy; the goal is elimination of immune-system-related myocardial damage.

Pathology and pathophysiology

Myocarditis of viral aetiology, particularly that due to Coxsackie B enterovirus, is believed to be the most common form of acute myocarditis, although viruses have never been unequivocally identified in human myocardium. Patients rarely die during the acute illness; the morphological alterations in patients who come to autopsy examination at a later date are primarily those of increased fibrous tissue in the myocardial interstitium. Other forms of infective myocarditis are commonly encountered in im-munosuppressed patients, where inflammatory cells or even focal myocar-dial abscesses may be seen at postmortem examination. Some forms of infective myocarditis have characteristic abnormalities; for example, in Chagas' disease, there is preferential involvement of the cardiac conduction system and of the apices of the cardiac ventricles, which typically become scarred and aneurysmal. Specific micro-organisms and parasites may also be identified in the myocardium, some producing an inflammatory response, others causing myocardial abscesses etc.

It is not known whether the actual infection or an autoimmune response to myocardial damage by the infecting organism is responsible for the subsequent abnormalities of myocardial structure and function. Many parasitic infections are characterized by sizeable myocardial cysts which may interfere with cardiac function by tissue compression or may cause abnormalities of valve function.

Specific common aetiologies of myocarditis[7–13]

Myocarditis is the major cause of death in patients with diphtheria, with bundle branch block and subsequent complete atrioventricular (AV) block giving the ominous warning of cardiac failure. The availability of cardiac pacemakers has altered the previous virtually uniform fatality from the conduction disturbances. Electrocardiographic abnormalities regress with recovery from the myocarditis. Acute Coxsackie myopericarditis of the adult is typically a benign illness, although the pain and electrocardio-graphic abnormalities often engender confusion with acute myocardial infarction. The heart failure, arrhythmias, and pericarditis with effusion typically resolve without residua. In Chagas' disease, the most common chronic cardiac disorder in many areas of the world, the major presentation

is of progressive congestive heart failure with frequent pulmonary embolization. Arrhythmias and conduction abnormalities are characteristic, and
death may either result from relentless congestive heart failure or be due to a
sudden cardiac arrhythmia. Left bundle branch block and left axis deviation
are the characteristic e.c.g. findings. There is usually evidence of systemic
echinococcosis in patients with echinococcal myocarditis. Cardiac manifestations may be due to obstruction to blood flow by the large cyst, to
pericarditis, or to heart failure. Eosinophilia is characteristic, and the cyst
may be delineated by both invasive and non-invasive procedures. Surgical
excision may be curative prior to cyst rupture.

Treatment

Management of the patient with acute infectious myocarditis includes
specific therapy for the underlying infection. The role of corticosteroid
hormone or other autoimmune suppressing agents remains controversial.
Antipyretic agents are indicated, and anticoagulant drugs are often required
for patients with significant congestive heart failure and cardiac arrhythmias. Supplemental oxygen may be of value. Alcohol use should be avoided
and adequate general nutrition is important. Control of congestive heart
failure involves activity restriction, improvement in myocardial contractility
by digitalis or the newer positive inotropic agents, decrease in fluid retention
by sodium restriction and diuretic use, management of tachyarrhythmias,
and often the use of vasodilator drugs. Temporary or permanent cardiac
pacing may be life-saving; and there appears to be increasing use of
temporary partial or total cardiopulmonary bypass and assisted circulation.

NEUROLOGICAL AND NEUROMUSCULAR DISORDERS[14]

Duchenne's progressive muscular dystrophy[15]

Clinical manifestations

Non-myotonic progressive muscular dystrophy is a recessively inherited
disorder which almost exclusively affects the male. Cardiomyopathy occurs
in more than half of all patients, and may be the initial manifestation of the
illness; its severity is not related to the severity of the skeletal muscle disease.

These patients have large calves, a peculiar waddling gait and a typical
'climbing up the legs' phenomenon. The cardiomyopathy is characterized by
tachycardia and cardiac enlargement, with mitral regurgitant murmurs due
to papillary muscle dysfunction. Symptomatic heart failure is usually not
evident because of the patient's inactivity. Death is often due to respiratory
infection; alternatively, there may be a sudden arrhythmic death.

Laboratory data

The electrocardiographic abnormalities are the most distinctive feature of
the cardiomyopathy; tall R waves in the right precordial leads and deep Q

waves in the inferior limb leads and left precordial leads are encountered in 40–90% of patients; tachycardia is characteristic and there are non-specific conduction and repolarization abnormalities. Determination of heart size on the chest roentgenogram is complicated by thoracic deformities and diaphragmatic dystrophy. Serum creatinine kinase levels are increased. Echocardiographic delineation of a left ventricular posterior wall relaxation abnormality may best identify early cardiac involvement.

Pathology and pathophysiology

The characteristic morphological myocardial lesion, selective scarring of the posterobasal portion of the left ventricle and posteromedial papillary muscle, correlates well with the e.c.g. abnormalities. However, comparable e.c.g. abnormalities occur in asymptomatic female carriers. An arteritis of the small myocardial arteries, including those supplying the conduction system, may be the basis for some arrhythmias.

Treatment

The congestive heart failure responds to the usual management; but there is no specific therapy.

Friedreich's ataxia[16]

Clinical manifestations

Cardiomyopathy, manifest as arrhythmias, cardiac enlargement, and congestive heart failure is encountered in between a third and a half of patients with heritable progressive spinocerebellar degeneration. There is no relationship between the severity of the neurological and cardiovascular disorders. The major cardiovascular manifestations include palpitations and exertional dyspnoea, accompanying the skeletal deformities, ataxia, and scanning speech, which have their onset in adolescence. Hypertrophic cardiomyopathy may also occur, but the outflow gradient and murmurs disappear as the left ventricle progressively fails. There is increasing congestive cardiac failure, and this or an intercurrent infection is ultimately the cause of death.

Laboratory data

Electrocardiographic repolarization abnormalities mimic those of myocardial ischaemia. Atrioventricular and bundle branch blocks are encountered. Electrocardiographic disturbances tend to be comparable in family members and are more common with severe neurological disease. Vectorcardiographic abnormalities have even greater sensitivity. Echocardiography can document the development of hypertrophic obstructive cardiomyopathy.

Generalized cardiac enlargement and deformities of the thorax are evident on the chest roentgenogram.

Pathology and pathophysiology

Cardiac morphological abnormalities are virtually constant in Friedreich's ataxia and consist of myocardial fibrosis with compensatory hypertrophy of the remaining myofibres. There is variable fibrosis of the conduction system, which may explain the arrhythmias; and obliterative disease of the small intramural coronary arteries, which may contribute to the cardiomyopathy.

Treatment

Management is directed toward control of the congestive heart failure and arrhythmias.

Myotonia atrophica (Steinert's disease)[17]

Clinical manifestations

This hereditary disease is characterized by slow muscle relaxation after contraction, increased skeletal muscle tone, muscle atrophy, an expression-less face, premature frontal baldness, cataracts and gonadal atrophy; major manifestations occur in the third and fourth decades. Cardiac involvement with heart failure is typically a late feature in the course of the disease and is unrelated to the severity of the e.c.g. abnormalities or the muscular abnormalities. Patients describe dyspnoea and palpitations; the typical cardiac rhythms are sinus bradycardia or atrial flutter and fibrillation with high-grade AV block. Syncope and sudden death are probably due to ventricular fibrillation or complete heart block.

Laboratory data

The electrocardiogram is abnormal in over three-quarters of patients and is often the earliest evidence of cardiac involvement. It is characterized predominantly by atrioventricular and intraventricular conduction defects which are gradually progressive; abnormalities may mimic those of myocardial infarction. The chest roentgenogram is usually normal.

Pathology

The morphologic abnormalities include diffuse fibrosis and fatty infiltration; damage to the sarcoplasmic reticulum, defined by electron microscopy, has been believed to account for the conduction abnormalities.

Treatment

A permanently implanted cardiac pacemaker is indicated to control Stokes–Adams syncope.

Myasthenia gravis[18]

Tachycardia, arrhythmias, dyspnoea, and non-specific electrocardiographic abnormalities have been described in patients with myasthenia gravis, in association with the generalized muscle weakness. Myofibre necrosis with inflammatory myocardial infiltrates and interstitial and perivascular cellular aggregations are described. The electrocardiographic abnormalities are non-specific. The major concern in therapy is that cardiovascular drugs such as quinidine, procainamide and lidocaine may either intensify the myasthenia or interefere with neuromuscular transmission; this suggests that cardioversion is the management of choice for arrhythmias.

Other neuromuscular disorders[19–22]

Cardiac enlargement and non-specific electrocardiographic abnormalities have been described in other forms of non-myotonic muscular dystrophy. The patient with X-linked humeroperoneal neuromuscular disease has mild muscular disability but life-threatening cardiovascular complications. Progressive bradycardia, varying atrioventricular block and permanent atrial standstill with a junctional bradycardia warrant permanent pacing to avert the risk of sudden cardiac death.

The cardiomyopathy of Roussy–Lévy hereditary polyneuropathy mimics that of Friedreich's ataxia. Conduction disturbances and progressive AV block may occur with chronic progressive external ophthalmoplegia (Kearn's syndrome), and a prophylactic implanted pacemaker may avert sudden death. Patients with the Kugelberg–Welander syndrome, juvenile progressive spinal muscular atrophy, may also require pacemaker therapy for atrioventricular conduction abnormalities. Management for congestive heart failure is the therapy of choice in the progressive cardiomyopathy of familial centronuclear myopathy.

COLLAGEN VASCULAR DISEASES

This group of disorders is characterized by varying inflammatory involvement of the connective tissues, muscles and joints.

Lupus erythematosus[23,24]

Clinical manifestations

This disease most commonly affects women in the second and third decades. Cardiovascular abnormalities are more prominent in systemic lupus erythematosus than in the other collagen vascular diseases, and at times may be the presenting manifestations of the illness. Pericardial involvement, at times with effusion and tamponade, is the most frequent cardiac abnormality; the murmurs of valvular dysfunction related to Libman–Sachs endocarditis are frequent; and chest pain may be due to pericarditis or to intramural coronary artery involvement. Heart failure, as evidence of myocardial involvement, occurs in the minority of patients, typically in association with systemic hypertension. Arrhythmias and heart block are not common.

Laboratory data

Electrocardiogram is usually abnormal, but the changes are non-specific, save for those of pericarditis. The chest X-ray demonstrates cardiac enlargement, some of which may be due to pericardial effusion.

Pathology

In addition to the characteristic Libman–Sachs endocarditis and the pericarditis, lupus is manifest in the myocardium by interstitial and perivascular mononuclear infiltrates. The cardiac enlargement probably results from the hypertension and small vessel arteritis.

Treatment

Congestive heart failure may respond to the standard regimen, but corticosteroid hormones are typically indicated to treat severe or refractory heart failure. Azathioprine and cyclophosphamide may be added. Hypertension and arrhythmias respond to standard therapeutic measures, and pericardiectomy may be necessary for constrictive pericarditis or for the intractable pain of recurrent acute pericarditis.

Polyarteritis nodosa[25,26]

Clinical manifestations

This necrotizing vasculitis of unknown aetiology may produce a variety of cardiac manifestations; these reflect coronary arteritis with resultant myocardial infarction, myocarditis, or pericarditis; and some changes may relate to the hypertension secondary to renal involvement. The major clinical findings are tachycardia, fever, the pain and rub of pericarditis, chest pain which may represent myocardial ischaemia or infarction; congestive heart failure is a late occurrence. Arrhythmias are not prominent.

Laboratory data

The electrocardiographic changes are non-specific, but myocardial infarction may occasionally be evident. Left ventricular hypertrophy is common, as are bundle branch blocks and atrioventricular block. The roentgenogram of the chest shows generalized cardiomegaly.

Pathology

Coronary arteritis is common and may result in myocardial infarction. There is patchy inflammatory necrosis and fibrosis of the myocardium, the latter in part related to the hypertension. Conduction system abnormalities may be due to sinoatrial and atrioventricular node artery involvement. Changes of pericarditis and pericardial effusion, occasionally haemorrhagic, are described.

Treatment

Patients with cardiac involvement should be treated with corticosteroid hormone and other anti-inflammatory drugs, which are designed to reduce the progression of the disease and eliminate the pain and systemic toxicity. There is often dramatic improvement of otherwise refractory heart failure following the institution of steroid therapy. Immunosuppressive drugs should probably be continued even after the acute manifestations of the disease have subsided.

Rheumatoid arthritis[27,28]

Clinical manifestations

As the survival of patients with rheumatoid arthritis increases, rheumatoid heart disease may be increasingly encountered. This is the most common of the collagen vascular diseases and affects women predominantly; however, clinical cardiovascular disease is infrequent. Congestive heart failure, disproportionate to the severity of the aortic and mitral valve disease, is due to associated myocardial disease. Stokes–Adams syncope has been explained by rheumatoid nodular infiltration of the interventricular septum. Arrhythmias may be encountered, and there may be acute pericarditis, often with a rub, associated with effusion or tamponade; constrictive rheumatoid pericarditis is a late finding.

Laboratory data

The electrocardiographic changes are non-specific. Echocardiography may detect early pericardial thickening or effusion and mitral or aortic valve abnormalities.

Pathology

The anatomical basis for these findings is involvement of the myocardium, pericardium and heart valves with granulomas which are histologically similar to rheumatoid nodules. These occur anywhere in the epicardium or myocardium, and at the bases of the aortic and mitral valve cusps in up to 20% of patients. About the same percentage of patients have a non-specific interstitial myocarditis and/or diffuse coronary arteritis. The fibrofibrinous pericarditis is far more common morphologically than clinically, being evident in about 30% of patients at postmortem examination. The aortic and mitral valves are thickened and fibrosed, and calcific aortic stenosis may develop. The high incidence of rheumatoid morphological lesions contrasts sharply with the relatively uncommon severe cardiac manifestations. Cardiac amyloidosis may occur late in the course of the disease.

Treatment

Constrictive pericarditis may necessitate pericardiectomy and pacemaker therapy may be needed for the patient with complete heart block. Conventional management is recommended for heart failure and arrhythmias.

Ankylosing spondylitis[29,30]

Clinical manifestations

Cardiac disease is a late complication of ankylosing spondylitis, a disease which occurs almost exclusively in men, and the cardiovascular abnormalities are unrelated to the severity of the spondylitis. Both aortic regurgitation and conduction abnormalities are more frequent in older patients and in those with peripheral joint involvement. The cardiomyopathy may present with cardiac enlargement and congestive heart failure; atrioventricular block may progress to asystole or ventricular tachyarrhythmias.

Laboratory data

Electrocardiographic abnormalities of atrioventricular and intraventricular conduction often antedate the clinical evidence of valvular disease. A PR interval as long as 0.35–0.45 s may persist for many years; subsequent complete heart block is common.

Pathology and pathophysiology

About 20% of patients have anatomical abnormalities, but less than half have clinical cardiac manifestations. The aortic root and aortic valve demonstrate an inflammatory lesion with subsequent fibrosis, which may extend into the interventricular septum, replacing the atrioventricular bundle with fibrous tissue. Fibrosis may also extend to the base of the anterior leaflet of the mitral valve, producing mitral regurgitation. Pericarditis has been described.

Treatment

The aortic regurgitation is rarely of sufficient severity to warrant valve replacement. Heart failure and conduction abnormalities should be treated with standard therapeutic measures. Pacemaker therapy is recommended for complete atrioventricular block.

Scleroderma (progressive systemic sclerosis)[31,32]

Clinical manifestations

The clinical cardiovascular presentation of scleroderma may relate to the systemic arterial hypertension, the cor pulmonale, or to the myocardial disease; heart failure, arrhythmias, and myocardial infarction are described in almost half the patients. Exertional dyspnoea is common, and cardiac murmurs may reflect either the anaemia or papillary muscle dysfunction. Atypical chest pain and the pain of pericarditis are described. The apex impulse may be difficult to palpate because of sclerodermatous involvement of the chest wall. Pulsus paradoxus may be due either to the lung disease or to pericardial tamponade. In patients with significant pulmonary hypertension, there is an increased intensity of the pulmonic component of the second heart sound, at times with fixed splitting.

Laboratory data

The electrocardiographic findings are non-specific and include bundle branch and atrioventricular blocks. Low voltage may be a clue to the presence of pericardial fluid. The chest roentgenogram often shows an enlarged cardiac silhouette which may result either from myocardial disease with cardiac dilatation or pericardial effusion.

Pathology

There is fibrous replacement of the cardiac musculature in about half of the patients, varying from patchy fibrotic scars to major replacement of myocardium; the papillary muscles may be involved. The myocardial fibrosis is unrelated to the severity of either large or small artery occlusions. Focal, intermittent ischaemic myocardial injury, due to vascular spasm, has been suggested as aetiological. Pericarditis, often adhesive, with and without effusion, is described.

Treatment

There is no effective therapy for the underlying disease. Patients respond to the usual management for congestive heart failure and arrhythmias, and corticosteroid hormones may be indicated to control both the pericarditis and the pericardial effusion. The role of vasodilator therapy is not known.

Dermatomyositis

There are few clinical cardiovascular abnormalities; the electrocardiographic changes, although common, are non-specific. Oedema and myocardial degeneration are present; cor pulmonale has been described, as has pericarditis. There is no definitive therapy, and the indications for corticosteroid hormones have not been well defined.

NEOPLASTIC DISEASES[33-40]

Manifestations of myocardial tumours

A minority of all cardiac neoplasms are diagnosed clinically, because they produce no characteristic symptoms unless they interfere with cardiac function. The lack of symptoms may, in part, be attributed to the slow growth of many cardiac tumours which allows for compensatory cardiac changes. Benign and malignant primary cardiac tumours and metastatic cardiac tumours produce indistinguishable cardiac manifestations; however, metastatic tumours are far more frequent. The increased prevalence of metastatic cardiac tumours in recent years appears related to the increased survival of patients with systemic neoplasms because of intensive surgical treatment and radiation or chemotherapy. Metastatic tumours of the heart should be considered as a cause of otherwise unexplained cardiac signs or symptoms in a patient with a malignant neoplasm.

Myocardial tumours occur at all ages and with an equal sex incidence. However, metastatic tumours are more frequent after age 50. They are typically incidental findings at autopsy, with arrhythmias often the only clinical clue in those tumours diagnosed antemortem.

Impairment of rhythm or conduction is the most frequent clinical presentation of myocardial tumours. Atrial arrhythmias are common, possibly because the less mobile atrium is invaded more frequently. Atrial fibrillation and flutter suggest atrial tumours; and tumour invasion of the AV node or the ventricular septum may result in complete heart block with Stokes–Adams syncope, which may be the mechanism of death. Ventricular arrhythmias are seen with tumour invasion of the myocardium. Arrhythmias tend to respond poorly to standard management. The other major manifestation related to primary or metastatic myocardial tumours is progressive intractable cardiac failure with occasional angina pectoris. Obstruction of cardiac lymphatic drainage may increase the severity of the heart failure. Less commonly, myocardial tumours may produce ventricular outlet gradients; myocardial rupture has occurred from tumour infiltration.

Radiation and chemotherapy used in the treatment of patients with malignant neoplasms may potentiate the myocardial damage. There is no characteristic electrocardiographic finding, but abnormalities may mimic those of myocardial infarction. Radionuclide imaging techniques may help identify or localize a myocardial tumour, and occasionally echocardiography may aid in diagnosis.

107

Specific myocardial tumours

Lipomas, angiomas, malignant haemangioendotheliomas, rhabdomyomas, sarcomas, mesotheliomas and fibromas may involve the myocardium, as may all forms of metastatic disease. Leukaemic myocardial infiltration is discussed later in this chapter, under Haematological Disorders.

Primary malignant tumours of the heart are predominantly sarcomas. They usually occur on the right side of the heart, equally distributed between the atrium and the ventricle, but more commonly originate from the endocardium or pericardium than from the myocardium.

Pericardial metastases are also more frequent with metastatic tumour than are myocardial metastases. Metastatic tumour may reach the heart by embolic haematogenous spread, by lymphatic spread, or by contiguous growth in descending order of frequency. However, in general, cardiac metastases are infrequent; this may be because of the kneading action of the beating heart, the rapid coronary blood flow, the metabolic characteristics of cardiac muscle, the afferent lymphatic drainage from the heart and so forth. Cardiac metastases occur most frequently from bronchogenic carcinoma and carcinoma of the breast; malignant melanoma is the only tumour which selectively tends to metastasize to the heart. There is frequent cardiac infiltration by leukaemia and lymphoma.

Treatment

Cardiac tumours are treated by a combination of surgery, radiation and chemotherapy, depending on the aetiology.

METABOLIC DISORDERS

Amyloidosis

See Chapter 6

Haemochromatosis[41,42]

Clinical manifestations

This is a potentially treatable form of cardiomyopathy, due to excessive iron deposition in the myocardium, which is encountered predominantly in older age males. The classical clinical presentation is the tetrad of liver disease, diabetes mellitus, heart disease and skin pigmentation; heart disease can occur without skin pigmentation and diabetes. Cardiac failure is the major cause of death in patients with haemochromatosis, and occasional patients with the disorder initially present with cardiac symptoms. Cardiac involvement is characteristic of the haemochromatosis which develops in children or young adults. Dyspnoea, cardiomegaly, stasis, cyanosis, oedema and ascites are common. Arrhythmias, particularly paroxysmal atrial tachycardia and fibrillation, are frequent and are presumed due to deposition of iron in the atrium rather than in the conduction system; atrioventricular block also occurs. Despite considerable deposition of iron in the ventricles, ventricular arrhythmias are less common. There is unexplained precordial pain; the congestive heart failure is rapidly progressive and responds poorly to standard therapy.

Laboratory data

Electrocardiographic abnormalities, which may be the earliest evidence of cardiac involvement, include diminished QRS voltage, conduction disturbances, and non-specific repolarization changes. The heart is enlarged and hypokinetic. In the early stages of the disease, a thickened and poorly compliant left ventricle can be demonstrated by echocardiography, but the progression to a dilated congestive cardiomyopathy is rapid. The diagnosis can be confirmed by demonstrating excessive iron deposition in a bone marrow aspirate or a liver biopsy specimen. The serum iron level is elevated. HLA typing may differentiate between patients with idiopathic haemochromatosis and those with chronic hepatic disease.

Pathology and pathophysiology

The characteristic lesion is iron deposition in the myofibres, with associated myofibre fragmentation and decreased mitochondria. Iron deposition occurs in the heart only after other organs are saturated with iron; iron deposition is greater in the myocardium than in other muscles. There is extensive deposition of iron in the subepicardium of the ventricles, but it is not known how iron enters the myocardial cells, nor is the mechanism of cell damage known; there is poor correlation between myocardial iron deposition, associated fibrosis and cardiac functional impairment. Iron pigment is not deposited in the interstitial connective tissue, and there is little iron deposition in the conduction system. The early haemodynamic abnormalities may mimic a restrictive cardiomyopathy; however, all patients with grossly visible cardiac iron deposition develop a dilated congestive cardiomyopathy.

Treatment

Repeated venesection to remove iron is the accepted therapy (except in patients with chronic refractory anaemia), and regression of symptoms and of haemodynamic abnormalities has been reported. Permanent pacing has been life-saving in patients with complete heart block. These combined therapies may reverse the previous characteristic mortality within the year after the onset of cardiac symptoms. The role of chelation is unknown.

Acquired haemochromatosis, encountered in patients with refractory anaemias who require repeated transfusion, may respond to chelating agents, designed to remove excess iron.

Phaeochromocytoma[43,44]

Clinical manifestations

The findings in patients with this epinephrine-secreting tumour include tachycardia, arrhythmia, sweating, weakness, abdominal pain, hypertensive episodes and subsequent congestive heart failure; postural hypotension is characteristic. Many of these features characteristically occur episodically; hypertrophic obstructive cardiomyopathy is an associated abnormality.

Laboratory data

The electrocardiographic abnormalities are non-specific and often reversible by adrenergic blocking drugs; cardiac enlargement is present on the chest X-ray.

Pathology and pathophysiology

The lesion is a catecholamine-induced myocardial necrosis, related to the excessive metabolic demands on the myocardium, possibly coupled with the effects of the hypertension and of vasoconstriction of the smaller coronary arteries. There is resultant fibrosis. Postural hypotension appears related both to a catecholamine-induced hypovolaemia and to impaired sympathetic reflexes which result from the ganglionic blocking effects of catecholamine excess.

Treatment

Surgical removal of the tumour improves the haemodynamic, electrocardiographic and clinical manifestations. Adrenergic blocking agents, typically phenoxybenzamine and propranolol, given preoperatively may decrease the risk of surgery. Intraoperative hypotension is best managed with volume expansion.

Cardiac glycogenosis[45–47]

Clinical manifestations

Glycogen storage disease is an autosomal recessive disorder of carbohydrate metabolism characterized by the excessive accumulation of normal glycogen in cardiac muscle, skeletal muscle and other body tissues. It is due to absence of the enzyme α-glucosidase. Cardiomyopathy is most prominent in type II glycogenosis (Pompe's disease), with heart failure characteristically occurring within the first 6 months of life. The baby presents with difficulty in feeding, dyspnoea, tachycardia, cyanosis, sweating and massive cardiac enlargement in the early months of life. Generalized muscle weakness, a large tongue, hyporeflexia and other neurological deficits are present.

Hypertrophic cardiomyopathy may also be encountered. Death in infancy or early childhood is typically due either to a respiratory infection or to severe congestive heart failure; alternatively, there may be a sudden arrhythmic death.

Laboratory data

The characteristic electrocardiographic pattern is of enormous QRS voltage with a shortened PR interval; pre-excitation and right ventricular hypertrophy are also seen. There is massive cardiac enlargement with pulmonary congestion on chest X-ray, with huge thickening of the interventricular septum and free wall of the left ventricle, at times with systolic anterior motion of the mitral valve and outflow tract obstruction described at echocardiography. The massive thick-walled ventricle can also be delineated at angiocardiography.

Skeletal muscle biopsy is diagnostic, revealing an increased glycogen content and absence at α-glucosidase activity. Periodic acid–Schiff staining of the peripheral blood lymphocytes demonstrates glycogen granules; there is decreased lymphocyte acid maltase activity which further confirms the diagnosis.

Pathology and pathophysiology

There is massive ventricular hypertrophy with myofibre enlargement. The diffuse extensive vacuolation due to glycogen deposition is described as a 'lacework pattern'. Energy deprivation contributes to the cardiomyopathy.

Treatment

There is no definitive therapy. Digitalis may be harmful in patients with pre-excitation and/or outflow tract obstruction. Surgical intervention has not proved effective nor has administration of acid maltase, and death is characteristic within the first year of life.

McArdle's syndrome[48]

This hereditary myopathy is due to deficient muscle glycogen breakdown owing to lack of muscle phosphorylase. Electrocardiographic abnormalities are seen, but clinical cardiovascular disease is unusual, despite the profound skeletal muscle weakness.

Polysaccharide storage disease[46]

This disorder may present with cardiomyopathy and electrocardiographic abnormalities, presumed to be related to the deposition of neutral polysaccharide and abnormal glycogen in the myocardium.

Fabry's disease[49] (angiokeratoma corporis diffusum universale)

This inherited abnormality of glycolipid metabolism is due to a deficiency of the enzyme ceramide trihexosidase, causing abnormal glycolipid deposition in the myocardium and blood vessels. It occurs predominantly in the male. The patients have corneal opacities and angiokeratosis; fever and burning pain in the extremities occur during crises. Cardiomyopathy is common, as is hypertension, the latter usually secondary to renal failure. Angina pectoris and myocardial infarction may occur; the terminal event is typically congestive heart failure. The electrocardiographic abnormalities are those of left ventricular hypertrophy and myocardial infarction, and cardiac enlargement on the chest roentgenogram is characteristic. The echocardiogram confirms the increased myocardial thickness, presumably due to glycosphingolipid deposition. The myocardium shows glycolipid deposition with myofibre fragmentation and vacuolation; glycolipid may also be deposited in the coronary arteries, the conduction system and heart valves. There is no effective therapy, although enzyme replacement may be feasible.

Tay–Sachs disease[46]

A neurodegenerative disorder due to a hexosaminidase A deficiency, this has frequent electrocardiographic abnormalities but few cardiovascular symptoms. *Sandhoff's disease*[46], due to a hereditary deficiency of hexosaminidase A and B, resembles Tay–Sachs disease. In addition to the electrocardiographic abnormalities, frequent cardiovascular derangements are present, including endocardial fibroelastosis, mitral valve abnormalities and coronary arterial narrowing. There is resultant congestive heart failure, and murmurs of mitral regurgitation are common. Cardiac dysfunction is rare in patients with G_{MI} *gangliosidosis*[46], *Gaucher's disease*[50], and *Niemann–Pick disease*, despite myocardial morphological abnormalities.

In the infant with *isolated cardiac lipidosis*[51], lipoprotein infiltration in the central nervous system and the heart results in cardiac enlargement, heart failure, arrhythmias and conduction abnormalities, as well as central nervous system symptoms.

Despite few cardiac symptoms, the patient with *porphyria*[52] has major myocardial anatomical disruption, and the electrocardiogram may be abnormal.

Gout[53]

Patients with clinical gout may have arrhythmias and conduction abnormalities, as well as pericarditis, presumed due to urate deposition in the heart. Hypertension is due to renal disease. Urate deposits may involve the coronary arteries, pericardium and myocardium, and even the valvular endocardium, especially of the mitral valve. Arrhythmias, including AV block, have been reported to subside with uricosuric therapy, presumably due to resolution of the gouty deposit. This has also been encountered with gouty pericarditis.

Oxalosis[54]

Primary oxalosis is an hereditary defect characterized by calcium oxalate deposition in body tissues with resultant nephrolithiasis, nephrocalcinosis, and renal failure, with characteristic refractile, yellow, rosette-like crystals deposited in the myocardium, coronary arteries and conduction system. Congestive heart failure has been described, as well as cardiac arrhythmias and conduction abnormalities, including complete heart block. Pacemaker implantation may be needed. Pericardial effusion may also be present. Haemodialysis may decrease the extent of oxalate deposition in patients with uraemia and secondary oxalosis.

Ochronosis (alkaptonuria)[55]

Ochronic pigment granules are deposited in the collagen and fibrous tissue of the myocardium and in the coronary arteries, producing a grey-purple colour; this disorder is due to a deficiency of homogentisic oxidase. The dark urine is caused by urinary homogentisic acid. Despite the prominent anatomic alterations, the major cardiovascular manifestations are aortic and mitral valve murmurs, due to calcification of these valves, and aortic and left ventricular aneurysms. The therapy is restriction of dietary phenyl-alanine

Mucopolysaccharidoses[56,57]

This group of hereditary diseases is characterized by disturbances of mucopolysaccharide metabolism and systemic deposition of glycoproteins. Cardiovascular disease is most prominent in patients with Hurler's syndrome (gargoylism, mucopolysaccharidosis I), with clinical cardiovascular disease seen in the majority of patients. Although myocardial morphological changes occur in a number of the other mucopolysaccharidoses, clinical evidence of cardiovascular disease is unusual.

Clinical characteristics

The disease usually becomes manifest within the first 2 years of life, as soon as sufficient glycoprotein has accumulated in the tissues to result in skeletal deformities, dwarfed growth, mental retardation, hepatosplenomegaly and corneal opacities. The murmur of mitral regurgitation, secondary to valve deformity, and progressive congestive heart failure are observed. Calcification of the mitral annulus is common. Death during childhood is predominantly due to the progressive congestive heart failure.

Laboratory data

The electrocardiographic abnormalities are non-specific. X-ray examination shows cardiac enlargement with mitral annular calcification, the latter also demonstrable echocardiographically. Diagnosis can be made by the excess amounts of dermitan sulphate and heparitin sulphate in the urine.

Pathology

The myocardial and connective tissue cells are hypertrophied, with large vacuoles filled with a complex macromolecular glycoprotein; this storage material impairs myocardial contractility. In addition to the biventricular hypertrophy, there is thickening of the heart valves, particularly the mitral valve.

Treatment

There is no definitive therapy.

Refsum's syndrome[58]

This hereditary disorder of lipid metabolism, characterized by the accumulation of phytanic acid, due to an impairment of oxidative degeneration, is manifest as chronic polyneuropathy, cerebellar ataxia and retinitis pigmentosa. Cardiovascular involvement occurs in most patients, with more severe cardiac problems characteristic of patients who have associated ophthalmoplegia, ptosis and facial weakness. The major problems are arrhythmias and conduction abnormalities, the most serious of which result in Stokes–Adams syncope and sudden death. QT interval prolongation has been described. There is abnormal accumulation of phytanic acid in the myocardium, as well as in the myelin sheath of the autonomic nerves and conducting tissue. The management consists of restriction of phytanic acid in the diet, standard antiarrhythmic therapy, and pacemaker implantation as needed.

Primary xanthomatosis[59]

Cardiovascular manifestations of patients with familial hypercholesterol-aemic xanthomatosis (type II hyperlipoproteinaemia) reflect both classical, although premature, atherosclerotic coronary heart disease with myocardial infarction and xanthomatous infiltration of the myocardium, which may result in arrhythmias and conduction abnormalities. Acquired aortic stenosis with foamy macrophages and cholesterol clefts in the aortic valve may be present. Treatment consists of dietary and drug regimens to effect lowering of cholesterol.

Hand–Schüller–Christian disease[60]

The lipid accumulation in this disorder is presumed secondary to an abnormality of the reticuloendothelial cells. Patients have exophthalmos, diabetes insipidus and bony defects of the skull. The xanthomatous cardiovascular infiltrates are often more prominent than the symptoms. There is no specific therapy.

Fibrocystic disease of the pancreas (mucoviscidosis)

Although chronic cor pulmonale is the major heart disease in patients with this problem, myocardial fibrosis has also been described to result in cardiac enlargement, arrhythmias, congestive heart failure and e.c.g. abnormalities.

Hypokalaemia[61,62]

Despite the significant myocardial lesions in hypokalaemic cardiomyopathy, including myofibre vacuolation and fragmentation, loss of muscle striation and interstitial infiltration, there are few clinical manifestations. The electrocardiogram is grossly abnormal, with QU interval prolongation, ST segment displacement, widening and flattening of the T wave, prominent U waves, and conduction abnormalities; the latter are thought to represent electrophysiological rather than anatomical disturbances. There is no correlation between the serum potassium level and the extent of the e.c.g. changes. Potassium replacement is the therapy of choice and is particularly urgent in patients receiving digitalis in whom digitalis toxicity may relate to the hypokalaemia.

Uraemia[63]

Because many cardiovascular manifestations are associated with uraemia – including arrhythmias, pericarditis, left ventricular hypertrophy and congestive heart failure as a reflection of the hypertensive cardiovascular disease, atherosclerotic coronary artery disease, metastatic myocardial calcification, electrolyte imbalance, anaemia, fluid overload, the high-output state from the haemodialysis shunt etc. – question has been raised as to whether a true uraemic cardiomyopathy exists. There does, however, seem to be a uraemic cardiomyopathy related to the low protein diet therapy for chronic renal failure; these patients have massive cardiomegaly, decreased cardiac output, hypotension, pericarditis, arrhythmias etc. Uraemic pericarditis seems related to the severity of the azotaemia, and may subside with dialysis, although pericardial tamponade and constrictive pericarditis may occur; the latter is more common in patients undergoing haemodialysis. The high fat renal failure diet increases the likelihood of atherosclerotic coronary artery disease. Electrocardiographic abnormalities include arrhythmias, conduction abnormalities and repolarization disorders. Haemodialysis is the management of choice, and pericardiocentesis or pericardiectomy may be indicated for significant pericardial effusion or constriction respectively.

HAEMATOLOGICAL DISORDERS

Leukaemia and lymphoma[64,65]

Clinical manifestations

About a quarter of patients with leukaemia have clinical or electrocardiographic evidence of cardiovascular involvement, with myocardial invasion and cardiovascular symptoms often occurring early in the course of the disease. The patients may present with tachycardia, arrhythmias, pericarditis, cardiac enlargement and congestive heart failure. Electrocardiographic abnormalities are non-specific.

Cardiovascular signs and symptoms occur in patients with lymphoma, with and without cardiac involvement; cardiovascular manifestations may be due to anaemia, to mediastinal or pulmonary involvement, to radiation therapy etc.

Pathology

There is minimal relationship between the severity of the morphological cardiac involvement and the cardiovascular symptoms. Myocardial leukaemic infiltrates are seen in the majority of patients dying of leukaemia, particularly acute myelocytic leukaemia. Infiltration is more prominent as the peripheral leukocyte count increases and as the duration of patient survival increases. Not all cardiac manifestations are due to myocardial leukaemic infiltration; many may be accounted for by myocardial haemorrhage, hypoxaemia, anaemia, pericarditis etc. Cardiac infiltration occurs in one sixth of patients dying of lymphoma and is most prominent with reticulum cell sarcoma.

Sickle cell anaemia[66,67]

As with leukaemia, a number of problems may contribute to the cardiovascular abnormalities including the anaemia, cor pulmonale secondary to pulmonary arterial thromboses, and the myocardial disease due to thromboses of intracardiac arteries. The prominent symptom is exertional dyspnoea, with heart failure occurring late in the course of the disease. There are frequent cardiac murmurs, the heart is enlarged, and electrocardiographic abnormalities are non-specific. The anatomical changes are of biventricular hypertrophy and dilatation, as well as a proliferative and thrombotic arteritis. There is no specific therapy. Cardiomyopathy has also been described with sickle cell trait.

Other disorders

The major cardiovascular manifestation of polycythaemia vera is probably myocardial infarction, due in part to intravascular thrombosis; the contribution of systemic arterial hypertension is uncertain. Patients with myeloma[68] may develop cardiac tamponade and cardiac arrhythmias, and often have associated cardiac amyloidosis. Arrhythmias and conduction abnormalities have been described with thrombotic thrombocytopenic purpura, as well as anaphylactoid purpura[69]. Patients with the latter problem may also have heart failure, chest pain, and non-specific electrocardiographic abnormalities due to an arteriolar and capillary periangiitis; corticosteroid hormone therapy is recommended.

ENDOCRINE DISORDERS[70]

Thyrotoxicosis[71,72]

There is no apparent specific morphological myocardial lesion in thyrotoxicosis; the thyrotoxic heart is physiologically hyperactive, with an increased heart rate and myocardial oxygen consumption (a high cardiac output state), an enhanced inotropic state, but without structural alterations. The heart shares in the general tissue hypermetabolism, and the increase in cardiac work also reflects increased peripheral arteriovenous shunting.

The cardiovascular complications of atrial fibrillation and cardiac enlargement, often with associated congestive heart failure, are not due to a primary morphological abnormality in the myocardium. An excess of thyroid hormone produces myocardial hypertrophy. It also increases atrial conduction velocity and decreases the atrial refractory period, predisposing to arrhythmias.

The occurrence of heart failure in the thyrotoxic patient, primarily in the older age group, suggests that it reflects an increase in cardiac work superimposed on underlying organic heart disease. The treatment is that for the underlying disease; β-adrenergic blocking drugs may also slow the atrial fibrillation; conventional therapy is indicated for heart failure.

Myxoedema[73,74]

As in thyrotoxicosis, no specific myocardial lesion has been delineated in myxoedema, although myxoedema and the associated type III hyperlipoproteinaemia appear to predispose to coronary atherosclerosis.

The homogeneous mucoid myocardial infiltrate is histochemically different from the myxoedematous infiltrate in the skin and tongue; it appears reversible with thyroid therapy in the early stages of the disease. Neither the bradycardia nor the heart failure seem to reflect a primary anatomical abnormality of the myocardium. Cardiac output appears appropriate for the decreased peripheral tissue demand. Cardiomegaly, when present, is often due to pericardial effusion.

Thyroid replacement therapy results in reversal of the cardiovascular manifestations, but should be administered with caution if associated coronary atherosclerotic heart disease is suspected.

Acromegaly[75,76]

Cardiac enlargement, hypertension and congestive heart failure are the major cardiovascular manifestations of acromegaly. Disproportionate cardiac enlargement is almost universal, although the component due to the associated hypertension is not known. Cardiac failure occurs in about one fourth of patients. Diabetes mellitus and coronary atherosclerosis may be contributory. Dyspnoea is the most prominent cardiac symptom, with weakness, palpitations and syncope also described. Cardiovascular complications are frequently the cause of death.

The electrocardiographic abnormalities are frequent but non-diagnostic, with changes of left ventricular hypertrophy most common, and arrhythmias and conduction abnormalities also described. There is cardiac enlargement on the chest X-ray, disproportionate to the increased somatic growth.

The myocardial morphological changes are of pronounced hypertrophy, particularly of the left ventricle, with the heart often weighing in excess of 500 g. Severe coronary atherosclerosis is frequent, at times associated with myocardial infarction. The chronic congestive heart failure is presumed secondary to dysfunction of the hypertrophied myofibres, to impaired contractility and impulse transmission due to fibrosis, and to the associated coronary atherosclerosis. The myocardial hypertrophy probably reflects both the generalized organomegaly due to an excess of growth hormone and the excessive cardiac work required to supply blood to an enlarged body. The treatment is that of the underlying disorder.

Cushing's syndrome[77]

This disorder predominates in women. The cardiovascular manifestations depend on the excessive secretion of cortisol, aldosterone and androgen; the relative contributions of hypertensive and atherosclerotic disease tend to overshadow those of primary myocardial dysfunction. Congestive heart failure occurs in about a quarter of patients and characteristically responds poorly to conventional therapy.

The cardiac enlargement is predominantly due to the hypertension and the major myocardial morphological alterations reflect the associated hypertension and atherosclerotic coronary heart disease.

The treatment is that of the underlying disorder.

Addison's disease[78]

The cardiocirculatory manifestations of primary adrenal insufficiency are due to hyposecretion of cortisol and aldosterone and include systemic arterial hypotension, postural hypotension, hypovolaemia and a decreased heart size. Electrocardiographic abnormalities are common but non-specific, and the heart is hypodynamic at fluoroscopy.

The small cardiac size may reflect a loss of body weight, decreased cardiac work, systemic hypotension or hypovolaemia. Myocardial contractility is often impaired; there is no characteristic myocardial morphological abnormality.

The management is hormonal replacement therapy.

NUTRITIONAL DISORDERS[79]

Beriberi[80,81]

Clinical manifestations

Oriental (Shoshin) beriberi is usually caused by malnutrition and is characterized by high cardiac output failure, often associated with syncope and shock, progressing rapidly to fatality. In the Western hemisphere, the so-called occidental beriberi is encountered most commonly in alcoholic men; the hyperkinetic features are typically absent, and the major presentation is of biventricular congestive heart failure. The presenting symptoms include fatigue, dyspnoea, orthopnoea, palpitations and oedema; the condition may be misdiagnosed as a cardiomyopathy.

In the high cardiac output stage, in addition to the neurological abnormalities, the prominent features are sinus tachycardia, tachypnoea, a wide pulse pressure, peripheral vasodilatation, elevation of the jugular venous pressure, cardiac enlargement, systolic murmurs and gallop rhythm, pulmonary congestion, hepatomegaly, serous effusions and oedema. The congestive heart failure is most prominent in those patients able to be active, i.e. those with minimal neurological involvement.

Beriberi should be considered as aetiological in patients either with known alcoholism or malnutrition who have unexplained heart failure.

Laboratory data

The electrocardiographic abnormalities of sinus tachycardia, low QRS voltage and non-specific repolarization changes, at times with QT interval prolongation due to hypokalaemia, often resolve with thiamine therapy. The heart is enlarged on X-ray. Anaemia and hypoproteinaemia are common. High-output cardiac failure may be noted at cardiac catheterization in the early stages of the disease.

Pathology and pathophysiology

The anatomical changes are of biventricular dilatation and hypertrophy with myofibre degeneration and interstitial and intracellular oedema. There is a notable absence of inflammation and necrosis.

The cardiovascular manifestations are presumed due to a derangement of carbohydrate metabolism, with inability of the myocardium to use oxygen; myocardial energy production is impaired by lack of cocarboxylase so that fats must provide the major source of energy. The high-output cardiac state imposes an additional workload on the heart with this metabolic handicap. In the later stages of the disease, biventricular failure with a decreased cardiac output and normal peripheral vascular resistance, rather than the decreased peripheral vascular resistance of the high cardiac output state, are present.

Treatment

The major components of management include thiamine and other vitamin administration, adequate diet, prolonged rest, sodium restriction, and diuretic drugs. Digitalis alone cannot control the heart failure, as the abnormality of myocardial energy production must be reversed. On occasion, when the systemic vascular resistance acutely returns to normal, systemic hypertension and pulmonary oedema may develop, due to return of fluid to the intravascular space prior to the restoration of normal ventricular function.

Pellagra[82]

Patients with pellagra describe palpitations, tachycardia, exertional dyspnoea, and oedema. These are associated with the typical erythematous skin lesions, diarrhoea and dementia. Electrocardiographic abnormalities are non-specific and may regress with therapy. The cardiovascular manifestations have been attributed both to nicotinic acid deficiency and to the frequently associated beriberi. There are no specific anatomical myocardial lesions. Niacin replacement is the specific therapy, but multivitamin administration is generally recommended.

Scurvy[83]

Patients with scurvy may have chest pain, dyspnoea and electrocardiographic abnormalities; sudden death of uncertain mechanism has been described. There is fatty degeneration of the myocardium. The diagnosis should be considered as a medical emergency requiring intravenous ascorbic acid therapy, which may reverse the e.c.g. abnormalities.

Hypervitaminosis D[84]

Patients with this condition have gross and microscopic calcium deposition in the myofibres. Electrocardiographic abnormalities of hypercalcaemia, a shortened QT interval, and ST–T changes of myocardial damage may be present.

Kwashiorkor[85]

Clinical manifestations

This disease predominates in urbanized South Africa, affecting persons who consume a high carbohydrate, low protein diet. The characteristic findings include tachycardia, cardiomegaly and low cardiac output failure, with extreme oedema and skeletal muscle wasting. Pulmonary and peripheral emboli are common, as is sudden death; the latter often occurs during the initial week of therapy.

Laboratory data

Non-specific repolarization abnormalities are the most common electrocardiographic changes, with low QRS voltage and prominent U waves; these are typically reversed with potassium therapy. The electrocardiogram returns to normal in most patients who recover. The heart is small on roentgenographic examination.

Pathology

The striking morphological abnormalities include atrophy and disintegration of the conduction system, which may account for the arrhythmias and conduction disturbances. Biventricular dilatation and hypertrophy, myofibre oedema and atrophy, and endocardial mural thrombosis are present, the latter presumed to be the basis for the thromboembolic complications.

Treatment

The patients respond to adequate diet and bed rest, but relapse may occur with resumption of physical activity and an inadequate diet.

CHEMICAL AND DRUG EFFECTS[86]

Cobalt (beer-drinker's) cardiomyopathy[87,88]

Clinical manifestations

This fulminant cardiomyopathy was described primarily among men drinking excessive quantities of beer. The epidemic occurrence of this disease in several cities coincided with the addition of cobalt sulphate as a frothing agent to beer and subsided when this practice was discontinued. The clinical presentation was initially of anorexia, nausea and vomiting; there was subsequent severe cardiac failure characterized by dyspnoea, cough, epigastric discomfort, agitation and oedema. The breathlessness was disproportionate to the degree of lung rales. Almost half of the patients with severe manifestations died of clinical shock within the first 24 hours. On physical examination there was a peculiar cyanosis limited to the face and trunk, tachycardia, elevation of the jugular venous pressure, hypotension, hepatomegaly and oedema.

Laboratory data

The electrocardiogram showed sinus tachycardia, low QRS voltage, bizarre P wave configuration, and non-specific repolarization changes. On chest X-ray there was cardiac enlargement with poor cardiac pulsations; pericardial effusion was often present. There was associated polycythaemia and severe acidosis. At cardiac catheterization, the cardiac output was decreased, peripheral resistance was normal and there was evidence of decreased ventricular compliance.

Pathology and pathophysiology

Cobalt toxicity depresses myocardial contractility by interfering with myocardial cellular respiratory enzymes. Although the amount of cobalt in the beer was subtoxic, presumably the setting of a patient with protein malnutrition, often an underlying alcoholic cardiomyopathy, and an individual doing heavy physical work, seemed to potentiate the problem. The morphological changes included myofibre, dystrophy, vacuolar degeneration and interstitial oedema; on electron microscopy the myofibrils were fragmented with damage of the contractile elements, the mitochondria were shrunken and there was increased lipid accumulation.

Treatment

The routine management for congestive heart failure, administration of vitamins and an adequate diet, and abstinence from cobalt-containing beer produced a gradual return to normal of the heart size and cardiovascular haemodynamics. Electrocardiographic abnormalities regressed somewhat more slowly. There was a high recovery rate among the survivors. The disease did not recur among patients who resumed beer-drinking once the cobalt additive had been removed.

Emetine and chloroquine[89]

Clinical manifestations

Cardiovascular toxicity is evident in most patients receiving these drugs for the management of amoebiasis and schistosomiasis. Dyspnoea and precordial pain are described, as well as arrhythmias and tachycardia. Arrhythmic, hypotensive, sudden deaths are described with emetine therapy.

Laboratory data

During the first week of emetine therapy there is the characteristic appearance of QT prolongation and T wave abnormalities on the electrocardiogram; these occasionally appear only after completion of a course of therapy. Arrhythmias and conduction disturbances have also been described, but typically regress after cessation of therapy. Electrocardiographic abnormalities are less pronounced with dehydroemetine and chloroquine. The chest X-ray is typically unremarkable. Cardiac serum enzyme levels may be elevated.

Pathology and pathophysiology

Although myofibre degeneration and selective mitochondrial damage on electron microscopy have been described, the latter appear to reverse after the cessation of therapy. Therefore, functional abnormalities are considered to predominate and e.c.g. changes appear reversible by potassium administration. However, since emetine inhibits mitochondrial oxidative phosphorylation, this feature may partially explain the cardiotoxicity.

Treatment

The patient should be at bed rest during therapy with these drugs, with continuous electrocardiographic monitoring and serial evaluation of the clinical features. Emetine should be avoided in patients known to have heart disease. The appearance of cardiovascular abnormalities should be an indication to terminate emetine therapy.

Phenothiazine drugs[90,91]

Clinical manifestations

Arrhythmias and syncope have occurred in patients receiving these psychotropic drugs, and their use is relatively contraindicated in patients known to have cardiovascular disease, particularly atherosclerotic coronary heart disease. Clinical manifestations are most prominent in the setting of drug overdosage.

Laboratory data

About half of all patients receiving phenothiazine drugs have repolarization abnormalities on the e.c.g. typically dose- and duration-related; QT prolongation appears most prominent with excessive dosage. U waves are prominent. The electrocardiogram characteristically returns to normal after cessation of therapy; potassium administration may normalize the electrocardiographic abnormalities even in the absence of hypokalaemia.

Pathology and pathophysiology

Focal interstitial myocardial necrosis is described. Phenothiazine drugs alter myocardial catecholamines; the increased circulating norepinephrine may precipitate cardiac arrhythmias, and cardiac catecholamine depletion may depress myocardial contractility. The hypotensive effect of the phenothiazine drugs is probably due to inhibition of centrally mediated pressor reflexes or to α-adrenergic blockade. In addition, the quinidine-like effect of these drugs enhances the likelihood of re-entrant tachyarrhythmias.

Treatment

Most abnormalities subside with discontinuation of psychotropic therapy. Serious arrhythmias may be managed with lidocaine; alternatively, pacing with overdrive suppression may be effective. Electrocardiographic monitoring is warranted in patients with drug overdosage until the QT interval has returned to normal; quinidine and procainamide are not recommended as antiarrhythmic drugs as they may re-enforce the arrhythmia.

Tricyclic antidepressant drugs[91,92]

Clinical manifestations

Hypertensive crises, unresponsiveness to antihypertensive therapy, arrhythmias, heart failure, myocardial infarction and sudden death have been described. Electrocardiographic abnormalities include conduction disturbances and arrhythmias.

Pathology and pathophysiology

The cardiovascular abnormalities may be caused by the anticholinergic activity, by direct myocardial depression, or by the effect of these drugs on adrenergic neurons. Tricyclic antidepressant drugs block norepinephrine reuptake at neuronal endings. High doses of the tricyclic antidepressant drugs may depress myocardial contractility. The drugs also have a quinidine-like antiarrhythmic effect.

Treatment

It seems unwise to administer these drugs to patients with cardiac disease, and they present an increased risk in elderly patients. Lidocaine is recommended to manage the arrhythmias. Dialysis is ineffective with drug overdosage. Digitalis should be used cautiously as it may increase the incidence of arrhythmias, and β-blocking drugs may potentiate myocardial depression.

Daunorubicin and doxorubicin (Adriamycin)[93,94]

Clinical manifestations

Myocardial toxicity is the major feature limiting the use of these antineo-plastic agents; rapidly progressive biventricular failure may occur within the first 6 months after the completion of chemotherapy. Intractable biventricular failure is rapidly followed by cardiac death.

Laboratory data

Electrocardiographic abnormalities, including arrhythmias and repolarization changes, often occur in the early days of drug administration, but are neither dose-dependent nor related to the subsequent cardiomyopathy. The QRS voltage decreases prominently with the clinical onset of cardiomyopathy, but the e.c.g. is insensitive in detecting early myocardial dysfunction.

There is rapid cardiac dilatation and pulmonary vascular congestion on chest X-ray. Serial measurement of systolic time intervals and echocardiographic parameters seem insensitive in detecting early cardiomyopathy in time to permit cumulative dose restriction.

Pathology and pathophysiology

The mechanism of toxicity appears related to the binding of the drug to DNA in nuclei and mitochondria; once bound, the drug is slowly liberated from the cell. Inhibition of protein synthesis interferes with normal protein regeneration; this could explain the delayed toxicity and the greater vulnerability in adults, particularly the elderly, as compared with children. There is myocardial interstitial fibrosis with myofibre loss and fragmentation, and loss of contractile substance with mitochondrial swelling and distortion on electron microscopy. The gross morphological changes include cardiac enlargement and mural thrombosis.

Treatment

Restriction of antineoplastic drug dosage may limit the degree of cardiomyopathy. Endomyocardial biopsy appears the most sensitive means of detecting early cardiomyopathy. The roles of radionuclide studies and nuclear magnetic resonance evaluation are being assessed. There seems to be a synergistic effect between radiation, other antineoplastic agents, and daunorubicin or doxorubicin in producing cardiotoxicity. Once cardiomyopathy is evident, there is minimal response either to positive inotropic drugs or mechanical ventricular assistance.

Cyclophosphamide[95]

This antineoplastic agent in large doses produces major myocardial necrosis and haemorrhagic myocarditis. The clinical presentation is of heart failure with pulmonary oedema and a low cardiac output state, essentially unresponsive to therapy. Electrocardiographic abnormalities are non-specific, and cardiac serum enzyme levels are elevated. Intensive dosage regimens should be avoided.

Methysergide

This drug is used to treat migraine and has been reported to cause endocardial fibroelastosis, coronary ostial stenosis, retroperitoneal fibrosis and pleuropulmonary fibrosis, in addition to the myocardial disorder. Methysergide is chemically similar to serotonin, which may explain the similarity of the cardiac lesions to those of the carcinoid syndrome; however, methysergide preponderantly affects the left side of the heart. The patients may develop valvular stenosis and insufficiency, which often regresses with cessation of therapy. The drug should be restricted in dosage or given only intermittently and seems contraindicated in patients with known atherosclerotic coronary heart disease, valvular disease or cardiac dysfunction.

Arsenic[96]

Acute interstitial myocarditis has been described during chronic arsenical therapy of syphilis, causing heart failure and non-specific electrocardiographic abnormalities.

Acute arsenic poisoning, usually due to arsenic trioxide, is the most common cause of acute heavy metal poisoning. There are no cardiovascular symptoms; the electrocardiographic changes, which typically disappear in patients who recover, are those of myocardial ischaemia and QT interval prolongation. Arsenic interferes with the function of respiratory system enzymes and may produce myocardial hypoxaemia. BAL (British antilewisite) may enhance the speed of recovery.

Acute poisoning with arsine gas causes red blood cell haemolysis, decreases the oxygen-carrying capacity of the blood, and may produce myocardial hypoxaemia; the major cardiovascular manifestation is electrocardiographic T wave abnormalities. There is no specific therapy.

Antimony[97]

Antimony compounds, used to treat schistosomiasis, frequently produce myocardial damage in addition to the common hepatic toxicity. Chest pain has been described, and sudden death appears due to arrhythmia. Electrocardiographic abnormalities are virtually constant by the end of the course of therapy, particularly non-specific repolarization changes and a prolonged QT interval; these commonly regress after the cessation of therapy.

Sympathomimetic amines[98]

Epinephrine, isoproterenol and angiotensin may produce myocardial lesions similar to those seen in patients with phaeochromocytoma; chest pain and e.c.g. changes of myocardial ischaemia have been described. Focal myocardial necrosis is present. Although pretreatment of animals with antiplatelet agents decreases sympathomimetic amine-induced myocardial necrosis, the clinical role of these drugs remains controversial.

Carbon monoxide[99]

The clinical manifestations include chest pain, dyspnoea and palpitations, with occasional pulmonary oedema and cardiovascular collapse. The electrocardiographic alterations of myocardial ischaemia are usually transient and arrhythmias may be encountered. Echocardiography has shown wall motion abnormalities and occasional mitral valve prolapse, the latter possibly reflecting the papillary muscle lesions of carbon monoxide poisoning. Myocardial damage from acute and chronic carbon monoxide poisoning is due both to the hypoxaemia resulting from a diminished oxygen transport capacity of the blood and to a direct toxic effect on myocardial fibre mitochondria. Carbon monoxide replaces oxygen in oxyhaemoglobin and decreases the tissue dissociation of oxyhaemoglobin. The morphological lesions are those of myocardial haemorrhage and necrosis, with a predilection for the papillary muscles and the subendocardium of the left ventricle. Management includes oxygen administration, with hyperbaric oxygen of possible additional value. Electrocardiographic monitoring and activity limitation are indicated when there is evidence of myocardial damage.

Fluorinated hydrocarbons[100]

Aerosol inhalation toxicity may occur from the fluorocarbon compounds used as aerosol propellants. The severe pneumonia and central nervous system toxicity may mask the cardiovascular symptoms, which are predominantly those of left ventricular failure, hypotension and arrhythmias. The depression of myocardial contractility appears dose-related. Electrocardiographic changes include sinus bradycardia, which may progress to AV dissociation and terminate in asystole or ventricular fibrillation; this is the probable mechanism of sudden death in glue-sniffing. Management includes supportive therapy and antiarrhythmic agents; caution is warranted if epinephrine is considered to reverse the cardiocirculatory failure.

127

Phosphorus[101]

Ventricular fibrillation or peripheral vascular collapse indicate a grave prognosis in patients with phosphorus ingestion, as death in the first 12–24 h is usually cardiovascular in origin. Electrocardiographic abnormalities occur in about half of all patients and appear dose-related; these include non-specific repolarization changes and QT interval prolongation, which typically regress with clinical improvement.

Phosphorus inhibits amino acid incorporation into myocardial proteins; there is also a direct toxic effect of phosphorus on the myocardium and on the peripheral blood vessels; this decreased cardiac output and lowered systemic vascular resistance are unresponsive to adrenergic agents. There is no specific therapy.

Lead[102]

Clinical and e.c.g. evaluation for evidence of myocardial dysfunction should be part of the assessment of all patients with chronic lead poisoning; myocardial damage may be due to a direct toxic effect of lead or to hypertensive changes secondary to lead nephropathy. Chest pain and congestive heart failure have been described; electrocardiographic conduction and repolarization abnormalities have subsided after therapy with EDTA.

Scorpion venom[103]

The cardiovascular manifestations and myocardial morphological alterations resulting from scorpion sting are due to elevated catecholamine levels; myocardial toxicity is more common than neurotoxicity and is often the cause of death. The tachycardia, pulmonary oedema and peripheral circulatory failure are typically reversible in patients who survive. Electrocardiographic abnormalities occur in the majority of patients, with changes often mimicking myocardial infarction; myocardial serum enzyme levels may be elevated.

The myocardial lesions in patients who die resemble those of catecholamine excess, with prominent damage to the papillary muscle and subendocardium. Adrenergic blocking agents may limit the cardiovascular manifestations and prevent the cardiomyopathy.

Variable cardiomyopathy and electrocardiographic abnormalities have been described due to venom from stings and bites of the black widow spider, a variety of toxic snakes, and wasps. Toxic myocarditis with cardiac enlargement and cardiac failure has also been described after regression of the neurological changes in a patient with tick paralysis.

Hypersensitivity, anaphylaxis, and serum sickness[104,105]

The drugs to be discussed generally produce direct damage to myocardial cells as a result of hypersensitivity; their effect may be directly on the myocardium or secondary to a coronary vasculitis. The associated electro-cardiographic abnormalities may reflect a direct effect on the myofibres or an alteration of the electrical activity of the heart.

Myocardial abnormalities may occur in *anaphylaxis*, independent of changes in coronary blood flow; typically, though, anaphylactic reactions to a variety of drugs are associated with profound hypotension. Non-specific e.c.g. abnormalities may reflect myocardial antigen–antibody reactions, the effects of drugs used to treat the anaphylaxis, myocardial hypoxaemia, effects of the mediator substances of anaphylaxis etc; since histamine is an important mediator of anaphylaxis, antihistamine therapy is generally effective.

Serum sickness may have as cardiac manifestations tachycardia or arrhythmia, hypotension, pericarditis, or chest pain compatible with myocardial ischaemia. The electrocardiographic changes are non-specific, but may mimic myocardial infarction. The morphological basis is a general-ized vasculitis and necrotizing arteritis; because the coronary and pericar-dial arteries are also involved, the clinical presentation may have variable cardiovascular components. Corticosteroid hormones are the treatment of choice.

Smallpox vaccine[106]

Myocarditis and pericarditis, presumably due to an antigen–antibody reaction, may occur 1–2 weeks after smallpox vaccination; the time lag suggests that this does not reflect a viraemia. Because the potential complications of vaccination are often more serious than the risk of smallpox infection in developed countries, smallpox vaccination is not currently routinely required.

The clinical manifestations are generally mild, with spontaneous recovery; but chest pain, dyspnoea and severe heart failure have been described. Death has occurred without premonitory cardiac symptoms. The electrocardiographic changes are non-specific.

Fatal smallpox myocarditis is characterized by acute myofibre degenera-tion, necrosis and oedema. The recommended management is corticosteroid hormone therapy and the usual treatment for congestive heart failure.

Allergic myocarditis has also been described after vaccination for cholera and tetanus.

Other drug hypersensitivity reactions

Allergic myocarditis has also been described after administration of aureomycin (chlortetracycline) and antituberculous drugs including streptomycin and para-aminosalicylic acid. With these drugs, as well as with phenindione, acetaminophen, reserpine, methyldopa and guanethidine, myocardial lesions are non-specific.

Lithium carbonate, used to treat manic-depressive illness, causes almost invariable T wave abnormalities on the electrocardiogram which characteristically subside after cessation of therapy. Lithium decreases intracellular potassium, prolonging repolarization and facilitating arrhythmias; arrhythmias may require discontinuation of the drug.

PHYSICAL CAUSES

Radiation[107]

Clinical manifestations

The increased survival of patients treated with potent sources of therapeutic radiation has increased the likelihood of clinical manifestations of high-dose radiation therapy to the thorax, which may potentially damage the heart and pericardium. Radiation-induced cardiac fibrosis should be considered in any patient who has received extensive radiation to the chest and who has unusual clinical cardiovascular manifestations or electrocardiographic abnormalities.

The clinical syndromes include chronic pericarditis, with and without constriction, and pericardial effusion, occasionally with tamponade. Radiation-induced pericardial effusion must be differentiated from that representing malignant involvement of the pericardium. Pacemaker therapy has been required for complete heart block with Stokes–Adams syncope.

Laboratory data

Electrocardiographic abnormalities are non-specific. Pericardial effusion, suggested on the chest roentgenogram, may be documented echocardiographically.

Pathology and pathophysiology

Radiation results in pericardial fibrosis, as well as occasional patchy myocardial fibrosis and necrosis. The coronary arteries may become thickened and hyalinized. Radiation may predispose to or accelerate coronary atherosclerosis, with vascular injury enhancing lipid deposition. Endocardial fibrosis and fibroelastosis may be the basis for cardiac murmurs, and fibrosis of the conduction system may be responsible for complete heart block.

Treatment

There is no specific therapy.

Other physical causes[108]

Electrocardiographic changes have been described with electric shock, and morphological myofibre damage secondary to heat stroke and hypothermia may be manifest by non-specific electrocardiographic abnormalities and conduction disturbances in patients who survive; there may be associated elevation of serum cardiac isoenzyme levels.

MISCELLANEOUS SYSTEMIC SYNDROMES

Reiter's disease[109]

Particularly after recurrent episodes of arthritis, urethritis and conjunctivitis, patients may develop pericardial, myocardial and valvular involvement. Acute pericarditis can be diagnosed by the pain and pericardial friction rub. Aortic regurgitation is a late complication of the disease. The electrocardiographic abnormalities include PR interval prolongation, which may progress to complete heart block. Pacemaker implantation may be required.

Cogan's syndrome[110]

About one third of patients with non-syphilitic interstitial keratitis and bilateral deafness develop cardiovascular manifestations which include cardiac enlargement, aortic regurgitation and congestive heart failure, the latter in part due to a myocardial arterial angiitis.

Behçet's disease[111]

The cardiac manifestations associated with the recurrent oral and genital ulceration and relapsing iritis include cardiac enlargement, heart failure, pericarditis and arrhythmias. Thrombophlebitis is also common. Corticosteroid therapy has been effective.

Rejection cardiomyopathy[112]

A decrease in exercise tolerance, the development of heart failure, fever and tachycardia may be the initial manifestations of rejection cardiomyopathy; however, three-quarters of patients with this problem remain asymptomatic. Decreased electrocardiographic voltage is a characteristic, but late, finding. Cardiac enlargement on the chest roentgenogram may be due to dilatation and/or pericardial effusion. Endomyocardial biopsy of the right ventricle provides the most reliable early identification of rejection cardiomyopathy. The anatomic alterations are necrotizing arteritis, fibrinoid necrosis, myocytolysis and a mononuclear cell infiltrate. Increasing doses of corticosteroid hormones, or administration of cyclosporine or other immunosuppressive therapy, may reverse the process.

Cardiomyopathy of ageing[113]

The major causes of myocardial abnormalities in the elderly are senile cardiac amyloidosis and degenerative calcification of the mitral and aortic valve cusps and rings. Additionally, increased myofibre vacuolation and neutral fat and lipofuscin deposition occur with ageing. The aged heart has a decreased cardiac output, presumably related to a lesser metabolic demand.

Marfan's syndrome

Patients with Marfan's syndrome, in addition to the aortic, valvular and coronary arterial disease, may also have myocardial abnormalities which contribute to the cardiac enlargement and heart failure.

Noonan's syndrome

In patients with Noonan's syndrome, left ventricular cardiomyopathy, both obstructive and non-obstructive, has been described, in addition to the congenital heart disease, most commonly valvular pulmonic stenosis.

Weber–Christian disease[114]

Cardiac involvement is unusual in Weber–Christian disease, relapsing febrile nodular non-suppurative panniculitis; nevertheless, myocardial nodules, identical to those seen in the skin, have been described, and cardiac enlargement and heart failure may occur.

Scleroedema of Buschke[115]

This is a self-limiting acid mucopolysaccharide skin infiltration; myocardial involvement has been characterized by pericardial effusion and heart failure. This cardiomyopathy also has a good prognosis, as the cardiac abnormalities and non-specific electrocardiographic changes subside as the skin infiltrate resolves.

Wegener's granulomatosis[116]

This allergic panarteritis is characterized by non-healing midline granulomas of the nose, pulmonary infiltrates and renal disease. Myocardial morphological abnormalities include a vasculitis, granulomatous lesions and an inflammatory cell infiltrate. The clinical cardiovascular presentation includes cardiac enlargement, congestive heart failure and pericarditis with effusion. Cytotoxic drugs, with and without corticosteroid hormones, appear of value.

Reye's syndrome[117]

This rapidly fatal disease of young children is of unknown cause and is characterized by encephalopathy, fatty visceral degeneration, and cardiac involvement, particularly bundle branch block and complete atrioventricular block. Aspirin administration for a viral infection has been implicated as contributing to this problem. Extensive morphological abnormalities of the conduction system have been described.

Lentiginosis[118]

All patients with prominent widespread lentigenes should be periodically evaluated for the development of cardiomyopathy. Cardiac enlargement and/or systolic murmurs may reflect hypertrophic cardiomyopathy. The atrioventricular septum progressively hypertrophies, often resulting in bilateral outflow tract obstruction. Propranolol therapy is suggested, and surgical septectomy has had variable success. Associated atrial myxoma is described.

Myocardial lesions have also been described in neurofibromatosis (von Recklinghausen's disease); patients may have myocardial and epicardial neurofibromas, as well as acquired fibromuscular stenosis of the right ventricular outflow tract and obstructive cardiomyopathy.

Diabetic cardiomyopathy

Heart failure in diabetic patients is typically due to a combination of atherosclerotic coronary heart disease and hypertensive cardiovascular disease. However, insulin-dependent diabetics, particularly women, seem to have a preponderance of biventricular failure. It is not known whether a microangiopathy or a metabolic defect in energy production underlies this cardiomyopathy.

Mulibrey nanism[119]

This hereditary disorder has commonly associated constrictive pericarditis, but myocardial fibrosis may also occur. There is heart failure of varying severity, and electrocardiographic abnormalities are non-specific. The pericardial thickening can be confirmed echocardiographically, and pericardiectomy may be indicated in sicker patients.

Ulcerative colitis[120]

Recurrent myopericarditis has also been described in patients with chronic ulcerative colitis, manifest by pleuritic chest pain and a pericardial friction rub, associated with non-specific electrocardiographic abnormalities. The cardiovascular abnormalities resolve with corticosteroid hormone therapy.

Whipple's disease[121]

Most patients with intestinal lypodystrophy have clinical cardiac findings, unrelated to the severity and duration of the Whipple's disease; these include cardiac murmurs, particularly from the mitral valve, pericardial friction rubs, and congestive heart failure. Electrocardiographic abnormalities are non-specific. The anatomical changes are those of large macrophages with PAS-positive granules, identical to those seen in the intestine, in the pericardium, myocardium and heart valves. Rod-shaped bodies, which may be bacteria, also are seen in the myocardium and heart valves. Antibiotic therapy is recommended.

Pseudoxanthomia elasticum (Grönblad–Standberg syndrome)[122]

Patients with this hereditary disorder of connective tissue have cardiac manifestations of heart failure, arrhythmias, cardiac murmurs and Stokes–Adams syncope, in association with the crêpe-like skin lesions and angioid streaks of the retina. There is no specific therapy.

Alcoholic heart muscle disease

Large quantities of alcohol taken over a long period (40 g daily for 10 years or more) can cause severe myocardial disease leading to dilated ventricles and reduced contractile function and a clinical picture of severe low output congestive heart failure. Heart failure may be preceded by episodic arrythmia; such as ectopic beats or paroxsysmal atrial fibrillation. Hypertension may be associated.

The pathology is not specific, but lipid deposits are present in the myocardium.

The action of alcohol on the heart is a direct one; the ionic permeability of myocardial cells is altered; electrolytes are depleted and lipid transport is abnormal. Free fatty acid uptake is reduced. Acetaldehyde may increase myocardial damage.

The diagnosis depends upon a clinical picture resembling dilated cardiomyopathy in a patient with a history of heavy and prolonged alcohol intake and no other cause for congestive heart failure.

Laboratory studies are not diagnostic, but an increased mean corpuscular volume of the erythrocyte and raised gamma glutamyl transpeptidase are pointers, as are increased levels of triglycerides and uric acid. Blood alcohol estimations may be of value.

Specific cardiac investigations do not reveal any diagnostic evidence, indicating dilatation and reduced contraction of the left ventricle, generalized cardiomegaly and non-specific repolarization changes on the electrocardiogram.

The early stages of alcoholic heart muscle disease may be revealed by arrythmias and by echocardiographic changes indicating reduced systolic function, such as a decrease in the velocity of fibre shortening of the left ventricle, together with increased systolic and diastolic dimensions. Treatment essentially consists of complete withdrawal of alcohol, adequate diet with vitamin supplements and treatment for heart failure and arrythmia.

Acknowledgement

With appreciation to Jeanette Zahler for help in preparation and typing of the manuscript.

References

1. Goodwin, J.F., Roberts, W.C. and Wenger, N.K. (1982). Cardiomyopathy. In Hurst, J.W. (ed.) *The Heart*. 5th Ed. p. 1299. (New York: McGraw-Hill)
2. Perloff, J.K., Lindgren, K.M. and Groves, B.M. (1970). Uncommon or commonly unrecognized causes of heart failure. *Prog. Cardiovasc. Dis.*, **12**, 409
3. Wheeler, R.C. and Abelmann, W.H. (1972). Cardiomyopathy associated with systemic diseases. *Cardiovasc. Clin.*, **4**, 283
4. Roberts, W.C., McAllister, H.A. Jr. and Ferrans, V.J. (1977). Sarcoidosis of the heart. A clinicopathologic study of 35 necropsy patients (Group I) and review of 78 previously described necropsy patients (Group II). *Am. J. Med.*, **63**, 86
5. Fleming, H.A. (1974). Sarcoid heart disease. *Br. Heart J.*, **36**, 54
6. Wenger, N.K., Abelmann, W.H. and Roberts, W.C. (1982). Myocarditis. In Hurst, J.W. (ed.) *The Heart*. 5th Edn. p. 1278. (New York: McGraw-Hill)
7. Lansdown, A.B.G. (1978). Viral infections and diseases of the heart. *Prog. Med. Virol.*, **24**, 70
8. Walsh, T.J., Hutchins, G.M., Bulkley, B.H. and Mendelsohn, G. (1980). Fungal infections of the heart: Analysis of 51 autopsy cases. *Am. J. Cardiol.*, **45**, 357
9. Kean, B.H. (1964). *Parasites of the Human Heart*. (New York: Grune and Stratton)
10. Hirshman, S.Z. and Hammer, G.S. (1974). Coxsackie virus myopericarditis. A microbiological and clinical review. *Am. J. Cardiol.*, **34**, 224
11. Santos-Buch, C.A. (1979). American trypanosomiasis: Chagas' disease. *Int. Rev. Exp. Pathol.*, **19**, 63
12. Sanders, V. (1963). Viral myocarditis. *Am. Heart J.*, **66**, 707
13. Kawai, C., Matsumori, A., Kitaura, Y. and Takatsu, T. (1978). Viruses and the heart: Viral myocarditis and cardiomyopathy. *Prog. in Cardiol.*, **7**, 141
14. Perloff, J.K. (1972). Cardiac involvement in heredofamilial neuromyopathic diseases. *Cardiovasc. Clin.*, **4**, 333
15. Perloff, J.K., deLeon, A.C. Jr. and O'Doherty, D. (1966). The cardiomyopathy of progressive muscular dystrophy. *Circulation*, **33**, 625
16. James, T.N. and Fisch, C. (1963). Observations on the cardiovascular involvement in Friedreich's ataxia. *Am. Heart J.*, **66**, 164
17. Clements, S.D. Jr., Colmers, R.A. and Hurst, J.W. (1976). Myotonia dystrophica. Ventricular arrhythmias, intraventricular conduction abnormalities, atrioventricular block and Stokes–Adams attacks successfully treated with permanent transvenous pacemaker. *Am. J. Cardiol.*, **37**, 933
18. Gibson, T.C. (1975). The heart in myasthenia gravis. *Am. Heart. J.*, **90**, 389
19. Waters, D.D., Nutter, D.O., Hopkins, L.C. and Dorney, E.R. (1975). Cardiac features of an unusual X-linked humeroperoneal neuromuscular disease. *N. Engl. J. Med.*, **293**, 1017
20. Lascelles, R.G., Baker, I.A. and Thomas, P.K. (1970). Hereditary polyneuropathy of Roussy–Levy type with associated cardiomyopathy. *Guy's Hosp. Rep.*, **119**, 253
21. McCormish, M., Compston, A. and Jewitt, D. (1976). Cardiac abnormalities in chronic progressive external ophthalmoplegia. *Br. Heart J.*, **38**, 526
22. Tanaka, H., Uemura, N., Toyama, Y., Kudo, A., Ohkatsu, Y. and Kanehisa, T. (1976). Cardiac involvement in the Kugelberg–Welander syndrome. *Am. J. Cardiol.*, **38**, 528
23. Bulkley, B.H. and Roberts, W.C. (1975). The heart in systemic lupus erythematosus and the changes induced in it by corticosteroid therapy. A study of 36 necropsy patients. *Am. J. Med.*, **58**, 243

24. James, T.N., Rupe, C.E. and Monto, R.W. (1965). Pathology of the cardiac conduction system in systemic lupus erythematosus. *Ann. Intern. Med.*, 63, 402
25. Holsinger, D.R., Osmundson, P.J. and Edwards, J.E. (1962). The heart in periarteritis nodosa. *Circulation*, 25, 610
26. Fauci, A.S., Haynes, B.F. and Katz, P. (1978). The spectrum of vasculitis: Clinical, pathologic, immunologic, and therapeutic considerations. *Ann. Intern. Med.*, 89, 660
27. Bacon, P.A. and Gibson, D.G. (1974). Cardiac involvement in rheumatoid arthritis. An echocardiographic study. *Ann. Rheum. Dis.*, 33, 20
28. Weintraub, A.M. and Zwaiffler, N.J. (1963). The occurrence of valvular and myocardial disease in patients with chronic joint deformity. A spectrum. *Am. J. Med.*, 35, 145
29. Julkunen, H. (1962). Rheumatoid spondylitis – Clinical and laboratory study of 149 cases compared with 182 cases of rheumatoid arthritis. *Acta Rheum. Scand.*, 172 (Suppl. 4), 24
30. Bulkley, B.H. and Roberts, W.C. (1973). Ankylosing spondylitis and aortic regurgitation. Description of the characteristic cardiovascular lesion from study of eight necropsy patients. *Circulation*, 48, 1014
31. Bulkley, B.H., Ridolfi, R.L., Salyer, W.R. and Hutchins, G.M. (1976). Myocardial lesions of progressive systemic sclerosis. A cause of cardiac dysfunction. *Circulation*, 53, 483
32. Bulkley, B.H. (1979). Progressive systemic sclerosis: Cardiac involvement. *Clin. Rheum. Dis.*, 5, 131
33. McAllister, H.A. Jr. and Fenoglio, J.J. Jr. (1978). *Tumors of the Cardiovascular System*. (Washington D.C.: Armed Forces Institute of Pathology)
34. Harvey, W.P. (1968). Clinical aspects of cardiac tumors. *Am. J. Cardiol.*, 21, 328
35. Goodwin, J.F. (1968). The spectrum of cardiac tumors. *Am. J. Cardiol.*, 21, 307
36. Prichard, R.W. (1951). Tumors of the heart: Review of the subject and report of one hundred and fifty cases. *Arch. Pathol.*, 51, 98
37. DeLoach, J.F. and Haynes, J.W. (1953). Secondary tumors of heart and pericardium. Review of the subject and report of one hundred and thirty-seven cases. *Arch. Intern. Med.*, 91, 224
38. Lockwood, W.B. and Broghamer, W.L. Jr. (1980). The changing prevalence of secondary cardiac neoplasms as related to cancer therapy. *Cancer*, 45, 2659
39. Berge, T. and Sievers, J. (1968). Myocardial metastases. A pathological and electrocardiographic study. *Br. Heart J.*, 30, 383
40. Smith, L.H. (1976). Secondary tumors of the heart. *Rev. Surg.*, 33, 223
41. Buja, L.M. and Roberts, W.C. (1971). Iron in the heart. Etiology and clinical significance. *Am. J. Med.*, 51, 209
42. Arnett, E.N., Nienhuis, A.W., Henry, W.L., Ferrans, V.J., Redwood, D.R. and Roberts, W.C. (1975). Massive myocardial hemosiderosis: A structure-function conference at the National Heart and Lung Institute. *Am. Heart J.*, 90, 777
43. Garcia, R. and Jennings, J.M. (1972). Pheochromocytoma masquerading as a cardiomyopathy. *Am. J. Cardiol.*, 29, 568
44. Van Vliet, P.D., Burchell, H.B. and Titus, J.L. (1966). Focal myocarditis associated with pheochromocytoma. *N. Engl. J. Med.*, 274, 1102
45. Ehlers, K.H., Hagstrom, J.W.C., Lukas, D.S., Redo, S.F. and Engle, M.A. (1962). Glycogen-storage disease of the myocardium with obstruction to left ventricular outflow. *Circulation*, 25, 96
46. Blieden, L.C. and Moller, J.H. (1974). Cardiac involvement in inherited disorders of metabolism. *Prog. Cardiovasc. Dis.*, 16, 615
47. Ockerman, P.A. and Berlin, S.-O. (1964). Biochemical studies in familial cardiomyopathy. With special reference to the differential diagnosis from known types of glycogen storage disease. *Acta Med. Scand.*, 176, 277
48. Ratinov, G., Baker, W.P. and Swaiman, K.F. (1965). McArdle's syndrome with previously unreported electrocardiographic and serum enzyme abnormalities. *Ann. Intern. Med.*, 62, 328
49. Ferrans, V.J., Hibbs, R.G. and Burda, C.D. (1969). The heart in Fabry's disease. A histochemical and electron microscopic study. *Am. J. Cardiol.*, 24, 95
50. Smith, R.R.L., Hutchins, G.M., Sack, G.H. Jr. and Ridolfi, R.L. (1978). Unusual cardiac,

renal and pulmonary involvement in Gaucher's disease. Interstitial glucocerebroside accumulation, pulmonary hypertension and fatal bone marrow embolization. *Am. J. Med.*, 65, 352

51. Deacon, J.S.R., Gilbert, E.F., Viseskul, C., Herrmann, J., Angevine, J.M., Opitz, J.M. and Albert, A.E. (1974). Familial cardiac lipidosis. *Birth Defects*, 10, 181

52. Eilenberg, M.D. and Scobie, B.A. (1960). Prolonged neuropsychiatric disability and cardiomyopathy in acute intermittent porphyria. *Br. Med. J.*, 1, 858

53. Virtanen, K.S.I. and Halonen, P.I. (1969). Total heart block as a complication of gout. *Cardiologia*, 54, 359

54. Pikula, B., Plamenac, P., Curcic, B. and Nikulin, A. (1973). Myocarditis caused by primary oxalosis in a 4-year-old child. *Virchows Arch. (Pathol. Anat.)*, 358, 99

55. Lichtenstein, L. and Kaplan, L. (1954). Hereditary ochronosis. Pathologic changes observed in two necropsied cases. *Am. J. Pathol.*, 30, 99

56. McKusick, V.A., Neufeld, E.F. and Kelly, T.E. (1978). The mucopolysaccharide storage diseases. In Stanbury, J.B., Wyngaarden, J.B. and Fredrickson, D.S. (eds.) *The Metabolic Basis of Inherited Disease*. 4th Ed. p. 1282. (New York: McGraw-Hill)

57. Schieken, R.M., Kerber, R.E., Ionasescu, V.V. and Zellweger, H. (1975). Cardiac manifestations of the mucopolysaccharidoses. *Circulation*, 52, 700

58. Campbell, A.M.G. and Williams, E.R. (1967). Natural history of Refsum's syndrome in a Gloucestershire family. *Br. Med. J.*, 3, 777

59. Glomset, J.A. (1982). Cholesterol metabolism. In Hurst, J.W. (ed.) *The Heart*. 5th Edn. p. 951. (New York: McGraw-Hill)

60. Miller, A.A. and Ramsden, F. (1965). Neural and visceral xanthomatosis in adults. *J. Clin. Pathol.*, 18, 622

61. Fisch, C., Knoebel, S.B., Feigenbaum, H. and Greenspan, K. (1966). Potassium and monophasic action potential, electrocardiogram, conduction and arrhythmias. *Prog. Cardiovasc. Dis.*, 8, 387

62. Surawicz, B. and Gettes, L.S. (1971). Effect of electrolyte abnormalities on the heart and circulation. In Conn, H.L. Jr. and Horowitz, O. (eds.) *Cardiac and Vascular Disease*. p. 539. (Philadelphia: Lea & Febiger)

63. Bailey, G.L., Hampers, C.L. and Merrill, J.P. (1967). Reversible cardiomyopathy in uremia. *Trans. Am. Soc. Artif. Intern. Org.*, 13, 263

64. Roberts, W.C., Glancy, D.L. and De Vita, V.T. (1968). Heart in malignant lymphoma (Hodgkin's disease, lymphosarcoma, reticulum cell sarcoma and mycosis fungoides): A study of 196 autopsy cases. *Am. J. Cardiol.*, 22, 82

65. Roberts, W.C., Bodey, G.P. and Wertlake, P.T. (1968). The heart in acute leukemia. A study of 420 autopsy cases. *Am. J. Cardiol.*, 21, 388

66. Uzsoy, N.K. (1964). Cardiovascular findings in patients with sickle cell anemia. *Am. J. Cardiol.*, 13, 320

67. Fleischer, R.A. and Rubler, S. (1968). Primary cardiomyopathy in nonanemic patients. Association with sickle cell trait. *Am. J. Cardiol.*, 22, 532

68. Atkinson, K., McElwain, T.J. and Mackay, A.M. (1974). Myeloma of the heart. *Br. Heart J.*, 36, 309

69. Imai, T. and Matsumoto, S. (1970). Anaphylactoid purpura with cardiac involvement. *Arch. Dis. Child.*, 45, 727

70. Christy, J.H. and Clements, S.D. (1982). The heart and endocrine disease. In Hurst, J.W. (ed.) *The Heart*. 5th Edn. p. 1547. (New York: McGraw-Hill)

71. DeGroot, L.J. (1972). Thyroid and the heart. *Mayo Clin. Proc.*, 47, 864 (56 references)

72. Levey, G.S. (1975). The heart and hyperthyroidism: Use of beta-adrenergic blocking drugs. *Med. Clin. N. Am.*, 59, 1193

73. Graettinger, J.S., Muenster, J.J., Checchia, C.S., Grisson, R.L. and Campbell, J.A. (1958). A correlation of clinical and hemodynamic studies in patients with hypothyroidism. *J. Clin. Invest.* 37, 502

74. Santos, A.D., Miller, R.P., Pathenpurakal, K.M., Wallace, W.A., Cave, W.T. and Himojora, L. (1980). Echocardiographic characterization of the reversible cardiomyopathy of hypothyroidism. *Am. J. Med.*, 68, 675

75. Savage, D.D., Henry, W.L., Eastman, R.C., Borer, J.S. and Gordon, P. (1979). Echocar-

diographic assessment of cardiac anatomy and function in acromegalic patients. *Am. J. Med.*, **67**, 823

76. Mather, H.M., Boyd, M.J. and Jenkins, J.S. (1979). Heart size and function in acromegaly. *Br. Heart J.*, **41**, 697

77. Kaplan, N.N. (1974). Adrenal causes of hypertension. *Arch. Intern. Med.*, **133**, 1001

78. Liddle, G.W. (1974). The adrenals: The adrenal cortex. In Williams, R.H. (ed.) *Textbook of Endocrinology*. (Philadelphia: Saunders)

79. Alexander, C.S. (1972). Nutritional heart disease. *Cardiovasc. Clin.*, **4**, 221

80. Brink, A.J., Lochner, A. and Lewis, C.M. (1966). Thiamine deficiency and beriberi heart disease. *S. Afr. Med. J.*, **40**, 581

81. Stefadouros, M.A., El Shahawy, M. and Witham, A.C. (1976). Shoshin in Georgia: A case of acute fulminant cardiac beriberi. *J. Med. Assoc. Ga.*, **65**, 149

82. Rachmilewitz, M. and Braun, K. (1945). Electrocardiographic changes and the effect of niacin therapy in pellagra. *Br. Heart J.*, **7**, 72

83. Sament, S. (1970). Cardiac disorders in scurvy. *N. Engl. J. Med.*, **282**, 282

84. Bauer, J.M. and Freyberg, R.J. (1946). Vitamin D intoxication with metastatic calcification. *J. Am. Med. Assoc.*, **130**, 1208

85. Swanepoel, A., Smythe, P.M. and Campbell, J.A.H. (1964). The heart in kwashiorkor. *Am. Heart J.*, **67**, 1

86. Buja, L.M., Ferrans, V.J. and Roberts, W.C. (1974). Drug-induced cardiomyopathies, *Adv. Cardiol.*, **13**, 330

87. Morin, Y. and Daniel, P. (1967). Quebec beer-drinkers cardiomyopathy: Etiological considerations. *Can. Med. Assoc. J.*, **97**, 926

88. Wiberg, G.S., Munro, I.C., Meranger, J.C., Morrison, A.B., Grice, H.C. and Heggtveit, H.A. (1969). Factors affecting the cardiotoxic potential of cobalt. *Clin. Toxicol.*, **2**, 257

89. Murphy, M.L., Bulloch, R.T. and Pearce, M.B. (1974). The correlation of metabolic and ultrastructural changes in emetine myocardial toxicity. *Am. Heart J.*, **87**, 105

90. Fowler, N.O., McCall, D., Chou, T., Holmes, J.C. and Hanenson, I.B. (1976). Electrocardiographic changes and cardiac arrhythmias in patients receiving psychotropic drugs. *Am. J. Cardiol.*, **37**, 223

91. Stimmel, B. (1979). *Cardiovascular Effects of Mood-Altering Drugs*. (New York: Raven Press)

92. Jefferson, J.W. (1975).A review of the cardiovascular effects and toxicity of tricyclic antidepressants. *Psychosom. Med.*, **37**, 160

93. Editorial (1974). Daunorubicin and the heart. *Br. Med. J.*, **4**, 431

94. Friedman, M.A., Bozdech, M.J., Billingham. M.E. and Rider, A.K. (1978). Doxorubicin cardiotoxicity. Serial endomyocardial biopsies and systolic time intervals. *J. Am. Med. Assoc.*, **240**, 1603

95. Mills, B.A. and Roberts, R.W. (1979). Cyclophosphamide-induced cardiomyopathy. A report of two cases and review of the English literature. *Cancer*, **43**, 2223

96. Glazener, G.S., Ellis, J.G. and Johnson, P.K. (1968). Electrocardiographic findings with arsenic poisoning. *Calif. Med.*, **109**, 158

97. Somers, K. and Rosanelli, J.D. (1962). Electrocardiographic effects of antimony dimercapto-succinate ("Astiban"). *Br. Heart J.*, **24**, 187

98. Haft, J.I., Gershengorn, K., Kranz, P.D. and Oestreicher, R. (1972). Protection against epinephrine-induced myocardial necrosis by drugs that inhibit platelet aggregation. *Am. J. Cardiol.*, **30**, 838

99. Corya, B.C., Black, M.J. and McHenry, P.L. (1976). Echocardiographic findings after acute carbon monoxide poisoning. *Br. Heart J.*, **38**, 712

100. Harris, W.S. (1973). Toxic effects of aerosol propellants on the heart. *Arch. Intern. Med.*, **131**, 162

101. Talley, R.C., Linhart, J.W., Trevino, A.J., Moore, L. and Beller, B.M. (1972). Acute elemental phosphorous poisoning in man: Cardiovascular toxicity. *Am. Heart J.*, **84**, 139

102. Freeman, R. (1965). Reversible myocarditis due to chronic lead poisoning in childhood. *Arch. Dis. Child.*, **40**, 389.

103. Gueron, M. and Yarom, R. (1970). Cardiovascular manifestations of severe scorpion sting. Clinicopathologic correlations. *Chest*, **57**, 156

104. Wenzel, D.G. (1967). Drug-induced cardiomyopathies. *J. Pharm. Sci.*, **56**, 1209

105. Harkavy, J. (1970). Cardiac manifestations due to hypersensitivity. *Ann. Allerg.*, **28**, 242

106. Matthews, A.W. and Griffiths, I.D. (1974). Post-vaccinial pericarditis and myocarditis. *Br. Heart J.*, **36**, 1043

107. Burch, G.E., Sohal, R.S., Sun, S.-C., Miller, G.C. and Colcolough, H.L. (1968). Effects of radiation on the human heart. An electron microscopic study. *Arch. Intern. Med.*, **121**, 230

108. Kew, M.C., Tucker, R.B.K., Bersohn, I. and Seftel, H.C. (1969). The heart in heatstroke. *Am. Heart J.*, **77**, 324

109. Collins, P. (1972). Aortic incompetence and active myocarditis in Reiter's disease. *Br. J. Vener. Dis.*, **48**, 300

110. Eisenstein, B. and Taubenhaus, M. (1958). Nonsyphilitic interstitial keratitis and bilateral deafness (Cogan's syndrome) associated with cardiovascular disease. *N. Engl. J. Med.*, **258**, 1074

111. Lewis, P.D. (1964) Behçet's disease and carditis. *Br. Med. J.*, **1**, 1026

112. Mason, J.W. and Billingham, M.E. (1980). Myocardial biopsy. In Yu, P.N. and Goodwin, J.F. (eds.) *Progress in Cardiology*. Vol 9. p. 113. (Philadelphia: Lea & Febiger)

113. Stead, E.A. (1982). Heart disease in the elderly. In Hurst, J.W. (ed.) *The Heart*. 5th Edn. p. 1545. (New York: McGraw-Hill)

114. Wilkinson, P.J., Harman, R.R.M. and Tribe, C.R. (1974). Systemic nodular panniculitis with cardiac involvement. *J. Clin. Pathol.*, **27**, 808

115. Johnson, M.L. and Ikram, H. (1970). Scleroedema of Buschke. An uncommon cause of cardiomyopathy. *Br. Heart J.*, **32**, 720

116. Saheta, N.P. (1967). Cardiomyopathy and mitral stenosis associated with Wegener's granulomatosis. *Indian Heart J.*, **19**, 144

117. Morales, A.R., Bourgeois, C.H. and Chulacharit, E. (1971). Pathology of the heart in Reye's syndrome (encephalopathy and fatty degeneration of the viscera). *Am. J. Cardiol.*, **27**, 314

118. Somerville, J. and Bonham-Carter, R.E. (1972). The heart in lentiginosis. *Br. Heart J.*, **34**, 58

119. Tuuteri, L., Perheentupa, J. and Rapola, J. (1974). The cardiopathy of mulibrey nanism, a new inherited syndrome. *Chest*, **65**, 628

120. Mowat, N.A.G., Bennett, P.N., Finlayson, J.K., Brunt, P.W. and Lancaster, W.M. (1974). Myopericarditis complicating ulcerative colitis. *Br. Heart J.*, **36**, 724

121. McAllister, H.A. Jr. and Fenoglio, J.J. Jr. (1975). Cardiac involvement in Whipple's disease. *Circulation*, **52**, 152

122. Huang, S., Kumar, G., Steele, H.D. and Parker, J.O. (1967). Cardiac involvement in pseudoxanthoma elasticum. Report of a case. *Am. Heart J.*, **74**, 680

6
Amyloid heart disease

C.M. OAKLEY

INTRODUCTION

Virchow gave amyloid its name because the material gives a colour reaction to iodine which is similar though not identical to that given by starch. Amyloid is an abnormal eosinophilic fibrillar protein whose chemical origin was for a long time unknown. Amyloid can be deposited in almost any organ of the body and occurs in many characteristically distinct forms in different clinical conditions and by several different pathogenetic mechanisms. The characteristic fibrillar deposits may be produced by different proteins or polypeptides and the corresponding differing forms of the amyloid fibrils are identified by distinctive light and electron microscopic appearances[1,2].

CLASSIFICATION

This is as follows.

(1) Amyloidosis associated with an immunocyte dyscrasia in which the amyloid is composed of immunoglobulin light chains. This type of amyloid is seen in:

    (a) Amyloidosis associated with lymphoroliferative disorders, usually myeloma, less often Waldenström's macroglobulinaemia and non-Hodgkin's lymphoma.
        This type of amyloid may either be organ limited occurring in the heart, bone marrow, kidney, peripheral nerves or skeletal muscle (either in one or several sites) or generalized and

    (b) 'Primary' amyloidosis in which the immunocyte dyscrasia cannot be identified.

(2) In the familial amyloidoses the major protein component of the amyloid varies but is not an immunoglobulin.

(a) Familial amyloidosis occurs in neuropathic (e.g. Portuguese type), cardiopathic and nephropathic (Balkan) forms and also in

(b) Familial Mediterranean fever.

(3) Reactive amyloidosis is associated with chronic suppuration (as in osteomyelitis), chronic infection (as in tuberculosis) or chronic inflammation (as in rheumatoid arthritis, ankylosing spondylitis and Reiter's syndrome). The heart is not usually involved.

In organ-limited and endocrine-associated amyloid (such as medullary carcinoma of the thyroid) the heart is not involved.

In *senile amyloid* the protein is different and unique to senile cardiovascular amyloid.

PATHOLOGY

Cardiac involvement is common both in primary amyloid and in amyloidosis associated with multiple myeloma. Patients with cardiac amyloidosis sometimes also have amyloid infiltration of skin and mucous membrane, tongue, skeletal muscle, peripheral nerves and gastrointestinal tract. In primary amyloid and in amyloidosis associated with multiple myeloma the amyloid fibrils are derived from immunoglobulin light chains usually of the lambda type. Since the amyloid associated with multiple myeloma is similar to that seen in primary cardiac amyloid it has been supposed that patients presenting with amyloid heart disease have an underlying plasmacytoma which may be silent or indeed solitary and which often remains cryptic even after an extensive search at postmortem. It has been suggested that in primary amyloidosis the monoclone producing the abnormal protein light chains may rarely be insufficient in size to be detected even by careful marrow examination and immunocytochemical staining. In amyloidosis associated with myeloma the neoplastic clone is more advanced but myeloma patients may present with serious cardiac amyloid at a time when the myeloma seems to be early[3].

The amyloid which is commonly found in the hearts of those dying in advanced old age differs both in substance and in amount from that found in cardiac amyloidosis[4] and is only rarely associated with any detectable clinical abnormality, although its presence along with other degenerative changes in the elderly heart may contribute to a diminished cardiac reserve in the elderly in whom heart failure may develop with seemingly little provocation. Cardiac failure and death have however been attributed to it[5].

Amyloid material is deposited in the walls of capillaries, small arteries and veins. Characteristically, amyloid stains apple green with congo red when viewed by polarized light and gives a metachromatic reaction to methyl violet. The staining reactions of primary amyloidosis may be atypical, the iodine reaction may be negative and even the histological stains may be negative. These stains may be negative on cardiac biopsy specimens and light microscopic examination may fail to reveal the underlying amyloid unless electromicroscopic sections are made in which the character-istic irregularly arranged fibrillary protein deposition is easily recognizable.

Years ago, intravenous injection of congo red was used as a diagnostic test for amyloid, the red pigment being removed from the plasma because of its physical affinity for the amyloid deposits. However, a positive test depended on massive amyloid deposits so that false negatives were common and, since allergic reactions as well as false negatives could occur, the test has long ago been abandoned.

Pathology of the heart

The heart is usually not enlarged but it is overweight and appears to show concentric hypertrophy involving both ventricles. The ventricular cavities are not dilated and may appear small. The heart is abnormally firm and rubbery and holds its shape on the postmortem table. The gross appearance of marked generalized hypertrophy with an exaggeration of the size of the papillary muscles and the trabecular architecture has often led to a mistaken preliminary diagnosis of hypertrophic cardiomyopathy and it is of interest that in a few older patients with hypertrophic cardiomyopathy clinical distinction from cardiac amyloid can also be difficult.

The amyloid heart may be surrounded by a pericardial effusion associated with focal deposits of amyloid in the pericardium. The outside of the heart may show petechiae and the cut surface may have a 'lardaceous' look. Typically the myocardium stains bluish black with iodine but a negative reaction is often seen in primary amyloidosis.

The endocardium is usually involved, there may be visible deposits and occasionally the valves are thickened. When mitral regurgitation occurs it is usually attributable to heavy infiltration of the papillary muscle. Irregularity of the endocardial surface may, rarely, predispose to thrombosis and embolism. Most of the amyloid mass is within the myocardium and is responsible for the gross thickening of the ventricular and even atrial walls. Microscopically the amyloid is found between the myocardial fibres separ-ating and compressing them and extensively in the blood vessels[6-8]. The walls of the intramural coronary arteries may be so heavily infiltrated that the lumen is compromised. Amyloid deposits in the conducting tissue explain the frequency of sinoatrial disorders and fascicular blocks on electrocardiogram (e.c.g.)[9,10] as well, perhaps, as apparent sensitivity to digitalis[11].

CLINICAL FEATURES

Cardiac amyloidosis is uncommon below the age of 50 and most patients are in late middle or old age. However in a personal series of 15 cases two patients with primary amyloidosis were in their early 40s. Cardiac amy-loidosis complicating familial Mediterranean fever may present with cardiac failure at a much younger age.

Patients with primary amyloidosis may present with a petechial rash because of amyloid infiltration of the skin; this may be almost confluent in the periorbital tissues and it is most common on the face and neck. Macroglossia is rather uncommon in cardiac amyloidosis but when seen it can be very striking, causing dysarthria, and the tongue typically shows 'moulding' from pressure against the teeth. It feels abnormally firm and rubbery to the touch.

The patient usually looks chronically sick. He may have lost weight and may have thin wasted skeletal muscles. Rarely the skeletal muscles show a pseudohypertrophy on account of diffuse amyloid infiltration. Perineural involvement may lead to presentation with a carpal tunnel syndrome or a mononeuritis. The lymph nodes may be enlarged. Infiltration of the gastrointestinal tract may cause bleeding, diarrhoea or constipation. The liver may be very large on account of a high venous pressure even in the absence of amyloid infiltration. The spleen is not usually enlarged.

Examination of the heart usually reveals signs of a low output state, cool extremities, peripheral cyanosis and low blood pressure. There may be a bradycardia due to a conduction fault or atrial fibrillation. Digitalis toxicity is common.

The patient with cardiac amyloidosis usually presents with heart failure[12-14], but in the 10% or so who also have a nephrotic syndrome from renal amyloid cardiac involvement may be obscured by diuretics given for the hypoproteinaemic oedema and the resulting hypovolaemia. Since the cardiac output in amyloid is usually very low by the time of presentation, seemingly non-specific complaints of fatigue are common as well as shortness of breath, oedema, syncope or angina. Syncope may also be caused by conduction defects or digitalis intoxication. Angina results from deposition in the walls of coronary arteries.

The systemic venous pressure is usually very high with a small amplitude of pulsation, but tricuspid regurgitation sometimes occurs. The cardiac impulse is quiet and usually impalpable. Typically there are neither murmurs nor added sounds, but occasionally either mitral or tricuspid regurgitant murmurs are heard and a right ventricular third sound may be heard when the venous pressure is high but then disappears with diuretics. A left ventricular third sound is usually conspicuously absent despite evidence of left ventricular failure seen on the chest X-ray.

INVESTIGATIONS

Electrocardiogram

The electrocardiogram typically shows very low voltage and this low voltage may first suggest the diagnosis[15]. Repolarization abnormalities are not invariable. Fascicular blocks are frequent and by increasing the voltage may tend to obscure the diagnosis. Occasionally the abnormality in the e.c.g. is inconspicuous as in Figure 6.1, which shows sinus rhythm with a very abnormal axis but little else of note at a time when the patient was in gross heart failure.

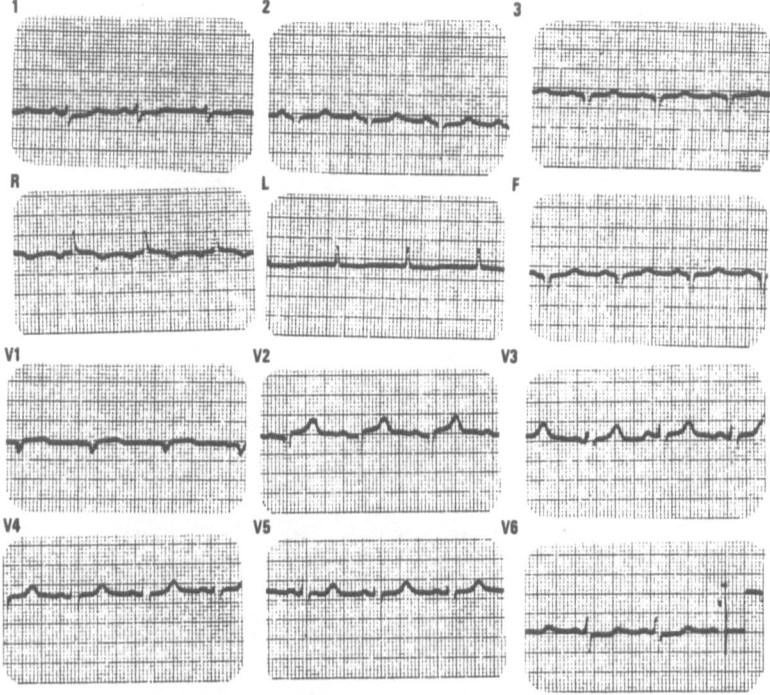

Figure 6.1 Electrocardiogram from 42-year-old man with primary cardiac amyloidosis showing bizarre deviation of the QRS axis but sinus rhythm and minimal repolarization abnormalities. The voltage is only slightly reduced

Radiography

The chest radiograph typically shows little or no cardiac enlargement but marked changes of pulmonary venous congestion. The superior vena cava and azygous vein shadows may be prominent, reflecting a high systemic venous pressure. A pericardial effusion when present may be sufficiently large to mimic gross cardiomegaly. Echocardiography quickly reveals the true situation.

Echocardiography

The echocardiographic features of amyloidosis are characteristic and usually diagnostic[16,17]. The M-mode echo reveals greatly reduced dimensions of the left ventricle with increased thickness of the right ventricle, the ventricular septum and the left ventricular posterior wall (Figure 6.2). A pericardial effusion may be seen. Diminished systolic thickening of the left ventricular wall can be recognized. The mitral valve usually appears normal or thickened but the aortic valve may reveal the shortened ejection time and low stroke volume with a tendency for the valve to drift towards closure during systole.

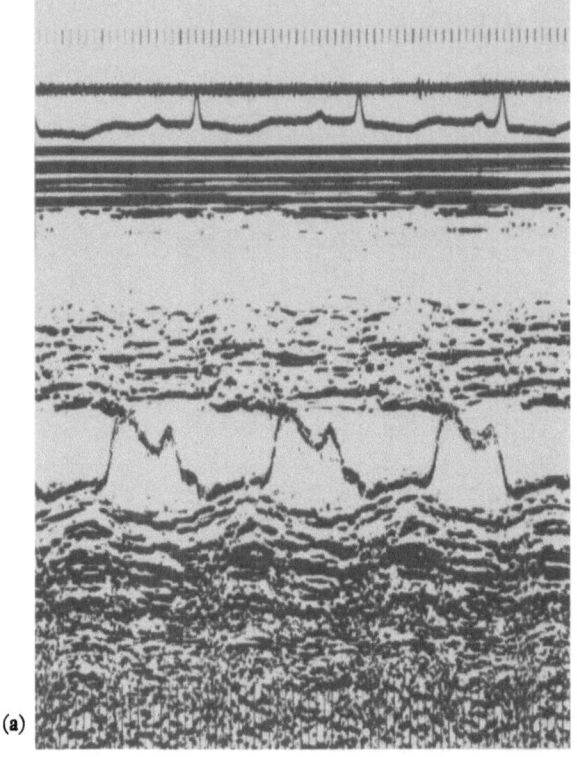

(a)

Cross-sectional echocardiography may be very striking, because of the abnormal texture of the myocardium from which the amyloid reflects the echoes giving rise to a so-called 'granular sparkle'. Unfortunately this is not totally specific, being seen also in hypertrophic cardiomyopathy and in other infiltrations such as haemochromatosis. However in hypertrophic cardiomyopathy the sparkle comes from the fibrous tissue and is typically most marked in the upper ventricular septum. In haemochromatosis the ventricular walls are not thickened and there may be left ventricular dilatation. The generalized thickening of the ventricular walls and small ventricular cavities are well appreciated on cross-sectional echo studies (Figures 6.3 and 6.4).

Haemodynamics

The findings at cardiac catheterization are characteristic. Stroke volume and minute output are very low. There may be moderate or, rarely, severe pulmonary hypertension. The diastolic pressures are high in both ventricles but the pressure is very much higher in the left ventricle than in the right ventricle. Although the diastolic contours may suggest a dip and plateau form, the diastolic pressure differs from that in constrictive pericarditis[13,18]

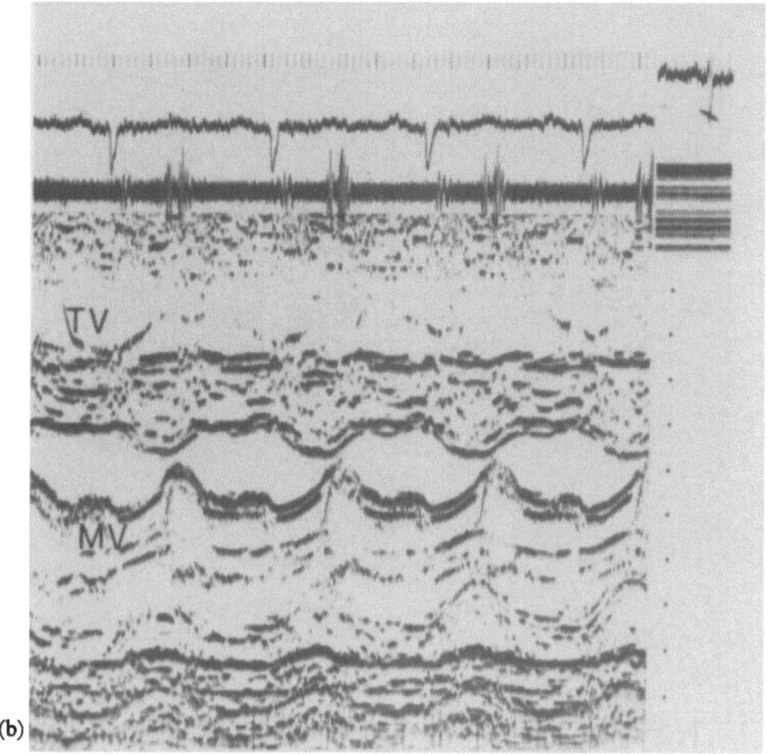

(b)

Figure 6.2 (a) and (b) M-mode echocardiograms showing very small left ventricular cavity with normal mitral valve and extremely thick septum and posterior walls. TV = tricuspid valve; MV = mitral valve. 1 cm marks on the right

because the beginning pressures are high and after an early rapid rise there is a continued slow rise, rather than a plateau, and there may also be a prominent a-wave (Figure 6.5). This difference may be masked unless the recording has been made on a fast paper speed.

Angiocardiography

The ventriculograms may mislead by looking remarkably normal but on close inspection the left ventricle may display a rather shaggy internal outline due to coarsened trabeculation and exaggerated papillary muscle indentations (Figure 6.6). The 'grey zone' is widened. The cavity is small and the ejection fraction may be normal or low but the end-diastolic volume is usually below normal. This accounts for the very low stroke volume and spurious impression of systolic competence. Both peak positive and peak negative dp/dt max. are abnormally slow reflecting the splinting of the myocardium by the masses within it. Mitral regurgitation is occasionally seen and not being associated with ventricular dilatation adds greatly to the

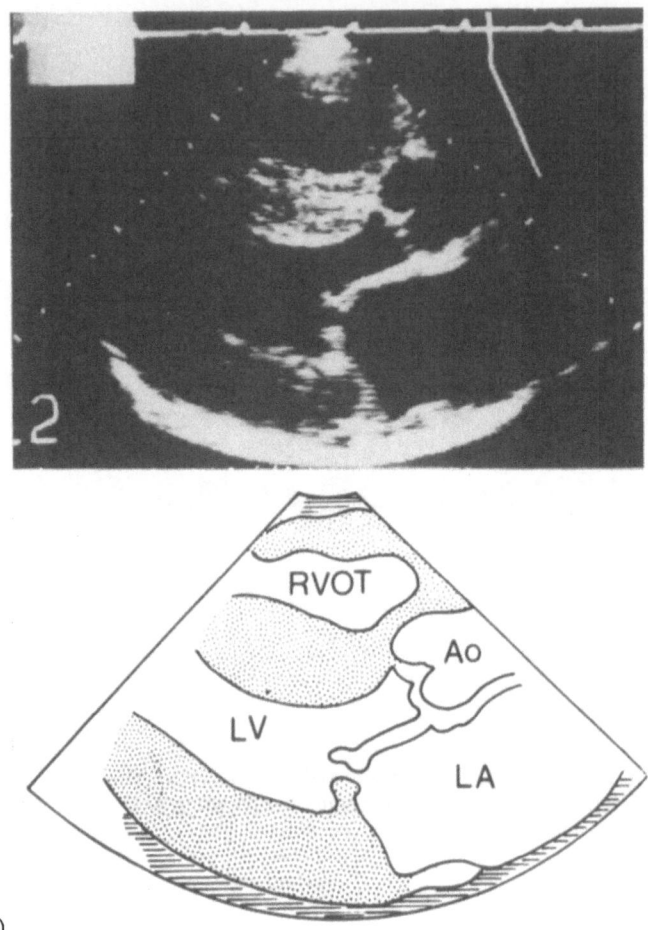

(a)

height of the left atrial pressure. There may be a pericardial effusion (Figure 6.6).

Cardiac biopsy

The diagnosis can be made by endomyocardial biopsy. Biopsies of rectum, gingiva or other tissue may also be positive in patients with cardiac amyloidosis, but not invariably so. Percutaneous per femoral venous biopsy of the right ventricle can be carried out very simply at the time of diagnostic cardiac catheterization and provides the diagnosis. Sampling errors are not a problem, because by the time cardiac amyloidosis becomes clinically important the disease is widespread without skip areas. It is important to realize that use of light miscroscopy alone may result in the diagnosis being

148

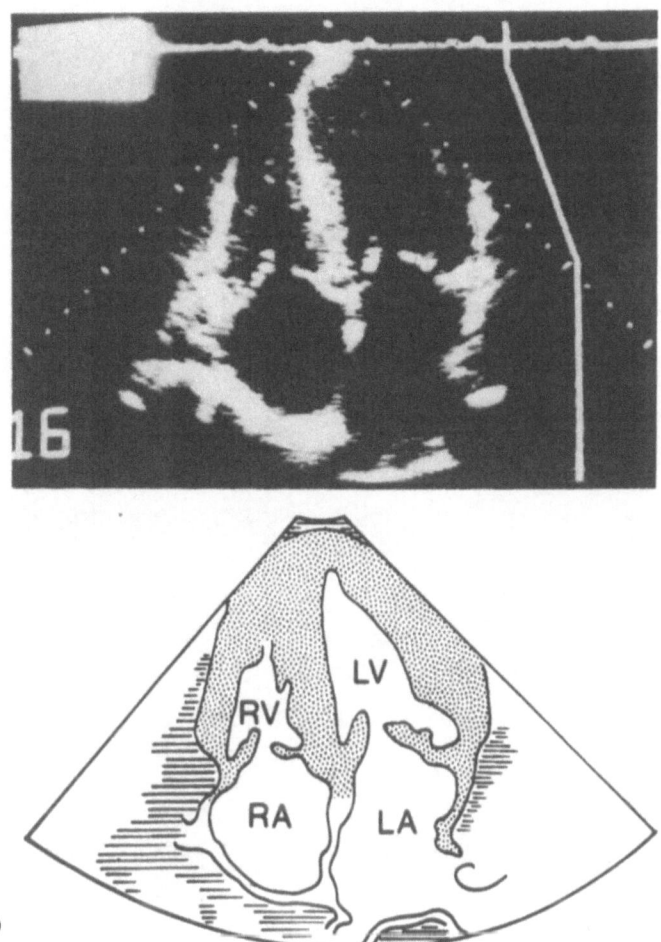

(b)

Figure 6.3 Cross-sectioned echocardiographic frames showing thickened ventricular walls and small cavities, (a) long axis view, (b) apical four-chamber view. In the line drawings RVOT = right ventricular outflow tract; LV = left ventricle; AO = aorta; LA = left atrium; RV = right ventricle; RA = right atrium. (I am grateful to Dr Petros Nihoyannopoulos for this figure.)

missed because of negative staining reactions. The most reliable method of diagnosing cardiac amyloidosis is by electron microscopy.

CARDIAC AMYLOID IN FAMILIAL MEDITERRANEAN FEVER

Familial Mediterranean fever, known also as recurrent polyserositis, is a genetic disorder in which bouts of abdominal pain and fever occur together usually with pleurisy and arthritis[19]. The disease is particularly seen in

149

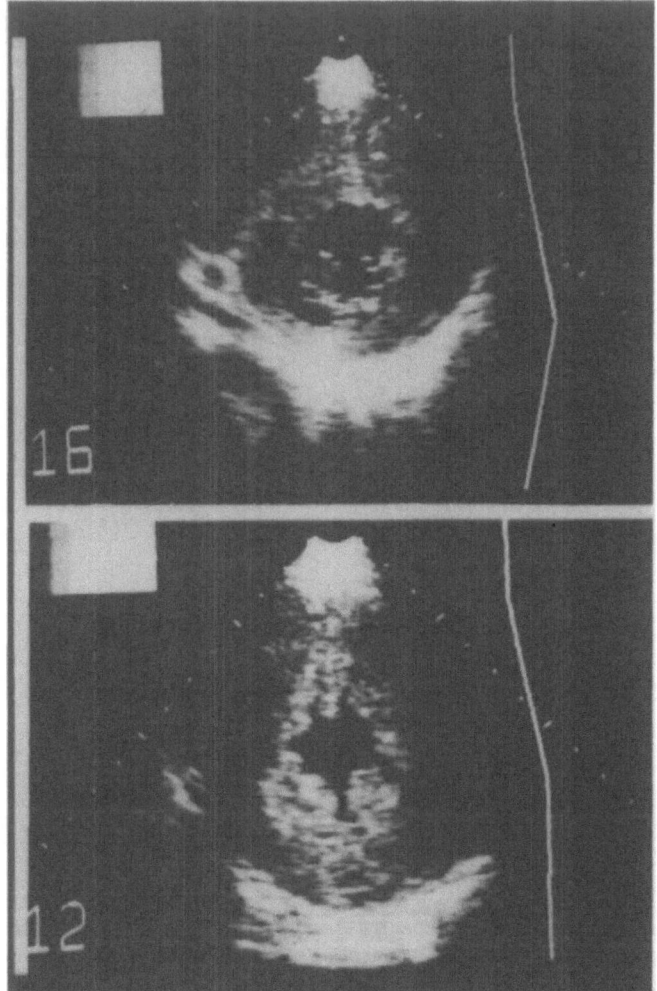

Figure 6.4 Short axis view of left ventricle, in diastole (*above*) and systole (*below*), showing the reduced size and movement of the greatly thickened LV and its markedly increased trabeculation. The increased echo reflectivity of the myocardium 'granular sparkle' is seen in each part of the figure. (I am grateful to Dr Petros Nihoyannopoulos for this figure.)

Arabs, Jews, Armenians and Turks and is inherited by an autosomal recessive gene. Skeletal myalgia may occur and attacks of pericarditis together with transient electrocardiography abnormalities. The most important complication of the disorder is amyloidosis whose incidence has been estimated at between 0 and 27% in reported series. The amyloid protein is of the reactive type seen in chronic inflammation. Renal amyloidosis is well known in this condition and may become complicated by renal vein thrombosis, renal failure and a need for haemodialysis and transplantation. Perivascular

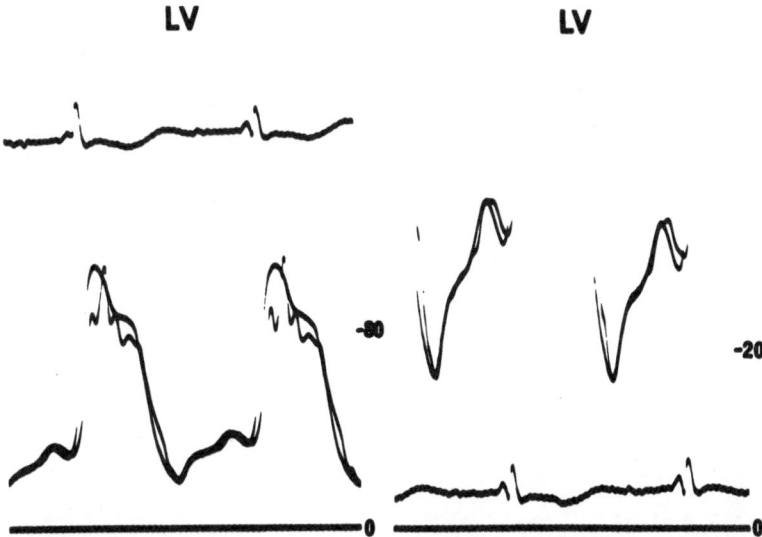

LV   **LV**

Figure 6.5 Left ventricular pressure contour (simultaneously recorded through fluid filled and manometer tipped catheter). On the left the low systolic pressure is seen and on the right at higher sensitivity the raised diastolic pressure, beginning at 15 mmHg and climbing through diastole to culminate in a prominent a-wave peaking at 40 mmHg with end-diastolic pressure 32 mmHg

amyloid deposits are widespread in all the organs including the heart, but clinically important cardiac amyloidosis is uncommon. I have seen only one case, which occurred in a young boy in his early 20s. He was the only patient with cardiac amyloidosis that I have seen who also had systemic hypertension and it was at first uncertain to what he owed his heart failure. He also had severe pulmonary hypertension. Cardiac investigations were typical of amyloidosis with all walls of the heart greatly thickened, with typical dense sparkling echoes seen on cross-sectional echocardiography, and with a positive cardiac biopsy.

The prognosis of familial Mediterranean fever has been greatly improved by the use of colchicine which prevents amyloidosis in this condition, although it is not yet known whether treatment with colchicine will lead to removal of already established deposits.

TREATMENT

There is still no effective treatment known for primary cardiac amyloidosis. The disorder is relentlessly progressive[20]; and most patients who present with symptomatic cardiac amyloidosis are dead within 2 years – and most of these within 1 year – of the diagnosis being made. Digitalis should not be used because it does not help the functional disorder and because of the enhanced risk of inducing excessive bradycardia and conduction defects. Diuretics should be used sparingly because reduction of the high venous

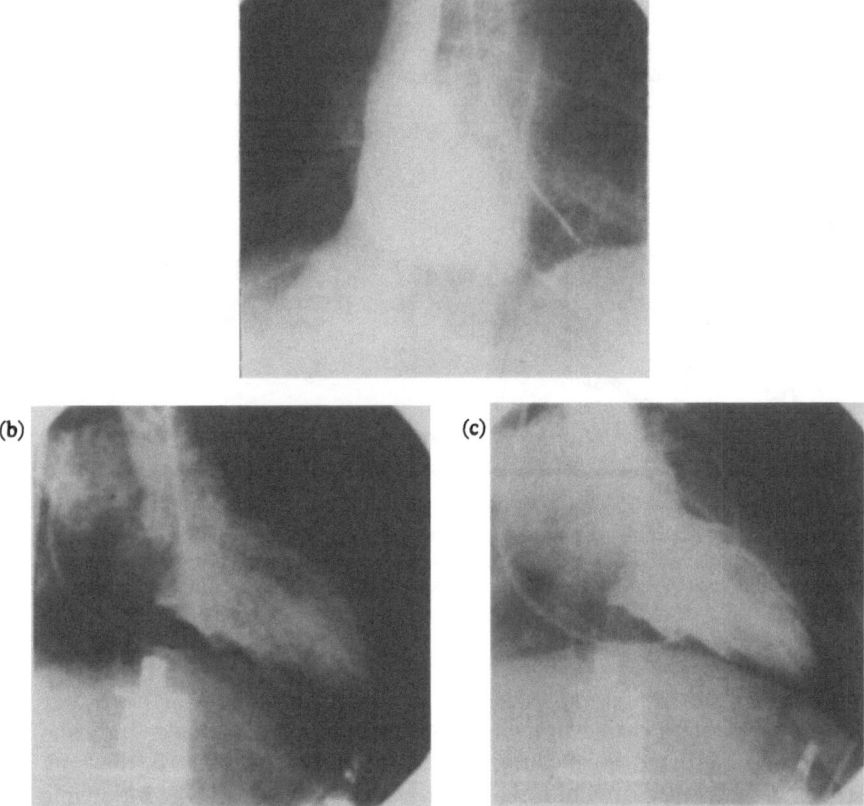

Figure 6.6 (a) Right atrial angiogram showing pericardial effusion, and (b, c) left ventricular angiograms showing normal size and contour apart from shaggy outline and reduced emptying

pressure tends to reduce forward output. Sufficient should be given only to relieve uncomfortable oedema. Vasodilators lead to a further fall in blood pressure and usually of output. Arterial unloading is met by hypotension and even syncope because of inability to increase stroke volume. Venodilators working much as diuretics may be followed by some fall in systemic and pulmonary venous pressure although at the usual expense of some loss in output. Conduction system involvement may need a pacemaker.

There is no evidence that cytotoxic drugs given for myeloma or colchicine have any influence on the progress of amyloid heart disease.

PROGNOSIS

The time course of deposition of amyloid is unknown. It may be extremely long, in which case cardiac transplantation might be justified in patients with primary cardiac amyloidosis who have no detectable involvement of other vital organs. So far there is no experience to call upon.

References

1. Glenner, G.G. (1980). Amyloid deposits and amyloidosis. *N. Engl. J. Med.*, **302**, 1283–1333
2. Kyule, R.A. and Baynd, E.D. (1975). Amyloidosis review of 236 cases. *Medicine*, **54**, 271
3. Isobe, T. and Osserman, E.F. (1974). Patterns of amyloidosis and their association with plasma cell dyscrasia monoclonal immunoglobulins and Bence–Jones proteins. *N. Engl. J. Med.*, **290**, 473
4. Westermark, P., Natuig, J.B. and Johansson, B. (1977). Characterization of an amyloid-fibril protein from senile cardiac amyloid. *J. Exp. Med.*, **146**, 631
5. Hodkinson, M. and Pomerance, A. (1977). The clinical significance of senile cardiac amyloidosis: a prospective clinico pathological study. *Q. J. Med.*, **46**, 677
6. Benson, R. and Smith, J.F. (1956). Cardiac amyloidosis. *Br. Heart J.*, **18**, 529
7. Brigden, W. (1957). Cardiac amyloidosis. *Prog. Cardiovasc. Dis.*, **7**, 142
8. Buja, L.M., Khoi, N.B. and Roberts, W.C. (1970). Clinically significant cardiac amyloidosis. *Am. J. Cardiol.*, **26**, 394
9. James, T.N. (1965). Pathology of the cardiac conduction system in amyloidosis. *Ann. Intern. Med.*, **65**, 28
10. Ridolfi, R.L., Bulkley, B.H. and Hutchins, G.M. (1977). The conduction system in cardiac amyloidosis, clinical and pathologic features of 23 patients. *Am. J. Med.*, **62**, 677
11. Cassidy, J.T. (1961). Cardiac amyloidoses. 2 cases with digitalis sensitivity. *Ann. Intern. Med.*, **55**, 989
12. Goodwin, J.F. (1964). Cardiac function in primary myocardial disease. *Br. Med. J.*, **1**, 1526
13. Chew, C., Ziady, G.M., Raphael, M.J. and Oakley, C.M. (1975). The functional defect in amyloid heart disease. *Am. J. Cardiol.*, **36**, 438–44
14. Oakley, C.M. (1983). Amyloid heart disease. In Symons, C., Evans, T. and Mitchell, A.G. (eds.) *Specific Heart Muscle Disease* pp. 13–23. (Bristol, London, Boston: Wright PSG)
15. Wessler, S. and Freedberg, A.S. (1948). Cardiac amyloidosis. Electrocardiographic and pathologic observations. *Arch. Intern. Med.*, **32**, 63
16. Child, J.S., Levisman, J.A., Abbas, A.S. and Macalpin, R.N. (1976). Echocardiographic manifestations of infiltrative cardiomyopathy. A report of seven cases due to amyloid. *Chest*, **70**, 726–31
17. Borer, J.S., Henry, W.L. and Epstein, S.E. (1977). Echocardiographic observations in patients with systemic infiltrative disease involving the heart. *Am. J. Cardiol*, **39**, 184–8
18. Tyberg, T.I., Goldyer, A.U.N., Hurst, V.W., Alexander, J. and Largon, R.A. (1981). Left ventricular filling in differentiating restrictive amyloid cardiomyopathy and constrictive pericarditis. *Am. J. Cardiol.*, **47**, 791–6
19. Ehrenfeld, E.N., Eliakim, M. and Rachmilewitz, M. (1961). Recurrent polyserositis. *Am. J. Med.*, **31**, 107
20. Brandt, K., Cathcart, E.S. and Cohen, A.S. (1969). A clinical analysis of the course and diagnosis of 42 patients with amyloidosis. *Am. J. Med.*, **44**, 955

with primary cardiac amyloidosis who have no detectable involvement of other vital organs, so far there is no experience to offer them.

References

Controversies in Cardiomyopathy

For many years the suggestion of Criley and colleagues that systolic gradients in the left ventricle in hypertrophic cardiomyopathy did not indicate an obstruction to outflow lay dormant, but was revived when diastolic disorders of function were found to be a major aspect of the disease, and when improved techniques of measuring blood flow and velocity became available. Much of the argument centres around semantics and the meaning of the word 'obstruction': perhaps, because it can be interpreted in different ways, 'obstruction' should be abandoned. Although intimate details of myocardial function are not fully understood, much is known about the haemodynamic and anatomical faults in hypertrophic cardiomyopathy: rapid powerful ejection with excessive ejection fraction; massive hypertrophy; contact between anterior mitral apparatus and septum; and regional and local impairment of relaxation and filling of the ventricles. These apsects are generally agreed, but the controversy about obstruction has important implications for surgical treatment by septal resection, and this is the main reason for choosing the topic for discussion in Chapter 7 (pp. 157–261).

Increasing accuracy in definition and diagnosis has revealed evidence of previous myocarditis in many cases of cardiomyopathy, although interpretation is still open to error. The idea that virus can infect the myocardium then disappear, but set up an autoimmune process that progressively damages the myocardium, is intuitively apealing but lacks proof. Because of its important implications for treatment with immunosuppressive and possibly even antiviral agents, this theory is discussed in Chapter 8 (pp. 263–84). Evidence is incomplete, controlled trials of treatment are needed, and methodology must be better standardised before the problem will be fully realised.

7.1
A non-obstructive view of hypertrophic cardiomyopathy

J.M. CRILEY and R.J. SIEGEL

INTRODUCTION

The presence of intracavitary left ventricular (LV) pressure gradients in patients without intraoperative or postmortem evidence of obstruction led Brock[1,2] to the concept of a 'functional obstruction of the left ventricle'. Although the precise site of the functional obstruction was initially thought to be a muscular bar, sphincter or 'contraction ring'[3–5], systolic anterior motion (SAM) of the anterior mitral leaflet resulting in apposition with the interventricular septum has been generally accepted as the anatomical basis for the pressure gradient and for an impediment to the egress of blood from the LV[6–8]. The temporal relationship between SAM–septal contact and the onset of the pressure gradient as well as the correlation between the duration of SAM–septal contact and the magnitude of the gradient have been cited as confirmation of the obstructing role played by the anterior mitral leaflet in hypertrophic cardiomyopathy (HCM)[8,9].

An alternative non-obstructive basis for the intracavitary pressure gradient in HCM grew out of the work of Gauer[10,11], who recorded LV gradients in experimental animals during haemorrhagic shock or the application of negative gravitational forces. Gauer postulated that continued isometric contraction after the ventricle was empty produced a high pressure in the obliterated cavity and a pressure difference between the contractile body and non-contractile outflow tract.

Hernandez[12] first documented a unique mode of LV ejection in patients with HCM which fit the Gauer concept – the LV ejected almost all of its stroke volume in the first half of systole. These investigators felt that the late systolic outflow cutoff could be explained by the ventricle ejecting down to its functional residual volume in little more than half of the available systolic ejection period. Since serial film angiocardiograms had demonstrated that the LV 'cavity was often ... completely obliterated'[13] and cineangiocardiograms revealed that this cavitary obliteration occurred

157

rapidly[14,15], Gauer's non-obstructive mechanism provided an explanation for pressure gradients in those instances where an obvious narrowing of the outflow tract could not be demonstrated by angiocardiography. Obliteration of the LV cavity also explained the 'sphincter' that had been eloquently described by surgeons whose fingers had been squeezed in the hyperdynamic ventricle[4,13].

Although most investigators continue to equate the presence of intracavitary pressure gradients with 'obstruction' in patients with HCM, Goodwin[16] stated that 'obstruction is a myth' and Shabetai[17] wrote that 'the evidence against true obstruction ... is overwhelming'.

It is therefore the purpose of this paper to restate and attempt to clarify the non-obstructive concept. It is important for the reader to keep in mind the definition of the term obstruction – an impediment or hindrance to passage.

EXPERIMENTAL STUDIES

Production of mechanical obstruction

When a mechanical impediment is produced experimentally in the LV outflow tract (Figure 7.1.1), there is an elevation of the LV pressure and a damping of the aortic waveform so that the rate of pressure rise is delayed and the magnitude of the pulse pressure is reduced, as seen in naturally occurring discrete forms of outflow tract obstruction. When the obstruction is made more severe, the LV responds by increasing its pressure. The LV empties more slowly and less completely in response to this hindrance to outflow.

Production of gradients without obstruction

When a *normal* canine ventricle is stimulated by systemic haemorrhage[10,17] or inotropic agents[18] (isoproterenol, amphetamines, glucagon, dobutamine etc) a pressure difference may be generated within the LV which has a contour different from that of mechanically induced obstruction (Figure 7.1.2). These pressure contours resemble the 'dynamic gradients' in HCM in which the LV and aortic pressures rise together in early systole, and as the aortic pressure falls the LV pressure rises to a late systolic peak.

The LV ejection dynamics during isoproterenol stimulation can be studied by placement of a flow velocity probe around the aortic root (Figure 7.1.2) or by recording LV cineangiograms before and after a pressure gradient is provoked by isoproterenol infusions in dogs. The flow-velocity profile reveals that the inotropically stimulated ventricle ejects most of its stroke volume in the first half of systole, and as the aortic pressure falls and the LV pressure rises, the outflow declines rapidly. This outflow profile is similar to that recorded in HCM[12,13].

Angiographic studies reveal that the canine ventricle empties more rapidly and more completely after the inotropic agent is given and the pressure

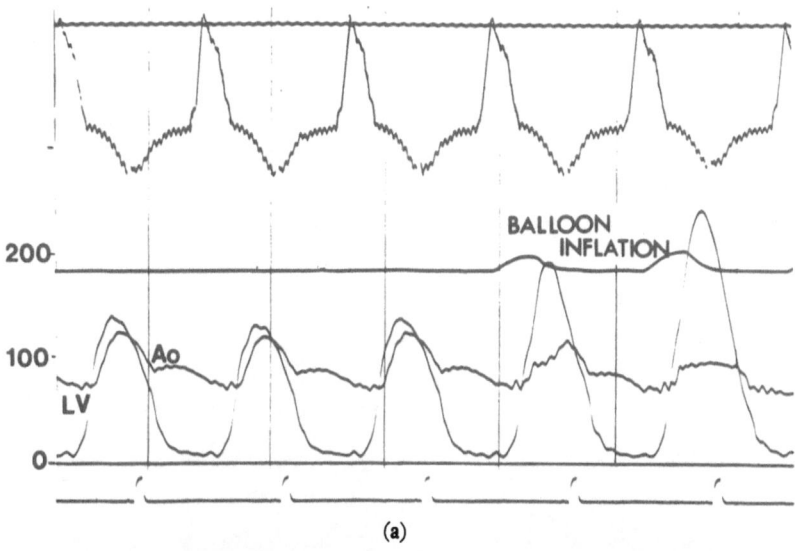

(a)

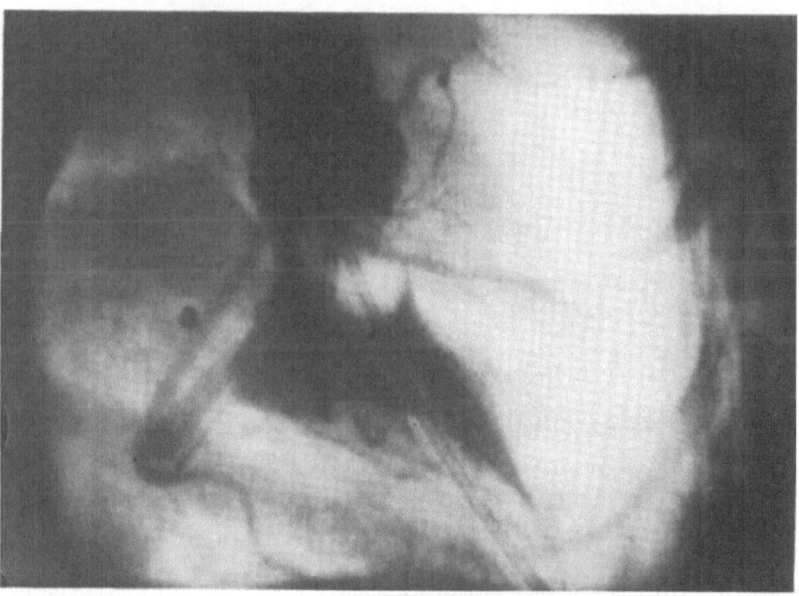

(b)

Figure 7.1.1 Experimental outflow obstruction in a canine left ventricle. **a,** A balloon catheter inserted through the left ventricular (LV) apex is abruptly inflated during the 4th and 5th systoles. With the first inflation, there is a marked increase in LV pressure, a delay in the aortic (**Ao**) upstroke, a pressure gradient of 80 mmHg, and a prolongation of the systolic ejection period. With a greater degree of inflation and obstruction on the 5th cycle, the LV pressure, gradient, and length of the systolic ejection period increase further. Greater degrees of obstruction cause an increase in the gradient predominantly through an increase in LV pressure. **b,** A left ventricular cineangiographic frame recorded at end systole demonstrates the radiolucent balloon in the outflow tract and moderate mitral regurgitation

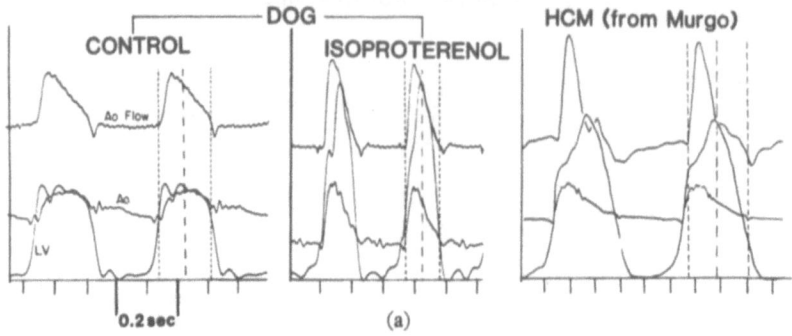

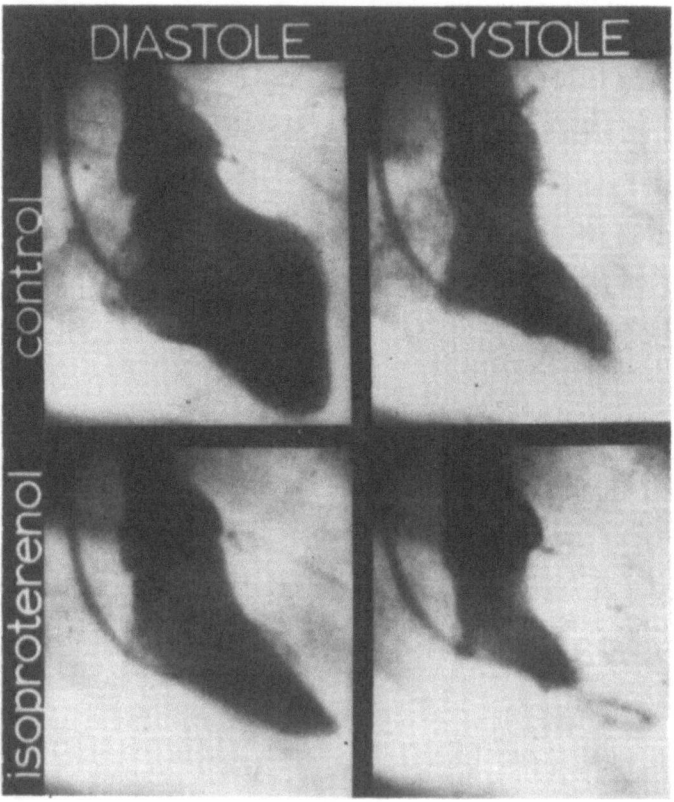

Figure 7.1.2 Dynamic gradient produced in a normal canine left ventricle with isoproterenol. **a,** A flow velocity probe has been placed around the aortic root and displays the ejection dynamics before and after an outflow tract gradient has been provoked by an isoproterenol infusion. During the control recording, 58% of the stroke volume is ejected in the first half of systole, and after isoproterenol, 70%. Unlike the obstructive gradient displayed in Figure 7.1.1, the gradient is largest in the last half of systole when the flow is decreasing. The relationships between pressure and flow in the isoproterenol-stimulated canine ventricle resemble those seen in HCM. **b,** Left ventriculography in the right anterior oblique (RAO) projection before and after isoproterenol induced a gradient of 65 mmHg. During the isoproterenol infusion, a loop of catheter recording high pressure is seen to be within the cavity in diastole and in the obliterated sinus portion of the LV cavity during systole

gradient is present than during the control angiograms performed without a pressure gradient[18]. This inotropically stimulated ventricle, in which there is no hindrance to outflow, therefore develops a gradient as a byproduct of its rapid emptying.

Dynamic pressure gradients can also be induced in experimentally *hypertrophic* canine ventricles by administration of vasodilator or inotropic agents[19-21]. When the LV is rendered hypertrophic by chronic subhypertensive norepinephrine infusions[21] or surgical creation of aortic coarctation[19,20], the haemodynamic, angiographic and anatomical features of HCM can be closely simulated.

When hypertrophy is induced by 4–12 weeks of norepinephrine infusion the LV has a thick walled small cavity with a high resting ejection fraction, and a dynamic pressure gradient can be induced by nitroglycerine administration (Figure 7.1.3). The aortic pressure develops a brisk upstroke and as the aortic systolic pressure falls a mid- and late-systolic pressure gradient results. Larger gradients can be induced with infusions of inotropic agents (Figure 7.1.3b). Angiography during the presence of the gradient reveals rapid emptying of the LV with a lucent line representing displacement of contrast medium by the distorted mitral valve leaflets in the small systolic cavity (Figure 7.1.3c). Mitral regurgitation may also be evident.

After hypertrophy is induced by surgical coarctation of the ascending aorta, dynamic gradients can be provoked by administration of nitroglycerine (Figure 7.1.4). These intracavitary gradients are superimposed upon the gradient within the aorta caused by the coarctation (Figure 7.1.4a). When there are spontaneous changes in the dynamic pressure gradient during respiration, the LV systolic pressure remains constant as the LV outflow tract and proximal aortic pressure rise with expiration and fall with inspiration (Figure 7.1.3b). This feature is characteristic of the respiratory changes in the pressure gradient seen in HCM[13]. This hypertrophic LV also empties rapidly and a lucent line, representing SAM of the mitral valve, may be seen (Figure 7.1.3c).

Thus in experimental animals there is a spectrum of haemodynamic and angiographic changes that can be induced when intracavitary gradients are produced. If the ventricle is normal, an inotropic stimulus (exogenous, or in the case of induced acute blood loss, endogenous) is usually required to produce a dynamic gradient. If the ventricle is hypertrophic, a gradient can be provoked with a vasodilator alone, and angiographic SAM can often be produced.

Non-obstructive gradients have also been induced in normal human subjects by combining the Valsalva manoeuvre with a postectopic beat[22].

Pressure gradients in hydrodynamic models

A simple and reproducible model capable of producing dynamic intracavitary gradients can be fabricated with a rubber surgical glove and two plastic catheters or drinking straws (Figure 7.1.5). The glove is filled with water and one catheter is placed in the thumb and the other in the palm of the

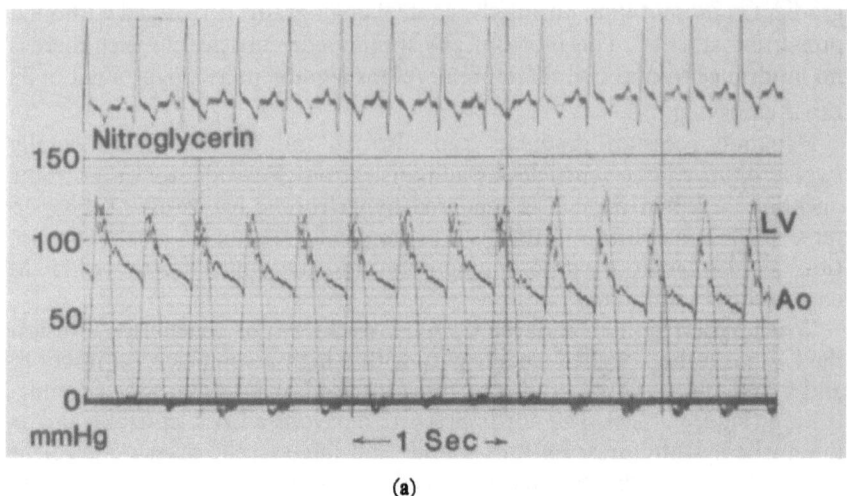

(a)

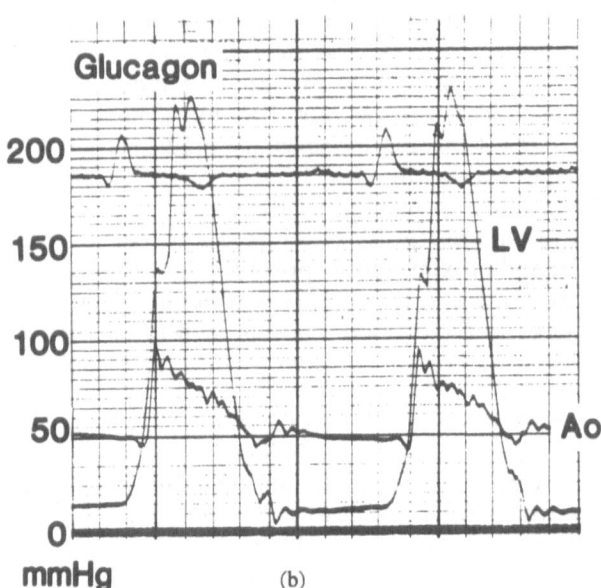

(b)

Figure 7.1.3 Dynamic gradient produced in a hypertrophic canine left ventricle. **a,** After a 12-week subhypertensive infusion of norepinephrine, nitroglycerine is administered and a mid- and late-systolic outflow tract gradient is induced. The LV pressure remains constant at 120–25 mmHg, while the aortic pressure falls to 100 mmHg to produce the gradient (time lines = 1 s). **b,** Glucagon provokes a larger gradient in the same animal. The increase in contractile force leads to a marked increase in LV pressure, while the aortic pressure remains constant at 100 mmHg. The pressure contours resemble those seen in HCM (time lines = 0.04 s). **c,** (facing), An RAO left ventriculographic frame in late systole demonstrates a horizontal radiolucent line representing systolic anterior motion (SAM) of the mitral valve during the presence of a 70 mmHg gradient. The dashed lines denote the diastolic contour of the left ventricle

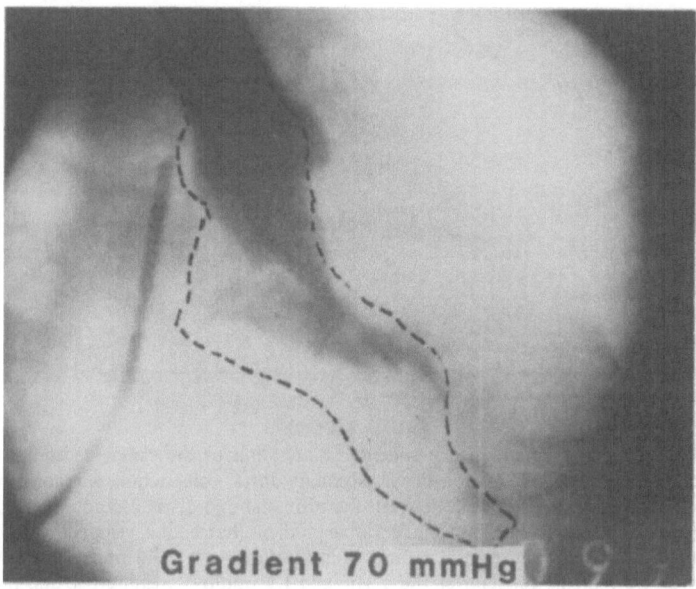

Gradient 70 mmHg

Figure 7.1.3   (c)

glove, with the proximal ends emerging from the cuff. The glove is then twisted on its cuff to prevent leakage of water.

If the thumb of the glove is then squeezed vigorously, water is ejected briskly from its catheter and merely trickles out of the catheter in the palm. Similarly, if pressure is recorded from the two catheters, the thumb has a considerably higher pressure than the palm. This pressure difference is not the result of an obstruction preventing egress of fluid from the thumb chamber nor is it due to compression or distortion of the catheter but rather to a vigorous contraction of the walls and the imparting of a high momentum (M) state to the fluid therein. Since force equals dM/dt and pressure equals force/area, there is a dynamic pressure difference established between the rapidly moving fluid in the thumb and the non-contractile palm. If the thumb is squeezed after the fluid has been expelled from its cavity, the pressure therein remains high as a result of the sustained isometric contraction.

Although this glove model is a caricature of the beating ventricle, there is a rough analogy between the thumb and the vigorous contracting sinus portion of the ventricle in HCM, and the palm and the non-contractile LV outflow tract. The outflow tract of the LV is largely membranous as it is bounded posteriorly and laterally by the anterior mitral leaflet, and is in free communication with the expanding aorta beyond. The angiogram illustrated in Figure 7.1.4c demonstrates the contrast between the vigorously contracting body of the LV and the expanding ascending aorta.

If a more sophisticated hydrodynamic model[18] of the LV is constructed (Figure 7.1.6) in which there are inflow and outflow valves as well as the

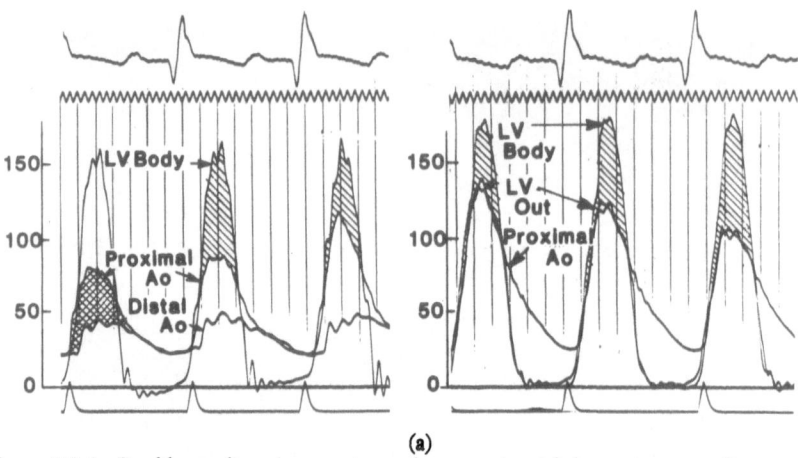

(a)

Figure 7.1.4 Double gradient in experimental coarctation of the canine ascending aorta. a, Six months after surgical creation of an ascending aortic constriction, a gradient (cross-hatched) of 40 mmHg was recorded between the proximal and distal ascending aorta. With administration of nitroglycerine, a second additive gradient (hatched) developed, which varied with the phase of respiration from 80 mmHg in inspiration (left) to 40 mmHg in expiration. The LV pressure remains constant as the aortic and LV outflow pressure rise and fall with respiration. b (facing), RAO left ventriculographic frames in diastole (*top*) and systole (*bottom*) recorded during the presence of a double gradient demonstrate a marked degree of cavitary obliteration and concomitant expansion of the ascending aorta. A radiolucent horizontal line representing SAM is seen in systole

capability of manipulating inflow volume, outflow resistance, and force of contraction, a closer simulation of the HCM ventricle results. In our model the latex ventricle contracts as a result of cyclic positive air pressure in the surrounding enclosure, and the outflow tract is prevented from contracting by the insertion of a semi-rigid sleeve immediately below the prosthetic aortic valve.

When the aortic resistance is lowered abruptly by removal of a hose clamp, a pressure gradient develops within the ventricle. As is seen in HCM and in the hypertrophic dog after administration of a vasodilator, the aortic and outflow tract pressures fall and the LV pressure remains constant to produce the gradient.

In this model, aortic outflow occurs predominately in early systole, and then progressively declines to zero in late systole. Concomitant with the decline in flow, a large pressure gradient develops, and this gradient persists after outflow ceases. This concurrence of a large pressure gradient and zero flow is clearly not a result of complete outflow tract closure or obstruction in this model which empties its cavity rapidly and completely (and is incapable of becoming obstructed), nor is the outflow in the face of a developing pressure gradient evidence that the ventricle is experiencing a progressive hindrance to ejection. In this model the degree of contractile force applied to the ventricle is greatly in excess of that required to expel its contents. This excessive contractile force is manifest as a pressure gradient

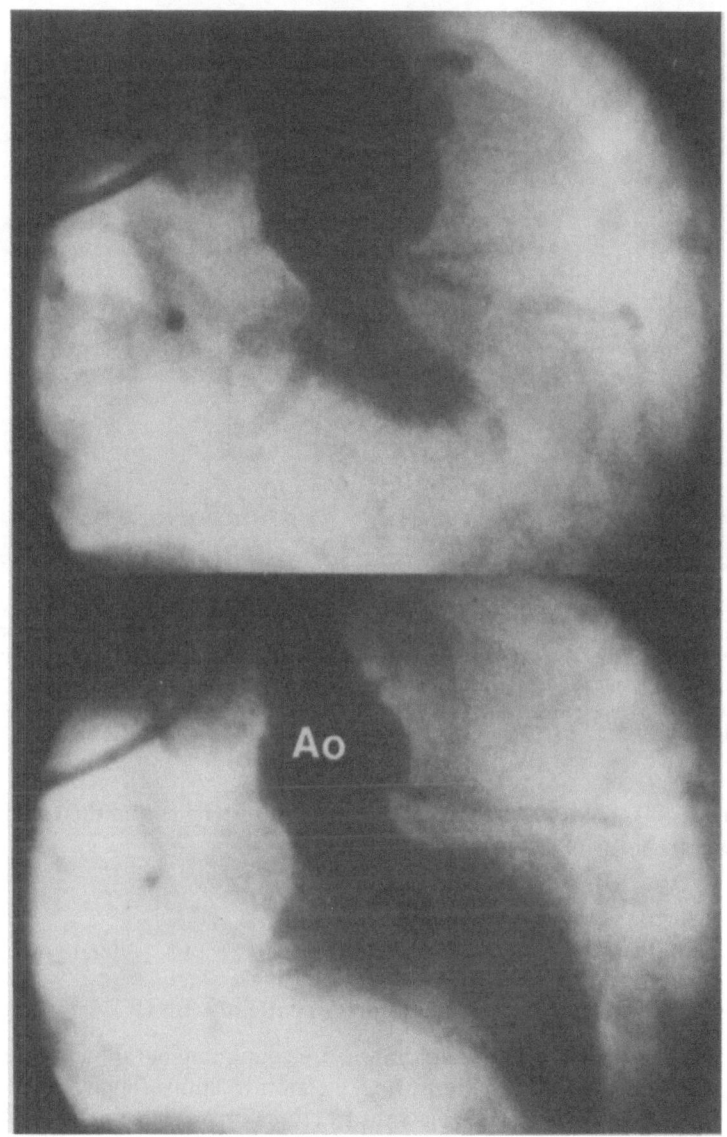

(b)

Figure 7.1.4

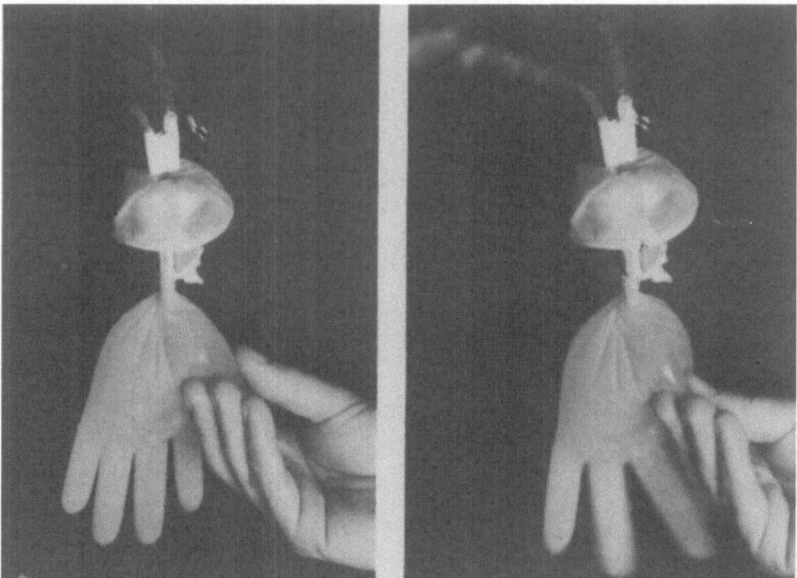

Figure 7.1.5 Dynamic pressure gradient in a surgical glove. The mechanism of cavitary obliteration pressure gradients is demonstrated in a water-filled surgical glove as the thumb is abruptly squeezed (right), causing the catheter therein to eject water while a catheter in the non-contracting palm of the glove samples a lower pressure. The thumb represents the hypercontractile sinus portion of the LV, while the palm represents the non-contractile aortic vestibule

and progressively less outflow as the ventricle approaches and then achieves its dead space or functional residual volume.

HUMAN STUDIES

Angiographic and haemodynamic studies in patients with HCM

The excessive degree of LV emptying is a striking angiographic feature in most patients with HCM. Supernormal ejection fractions (Figure 7.1.7) are usually present. When the LV ejection fractions of patients with HCM are grouped according to haemodynamic subsets, an interesting trend is seen: patients with resting pressure gradients have the highest ejection fractions, those with inducible gradients intermediate, and those HCM patients without resting or inducible gradients the lowest ejection fractions. When gradients are provoked, the ejection fraction increases.

An even more striking finding emerges when the rate of ventricular emptying[15] in HCM is examined (Figures 7.1.8–7.1.10). Despite the presence of a large gradient the HCM ventricle empties more rapidly and more completely than the normal ventricle (Figure 7.1.8). The HCM

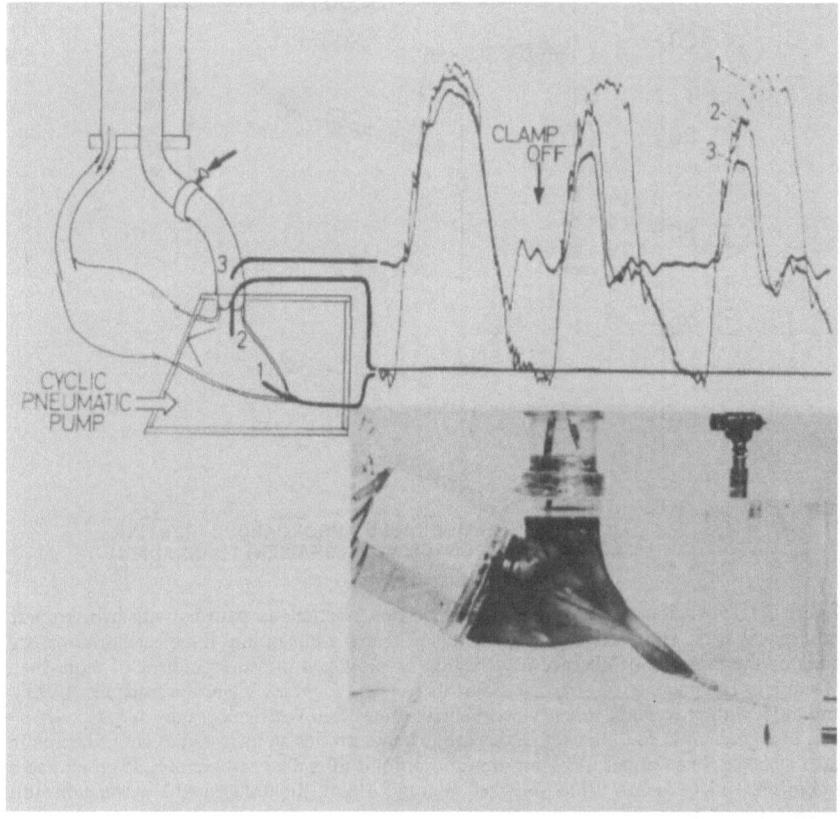

Figure 7.1.6 Dynamic pressure gradient in a hydrodynamic model of the left ventricle. A latex model of the LV is caused to contract by applying cyclic pneumatic pressure within a plastic enclosure. With three catheters in place as shown, the aortic resistance is abruptly diminished by removal of a hose clamp, and a dynamic mid- and late-systolic gradient occurs between the LV body (1) and outflow tract (2) catheters. A lesser early systolic 'flow' gradient develops between the outflow tract (2) and aortic (3) catheters. The LV (inset) develops cavitary obliteration

ventricle increases the rate and degree of emptying when a gradient is provoked by postextrasystolic potentiation (Figure 7.1.9) or vasodilator administration (Figure 7.1.10) in patients without resting gradients. Although varying degrees of mitral regurgitation are usually seen in HCM, the patients illustrated in Figures 7.1.8–7.1.10 had trivial (≤1+) mitral regurgitation.

A lucent line (Figure 7.1.11) can often be seen in lateral or left anterior oblique (LAO) angiocardiograms[23–25], and is considered to be the angiographic analogue of systolic anterior motion (SAM) of the mitral valve[25] with apposition with the interventricular septum. The time of appearance of this lucent line on LAO angiograms is indicated with arrows on Figures 7.1.8–7.1.10. There is no change in the slope of the curve of LV emptying

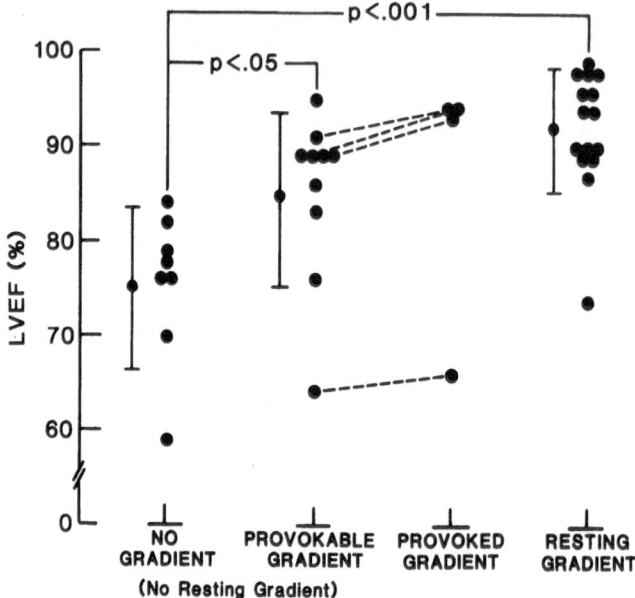

Figure 7.1.7 Angiographic left ventricular ejection fractions in patients with hypertrophic cardiomyopathy. Thirty-three patients with HCM are grouped into three categories on the basis of the presence or absence of a resting or provoked pressure gradient of more than 30 mmHg. The patients with resting gradients have the highest LV ejection fractions (LVEF), and those with provoked gradients intermediate values. Left ventriculography during provocation of a gradient in four patients in this group demonstrates an increased ejection fraction in each instance. The normal LVEF for our laboratory is 60 ± 8%, and each HCM group had a significantly higher mean value. (Brackets = mean ± 1 SD) (Reproduced with permission from *British Heart Journal*, 85, 283–91, 1985)

associated with SAM to suggest that an obstruction has occurred in these patients. SAM can therefore be explained as being a *result* of the convulsive emptying of the LV. Since SAM is often seen in the hypertrophic dog ventricle (Figures 7.1.3 and 7.1.4) in which a higher degree of LV emptying can be induced than in the normal ventricle, it appears to be the result of a more extreme degree of cavity obliteration with distortion of the mitral apparatus.

An argument which has been raised against cavity obliteration as an explanation of dynamic pressure gradients has been that the pressure just inside the mitral valve, measured with a transseptal catheter, is high. Ross has stated that 'the inflow tract of the left ventricle, that is, the area just downstream from the mitral valve, never empties completely' or stated in another way 'is never obliterated during systole'[23] in patients with HCM. Wigle and his associates concur with this view[26,27], and therefore both of these groups have used the inflow tract pressure to differentiate true obstruction from non-obstructive gradients. If the inflow tract pressure is higher than that in the outflow tract, true obstruction is present according to these investigators[23,26,27].

However the mitral valve sleeve is within the LV cavity and if a transseptal catheter is advanced through the valve sleeve it will record left atrial pressure until it emerges beyond the leaflet tips. In the right anterior oblique (RAO) projection, a catheter must be advanced well beyond a vertical line drawn anterior to the aorta in order to enter the LV cavity (Figure 7.1.12). Because of the systolic descent of the base of the heart, a catheter which is advanced just beyond the leaflet tips in diastole will be effectively withdrawn into the sleeve in systole, since the sleeve is pulled toward the apex during systole. Thus an RAO left ventriculogram that demonstrates obliteration of the entire LV cavity anterior to the aorta has obliterated the inflow tract (Figures 7.1.9 and 7.1.10).

Wigle introduced the concept of 'catheter entrapment' and equated it with cavity obliteration[26,27]. He has developed criteria to distinguish between true obstruction and catheter entrapment: an entrapped catheter does not eject blood from the proximal end during systole, and the declining LV systolic pressure crosses the aortic pressure *after* the dicrotic notch, whereas a catheter placed in the LV cavity proximal to an obstruction will eject blood and the pressure crossover occurs at or before the dicrotic notch (Figure 7.1.13). Wigle and co-workers have stressed the need to perform transseptal catheterization of the LV in order to measure the inflow tract pressure[26,27] and have stated that retrograde catheterization 'could not distinguish between true left ventricular outflow obstruction and cavity obliteration with catheter entrapment'[8].

In contrast to Wigle, we believe that catheter entrapment and cavity obliteration are different phenomena. The high pressure recorded from the obliterating LV cavity is not dependent on entrapment of a catheter, and as demonstrated in the glove experiment (Figure 7.1.5), there is ejection of fluid through the proximal end of the catheter during 'systole'. When cavity obliteration is produced in the hydrodynamic model (Figure 7.1.6) or in the LV of an experimental animal[18] (Figures 7.1.1–7.1.4), the LV pressure decline occurs at or before the central aortic dicrotic notch.

Wigle has correctly pointed out that catheter entrapment is a mechanism that can produce artifactual pressure gradients, and that the high systolic pressures recorded by an entrapped catheter decline late because the catheter is probably measuring intramyocardial pressure[27]. A falsely elevated pressure caused by catheter entrapment can be superimposed upon the high pressure recorded within the LV cavity and lead to an overestimation of the gradient. The catheter can be readily entrapped during a Valsalva manoeuvre, when the LV cavity size diminishes markedly, and it is important to scrutinize the timing of the LV pressure decline when assessing pressure gradients in patients with HCM.

Thus there are two non-obstructive mechanisms capable of producing a significant mid- and late-systolic pressure gradient within the ventricle: cavity obliteration, a true physiological phenomenon, and catheter entrapment, an artifact. As noted in the previous paragraph, these mechanisms may overlap and increase the magnitude of the pressure gradient. Another overlap of mechanisms may occur when the pressure gradient caused by a discrete

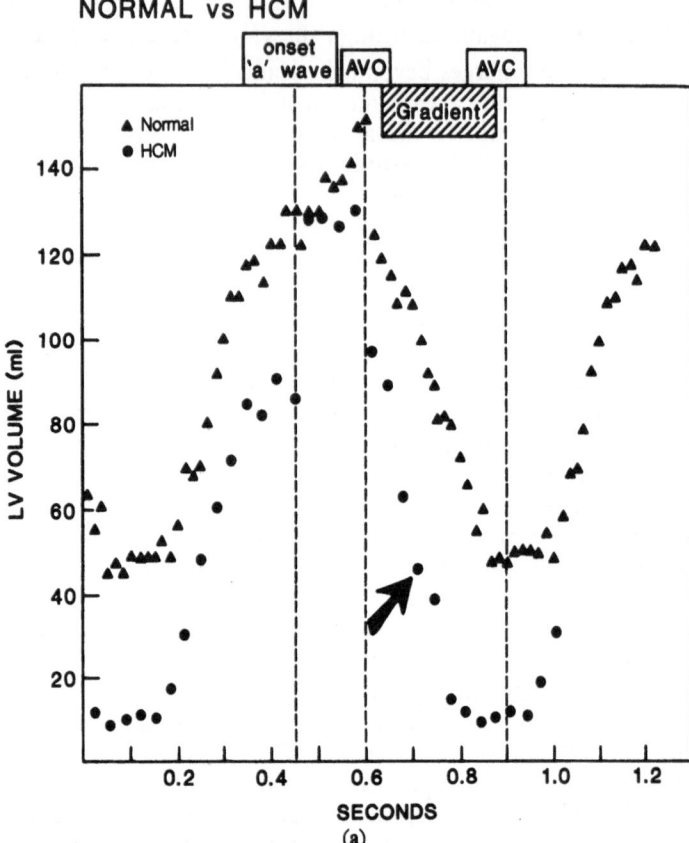

Figure 7.1.8 Left ventricular emptying rate in HCM. a, Frame-by-frame LV volume determinations in an HCM patient with a 90 mmHg gradient are compared with a normal patient's instantaneous volumes . The HCM patient (●) has a marked increase in LV volume at the time of atrial systole and empties more rapidly and completely than the normal patient (▲). The onset and duration of the gradient is indicated by the hatched bar and the time of SAM–septal contact, determined from the left anterior oblique (LAO) left ventriculogram is indicated by the arrow. The HCM patient was recorded at 30 frames per second (fps) and the normal patient at 60 fps. (AVO = aortic valve opening, AVC = aortic valve closure). b (facing), The RAO diastolic contour of the HCM patient's LV is superimposed on an end-systolic frame. There is extensive cavitary obliteration and trivial mitral regurgitation. c (facing), In comparison, the normal patient's left ventriculogram demonstrates uniform wall motion but a lesser degree of emptying

obstruction is elevated by concomitant cavity obliteration, which was demonstrated in Figure 7.1.4 and will be described in the next section.

Dynamic gradients in the presence of discrete obstruction

It has been known for over 20 years that dynamic gradients can also be found in patients with fixed obstructions of the LV outflow tract, particularly after relief of that obstruction[28,29]. Davies[28] found this phenomenon in

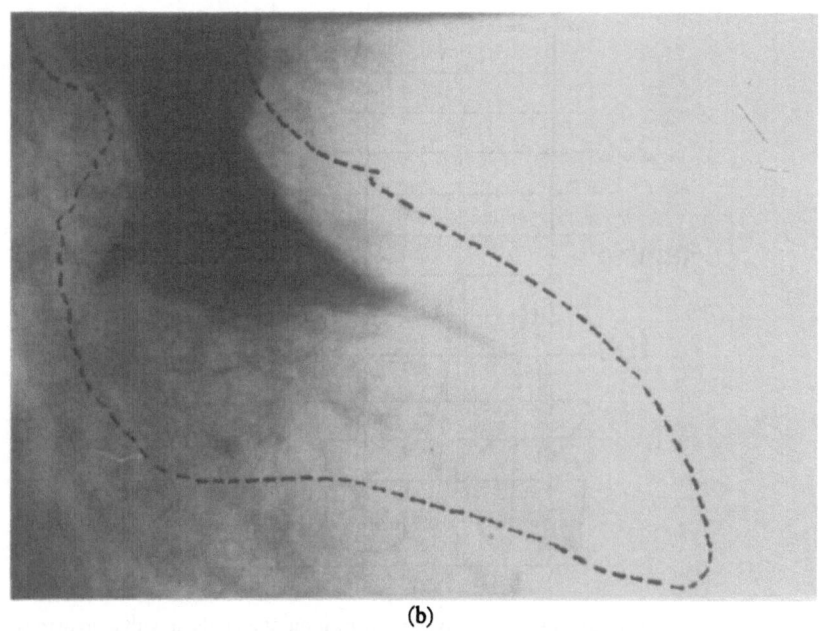

(b)

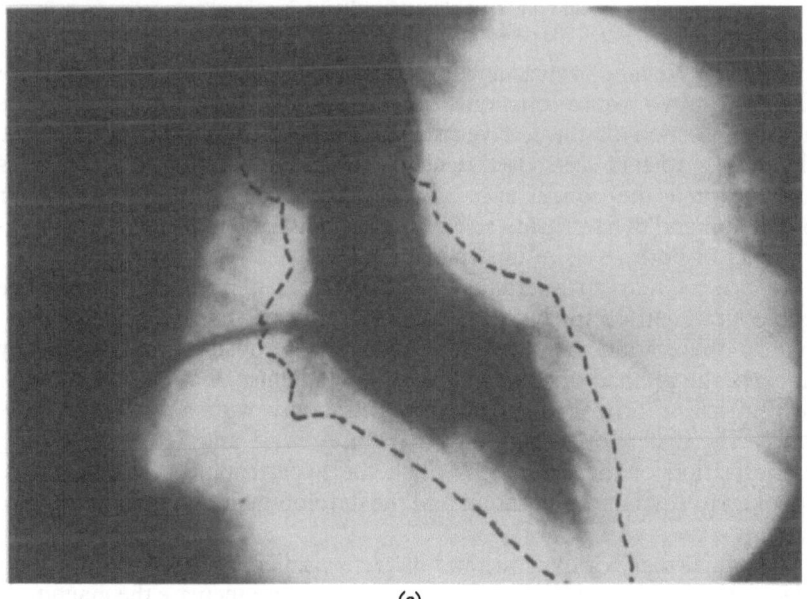

(c)

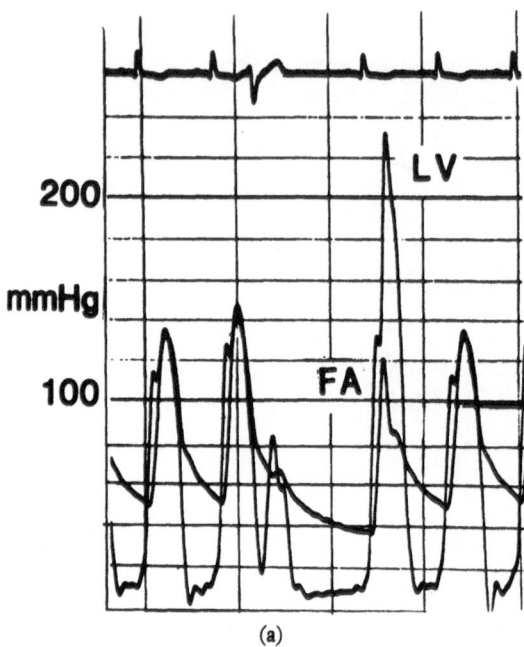

(a)

Figure 7.1.9 Left ventricular emptying in HCM: provocation of a gradient with a premature ventricular contraction. a, The LV and femoral artery (FA) pressure in a patient without a resting gradient demonstrates a 110 mmHg gradient following a premature ventricular beat. b (facing), The RAO left ventriculogram during the postextrasystolic (gradient present) beat demonstrates hyperkinesis and a small systolic cavity. (Reproduced with permission from *British Heart Journal*, 85, 283–91, 1985)

patients after relief of valvar aortic stenosis, and assumed that the pressure gradient resulted from a functional obstruction caused by contraction of the muscular portion of the left ventricular outflow tract, analogous to the subvalvar gradients seen after relief of valvar pulmonic stenosis. Others have reported the concurrence of two levels of stenosis, fixed valvar obstruction and dynamic subvalvar stenosis, and have recommended operative relief of both levels of obstruction[30].

We believe that an alternative explanation can be invoked for these double gradients, namely that a hypertrophied ventricle can develop cavitary obliteration early in systole either if the obstruction is surgically removed, the preload or afterload reduced by the use of a vasodilator, or if the ventricle is provoked to greater contractility with an inotropic substance. The hypertrophic dog model (Figures 7.1.3 and 7.1.4) serves as a demonstration of the ease with which the hypertrophic ventricle can be provoked to cavitary obliteration and the development of a non-obstructive gradient.

The concurrence of dynamic and discrete gradients can lead to considerable confusion, since they are additive and therefore increase the magnitude of the pressure difference between the LV and aorta. The patient illustrated in Figure 7.1.14 has discrete subaortic stenosis. The slow rate of aortic upstroke is diagnostic of a fixed obstruction, and the degree of stenosis was

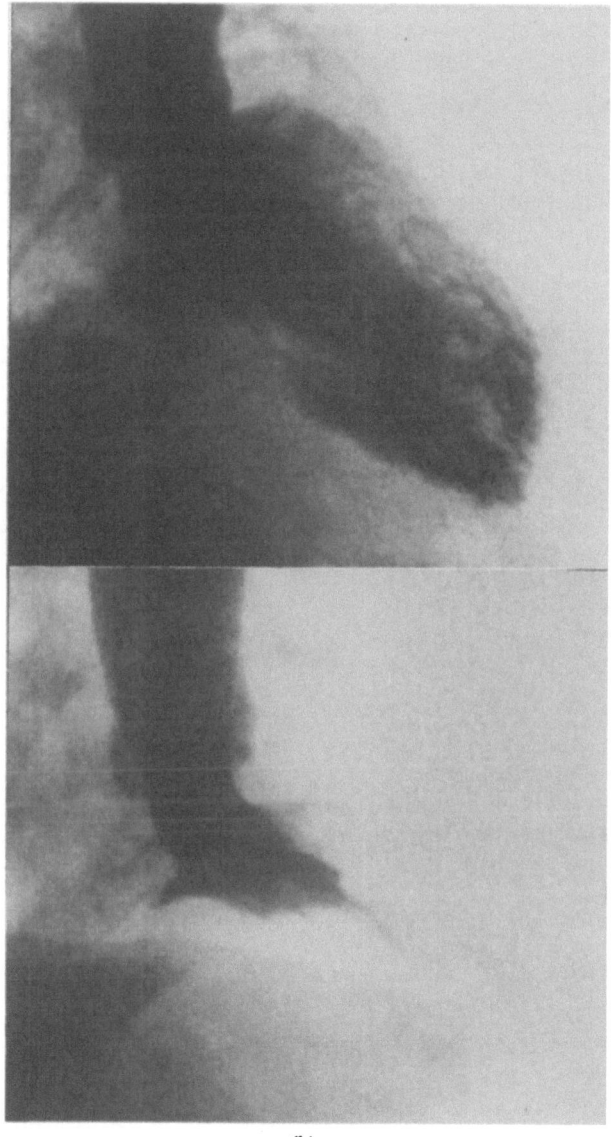

(b)

judged to be mild because of the modest pressure gradient in the presence of a normal cardiac output. She was given two sublingual nitroglycerine tablets for chest pain which occurred after the baseline measurements of pressure and flow had been obtained. Following administration of the vasodilator, she became hypotensive (90/66), and the pressure gradient rose from 40 to 90 mmHg (Figure 7.1.14b). A Valsalva manoeuvre caused the pressure gradient to rise further to 140 mmHg (Figure 7.1.14c). Her

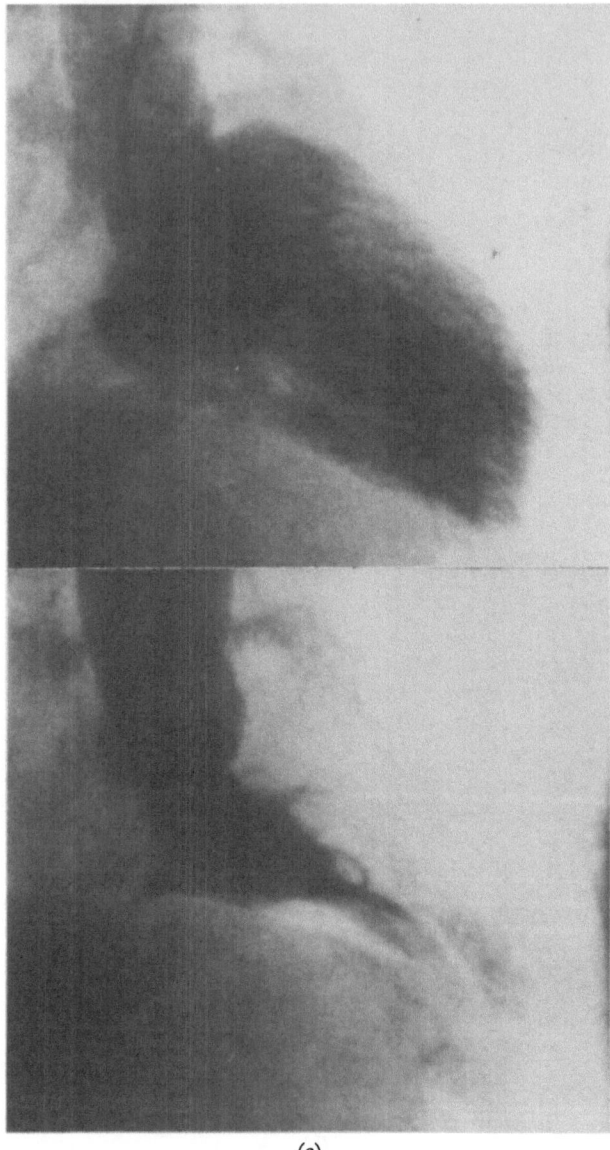

(c)

Figure 7.1.9 c, The RAO left ventriculogram during a normal (no gradient) beat demonstrates less complete emptying than was seen on postextrasystolic beat. d (facing), Frame-by-frame LV volume analysis demonstrates more rapid and complete emptying during the postextrasystolic beat in the presence of a gradient

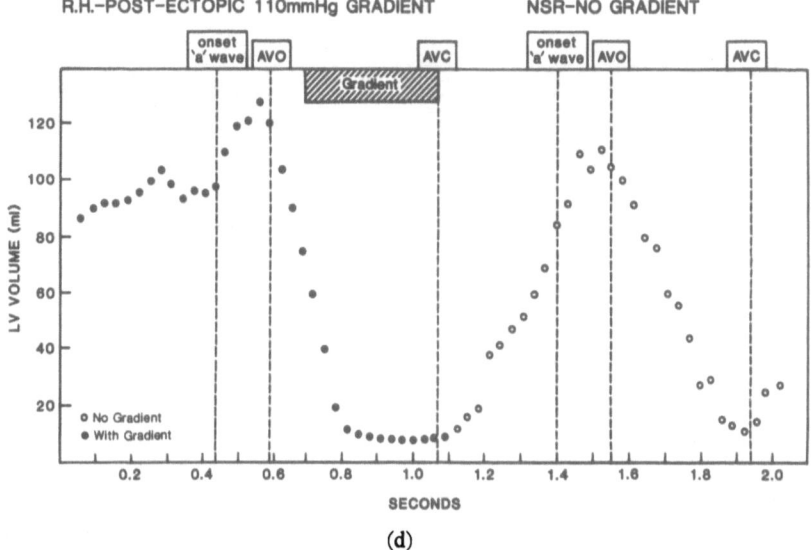

R.H.–POST-ECTOPIC 110mmHg GRADIENT   NSR–NO GRADIENT

(d)

pressures returned to baseline levels after elevation of her legs and infusion of fluids.

Although a repeat determination of cardiac output was not obtained during the brief period that she was hypotensive, it can be safely assumed that the output was markedly reduced during the Valsalva manoeuvre, and very probably reduced during the hypotensive episode. The increase in pressure gradient was therefore due to the superimposition of a dynamic pressure gradient on top of the modest obstructive gradient resulting from the fixed obstruction.

This case was chosen to illustrate the confusion that could result if the baseline pressure gradient were not known, and the overestimation of the magnitude of stenosis that might have resulted if the first gradient measured was the 90 mmHg gradient in the presence of a low cardiac output.

The further augmentation of the gradient with the Valsalva manoeuvre also deserves comment. It can be seen that the LV peak pressure rises during the strain phase from 170 mmHg to over 200 mmHg (Figure 7.1.14c). This immediate rise in LV peak pressure has been invoked as a proof of the presence of 'true obstruction' when it occurs in HCM, since 'an immediate increase in contractile force' must be invoked to explain the phenomenon, and such a change in contractility would not be expected in 'essentially empty portions of the ventricular cavity'[23]. An alternative explanation for the immediate increase in LV pressure is apparent when one looks at the *developed* LV pressure, or the total excursion from diastole to systole. The Valsalva manoeuvre increases the intrathoracic pressure by approximately 40 mmHg, and the entire LV pressure pulse is therefore displaced upwards by this amount. No immediate increase in contractile force need be invoked since there is no immediate increase in developed pressure. The increase in the pressure gradient results from the progressive decline in aortic pressure

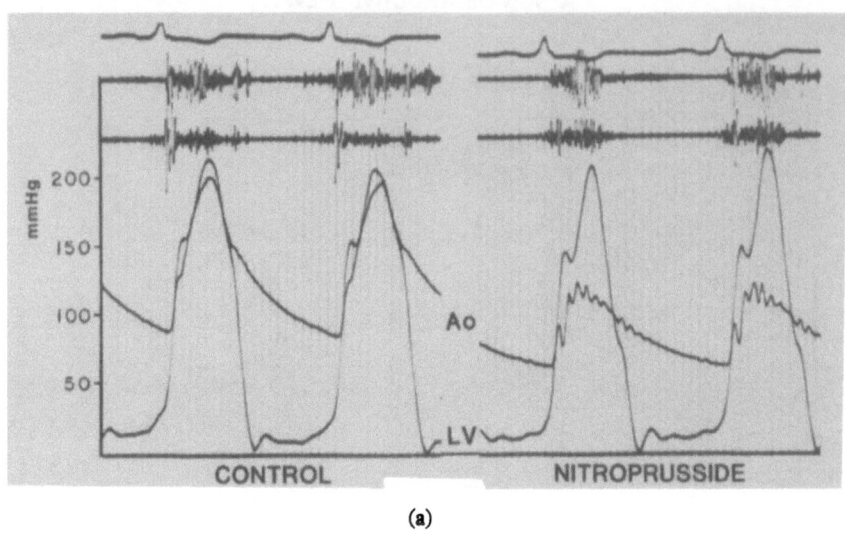

(a)

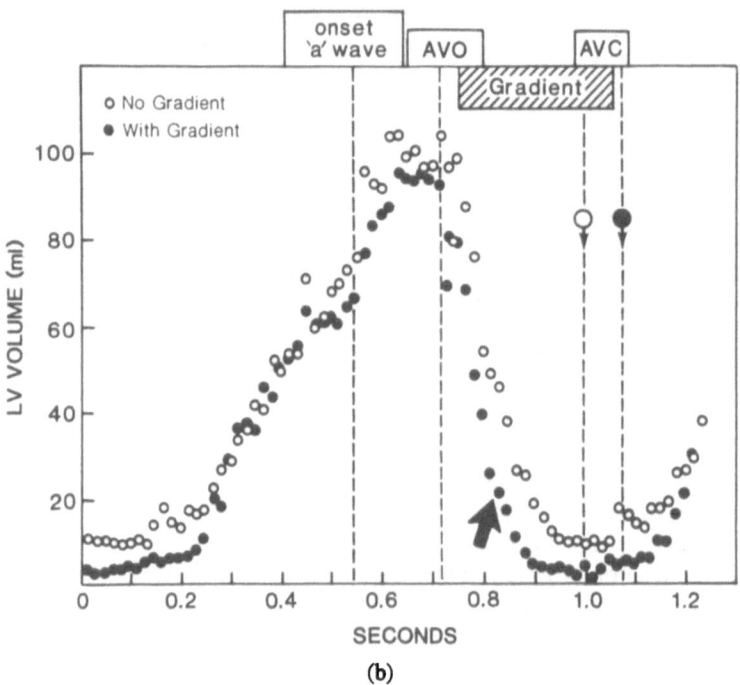

R.L.–CONTROL vs NITROPRUSSIDE

(b)

Figure 7.1.10 Left ventricular emptying in HCM: provocation of a gradient with nitroprusside. a LV and aortic pressures in a patient with HCM, before and after a gradient of 87 mmHg was induced by an infusion of sodium nitroprusside, demonstrate a constant LV pressure and a decrease in aortic pressure to result in a mid- and late-systolic gradient. b, Frame-by-frame LV volume analysis demonstrates more rapid and complete emptying in the beat with a pressure gradient. Aortic valve closure (solid dot and arrow) occurs later in the beat with a gradient because of delayed relaxation of the ventricle. (Reproduced with permission from *British Heart Journal*, 85, 283–91, 1985)

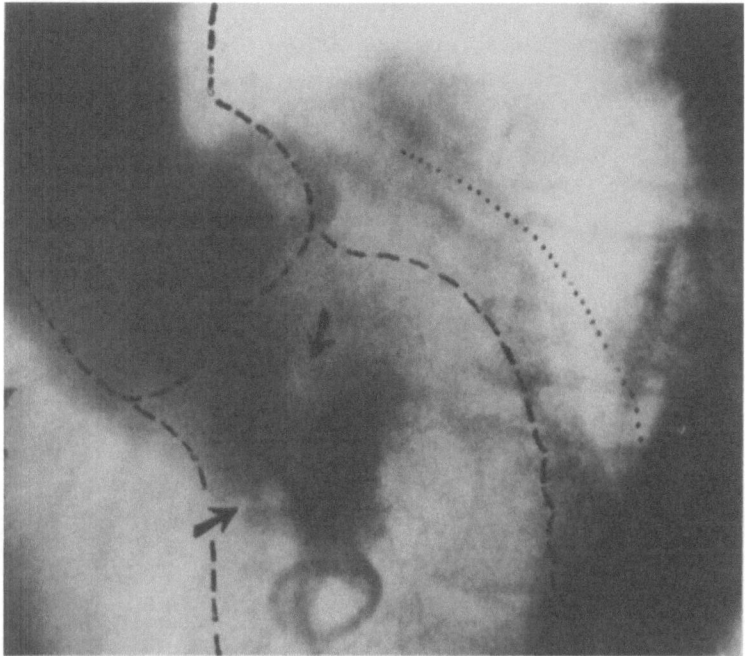

Figure 7.1.11 Angiographic depiction of systolic anterior motion in HCM. A left anterior oblique (LAO) end systolic left ventriculogram in a patient with a 70 mmHg gradient demonstrates a radiolucent line (arrows) comprised of both mitral leaflets compressed and distorted in the small cavity as a result of the vigorous thickening and inward motion of the posterolateral wall of the LV. The dashed line represents the diastolic contour and the dotted line the diastolic epicardial border. The LV is sufficiently emptied of its contents to reveal a loop of pigtail catheter in the obliterated cavity

which results from the progressive decline in LV inflow and resulting stroke volume.

Changing dynamic gradients

A unique feature of dynamic pressure gradients is that when spontaneous changes in the magnitude of the gradient occur without changes in contractile state of the LV, the LV developed pressure remains constant while the aortic pressure fluctuations are responsible for the changing gradient (Figures 7.1.4, 7.1.10 and 7.1.14). In contrast, when a hindrance to outflow is experimentally imposed, it is the LV pressure that rises to increase the magnitude of the gradient (Figure 7.1.1). A dramatic example of beat-to-beat changes in the magnitude of the pressure gradient can be seen when atrioventricular dissociation occurs as a result of heart block[31] or accelerated junctional or ventricular rhythm (Figure 7.1.15). In the example shown, the developed ventricular pressure remains almost constant, with some pulsus alternans, and there is a gradient of well over 100 mmHg on the

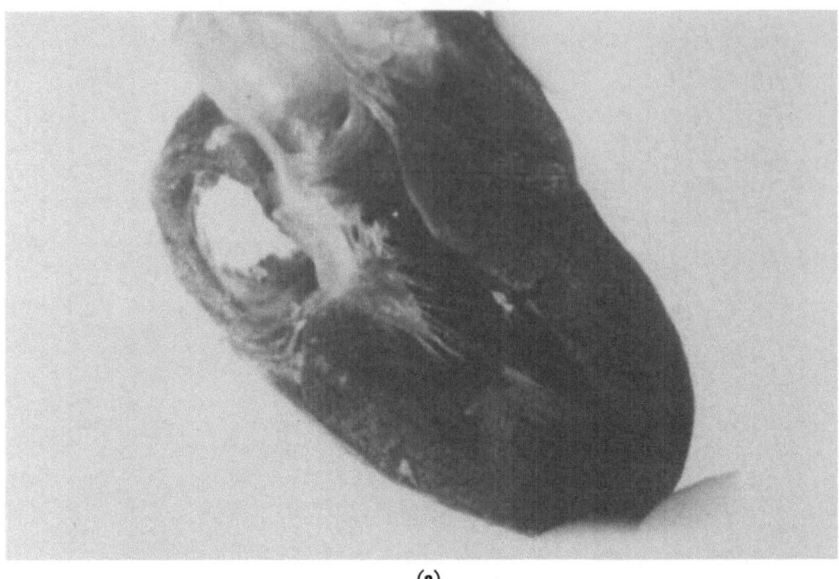

(a)

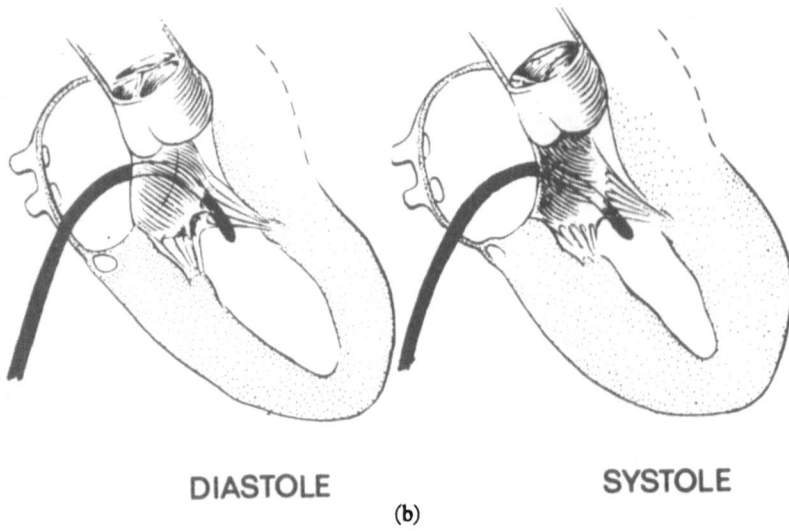

DIASTOLE   SYSTOLE

(b)

Figure 7.1.12   Transseptal catheterization of the left ventricular inflow tract in HCM. **a,** An anatomical dissection of the systolic LV in the RAO projection demonstrates the invagination of the flattened mitral valve sleeve into the LV cavity. **b,** The position of a catheter just inside the LV is seen to be anterior to the aorta in the RAO projection. **c** (facing) Transseptal (TS) and retrograde catheters in the left atrium (LA) and LV low pressure outflow region (star) are shown before and during injection of contrast medium through the LV catheter in a patient

178

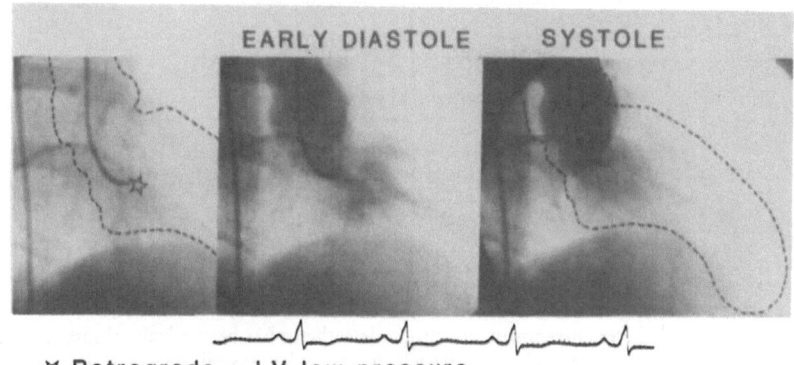

☆ Retrograde - LV low pressure

During Cine

TS -LA pressure

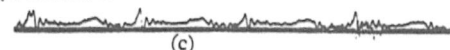

(c)

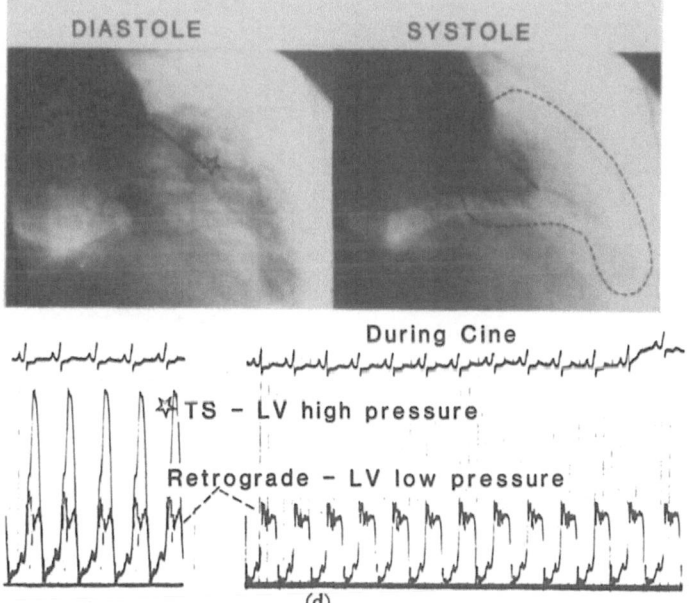

(d)

with HCM. Although the TS catheter is aligned with the anterior wall of the aorta in the RAO projection, it registers LA pressure (*bottom*) during cineangiography. The dashed line represents the end-diastolic LV silhouette. d, The transseptal catheter (star) has been advanced into the high pressure inflow tract where an injection of contrast medium demonstrates the RAO silhouette of the LV in diastole and systole. The catheter had to be advanced well into the silhouette of the LV in order to emerge from the mitral sleeve to record LV pressure. The bottom panels demonstrate the pressure recorded from the two catheters immediately before the injection (*left*) and from the retrograde catheter during the injection through the TS catheter (*right*)

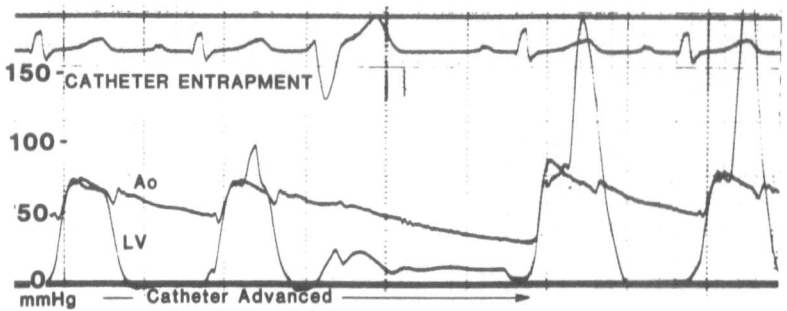

Figure 7.1.13 Catheter entrapment. A retrograde catheter has been advanced into a canine LV and records artifactually high pressures which reach a late systolic peak and descend after the aortic dicrotic notch

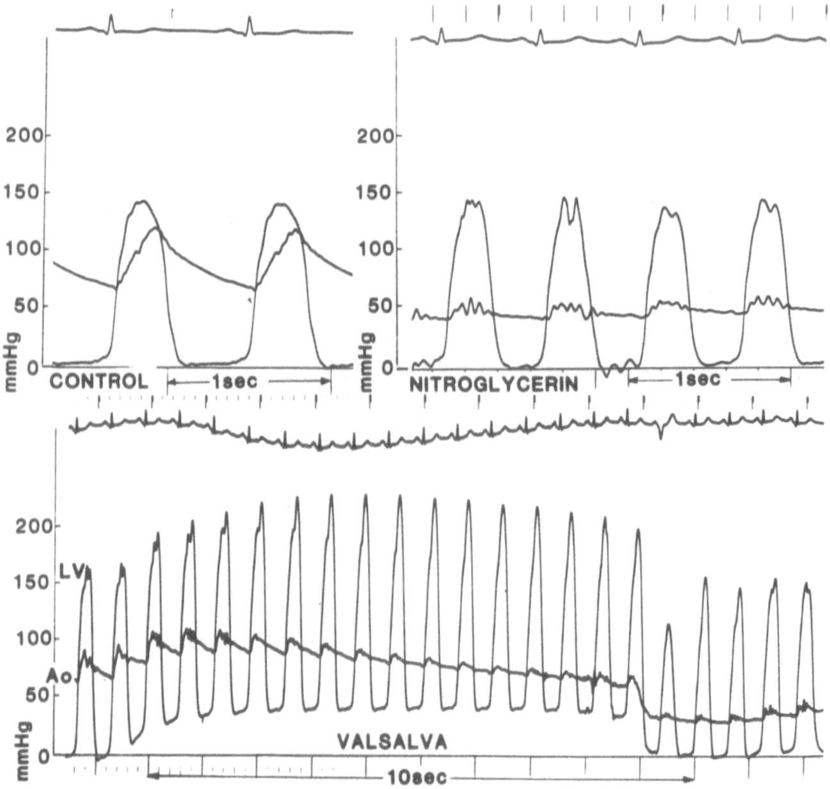

Figure 7.1.14 Augmentation of the gradient in discrete subaortic stenosis by vasodilatation and the Valsalva manoeuvre. A patient with mild discrete subaortic stenosis demonstrates a 40 mmHg gradient and a delayed aortic upstroke during a control recording. When nitroglycerine was administered, she became hypotensive and the gradient increased to 90 mmHg. With a Valsalva manoeuvre the gradient increased to 140 mmHg, with a constant LV pulse pressure (developed pressure) and a declining aortic pressure during the strain phase

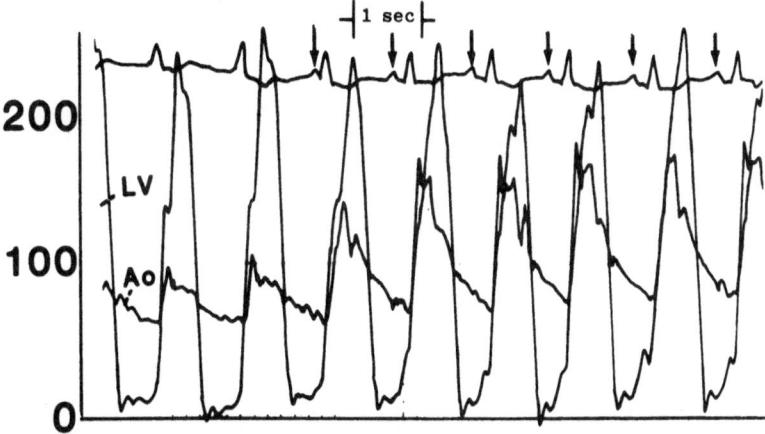

Figure 7.1.15 Variable gradient in HCM with atrioventricular dissociation. A patient with HCM and AV dissociation due to accelerated junctional rhythm has a gradient of 150 mmHg during cardiac cycles when ventricular filling is compromised by absence of properly timed atrial contractions, and diminishes the gradient when P waves (arrows) precede the QRS complexes. The *a*-wave 'kick' can be seen on the ventricular pressure pulses on the right. The magnitude of the gradient is a function of the aortic pressure, since the LV pressure remains nearly constant. The magnitude of the aortic pulse pressure is a function of ventricular filling and resulting stroke volume (Dr Rex MacAlpin kindly furnished the material for this figure)

left half of the figure. When the P waves precede the QRS complexes, the gradient is progressively diminished as the P–R interval progressively increases to approximately 0.20 seconds and the 'atrial kick' is seen on the LV pressure.

If the spontaneously variable gradient were due to differing degrees of obstruction, it would be anticipated that the LV pressure would increase and decrease as the degree of obstruction varied as seen in Figure 7.1.1. It would also be anticipated that the beats with the larger gradients would manifest a greater hindrance to emptying. Instead the LV develops a constant pressure and, depending on adequacy of ventricular filling, fluctuations in stroke volume lead to directionally similar variations in aortic pressure. The beats with gradients are accompanied by more rapid emptying because there is less to eject.

When spontaneous changes in the gradient occur as a result of changes in the contractile state of the LV as in a postextrasystolic beat (Figure 7.1.9 and 7.1.16), it is the increase in LV pressure that is responsible for the increase in the gradient. The failure of the aortic pulse pressure to rise in a postextrasystolic beat has been cited as evidence of increased obstruction[32]. However, in HCM there is little or no increase in the LV diastolic filling volume during the long diastolic pause, which obviates a significant increase in stroke volume. The LV increases its rate of emptying in the postextrasystolic beat[15,33] (Figure 7.1.9), belying the alleged sudden imposition of a severe obstruction. The gradient may therefore be a manifestation of the increased contractile force which is in excess of that which is needed to expel the blood from the ventricle. The failure of the pulse pressure to rise

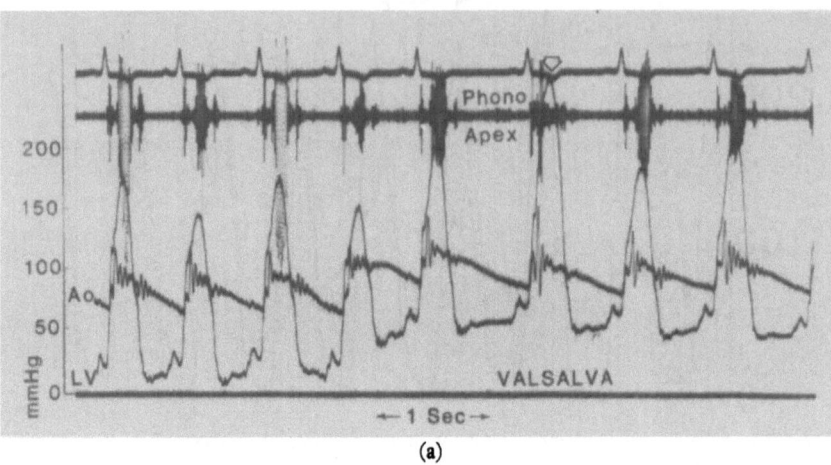

(a)

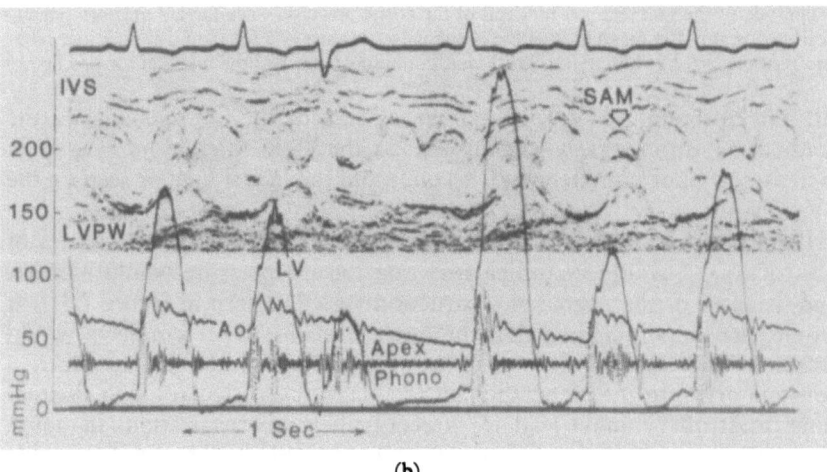

(b)

Figure 7.1.16 Phonocardiographic, echocardiographic and haemodynamic correlations in HCM. a, A Valsalva manoeuvre in a patient with a resting gradient of 55–70 mmHg (pulsus alternans) increases the gradient to >100 mmHg during the strain phase. The LV pulse pressure (developed pressure) remains constant and the gradient increases as a result of the decreasing aortic pressure, which is in turn a response to decreased LV filling and stroke volume. The contour of the late systolic murmur suggests a 'whoop' of mitral regurgitant origin. The beat marked with an arrow demonstrates an increase in developed LV pressure and a gradient of 130 mmHg in response to the longer preceding diastolic interval, and the murmur intensity decreases. b, Simultaneous pressure and echocardiographic recording in a patient with HCM demonstrates a resting gradient of 80 mmHg which increases to 175 mmHg after a premature ventricular contraction. There is a more vigorous excursion of the LV posterior wall (LVPW) and earlier systolic anterior motion (SAM) of the mitral leaflets with more prolonged septal contact in the postextrasystolic beat. Variations in murmur intensity do not correspond to changes in the magnitude of the pressure gradient, suggesting that the murmur is not a result of outflow obstruction

can be ascribed to the relatively fixed stroke volume[33] being ejected into an aortic bed that is more compliant as a result of the increased runoff time (the postextrasystolic pause) and/or an increase in the degree of mitral regurgitation.

Echocardiographic SAM in HCM

There is a positive correlation between the duration of SAM–septal contact and the dynamic pressure gradient in HCM in that the onset of SAM is earlier and the duration of septal contact longer when the pressure gradient is increased as with a postextrasystolic beat[8,9] (Figure 7.1.16). This correlation has been used to predict the presence and magnitude of pressure gradients by echocardiographic demonstrations of SAM[7], and has been used as an argument for the causation of the obstruction by SAM[7-9].

The correlation should not be viewed solely as a proof of the obstructing role of SAM since there is a more plausible alternative interpretation, namely, that the pressure gradient and SAM are both the result of rapid and complete LV emptying. In support of this alternative are the observations that although SAM occurs when a gradient is provoked, the rate of emptying of the LV is enhanced during the presence of the gradient and SAM (Figures 7.1.8–7.1.10).

Two-dimensional echocardiography permits viewing of the LV from multiple angles. Since it is a non-invasive technique and does not require the perturbation of an intracavitary injection to observe the LV cavity and its contents, it is well suited to the study of HCM.

Patients with resting pressure gradients in excess of 90 mmHg were studied in our laboratory by cardiac angiography and two-dimensional echocardiography, and each of the patients revealed comparable degrees of cavitary obliteration by both techniques[34].

Figure 7.1.17 diagrammatically depicts our two-dimensional echo-cardiographic findings in patients with HCM. The thick-walled LV contracts vigorously and rapidly eliminates the cavity up to the level of the submitral apparatus. The mitral leaflets are puckered and corrugated by the circumferential constriction of the mitral annulus, and SAM appears to result from the marked disproportion of the small ventricular cavity size and the crowded mitral valve. In serial short axis views, the cavity obliteration is confirmed.

The relationship of the high and low pressure zones in the ventricle to the long axis two-dimensional echocardiogram is also displayed in Figure 7.1.17. The high pressure is recorded from the rapidly eliminated cavity of the body of the ventricle, and the low pressure from the widely patent aortic vestibule which is in free communication with, and shares the same systolic pressure as, the aorta.

SUMMARY AND CONCLUSIONS

It has been the purpose of this paper to review and clarify the evidence against the presence of a significant hindrance or obstruction in the outflow

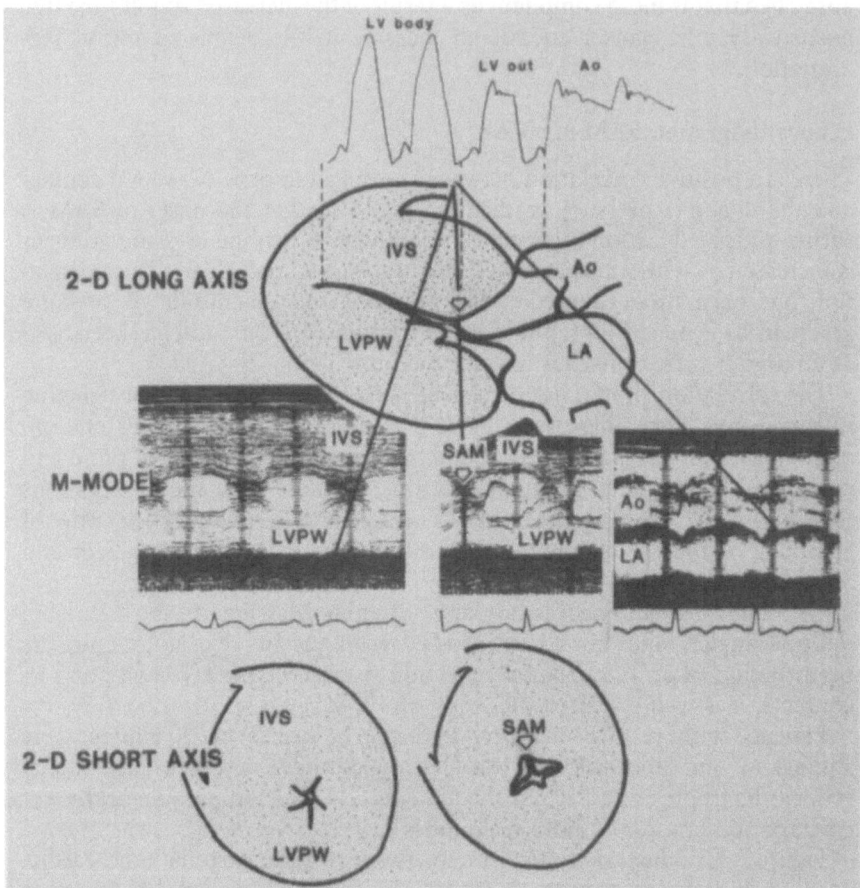

Figure 7.1.17 Echocardiographic and haemodynamic correlations in HCM. The pressure zones of the LV in HCM are vertically aligned by dashed lines with a diagram of the parasternal long axis two-dimensional echocardiographic view of the systolic LV. The high pressure is in the obliterated LV body and the low pressure in the non-contractile outflow tract which is isolated from the rapidly obliterating body, but in free communication with the aorta beyond and shares its systolic pressure. The mitral apparatus is compressed and distorted to produce SAM as a result of vigorous emptying of the LV. SAM is the site of the pressure transition because it forms the boundary between the contractile and non-contractile zones of the LV. The radial lines relate the two-dimensional long axis view to the M-mode echocardiograms of each region traversed by the lines. The short axis views of the systolic LV are aligned with the corresponding M-mode echocardiograms and demonstrate the obliterated LV cavity and the puckering of the mitral leaflets in the contracted inflow tract responsible for SAM. (Reproduced with permission from *British Heart Journal*, 85, 283–91, 1985)

tract of the LV in HCM. Our belief in the validity of a non-obstructive explanation of the pressure, flow, angiographic and echocardiographic findings in HCM is based on the basic observation that the ventricle ejects more rapidly and more completely than the normal LV[15,35] and increases the rapidity of emptying when the pressure gradient is increased.

The concept of dynamic pressure gradients resulting from cavity obliteration and not obstruction is supported by experiments in hydrodynamic models incapable of obstruction, and by the generation of non-obstructive gradients in experimental animals and man[22,36]. In each example production of the intracavitary gradient is associated with rapid and complete emptying, the antithesis of obstruction.

The unfortunate substitution and equating of the term 'catheter entrapment' for cavity obliteration[26,27], and the interchangeable usage of 'obstruction' and gradient have added greatly to the confusion that surrounds HCM. It is hoped that our efforts to clarify the mechanisms by which non-obstructive pressure gradients occur in hypercontractile ventricles will enhance the reader's understanding of this fascinating disorder.

Acknowledgements

The authors would like to thank Grace Fredrickson for typing the manuscript, and to acknowledge the extensive contributions of past co-investigators on the many projects that contributed to our understanding of 'gradients without obstruction': Robert I. White Jr., Richard S. Ross, Travis Meredith, W. Stanley Wilson, Arnold Nedelman, James Beazell, Daniel Garner and Bruce Ishimoto.

References

1. Brock, R. (1957). Functional obstruction of the left ventricle (acquired aortic subvalvar stenosis). *Guy's Hosp. Rep.*, 106, 221–38
2. Brock, R. (1959). Functional obstruction of the left ventricle (acquired aortic subvalvar stenosis). *Guy's Hosp. Rep.*, 108, 126–42
3. Morrow, A.G. and Brockenbrough, E.C. (1961). Surgical treatment of idiopathic hypertrophic subaortic stenosis, technique and hemodynamic results of subaortic ventriculomyotomy. *Ann. Surg.*, 154, 181–9
4. Dobell, A.R.C. and Scott, H.J. (1964). Hypertrophic subaortic stenosis: evolution of a surgical technique. *J. Thorac. Cardiovasc. Surg.*, 47, 26–32
5. Wigle, E.D., Heimbecker, R.O. and Gunton, R.W. (1962). Idiopathic ventricular septal hypertrophy causing muscular subaortic stenosis. *Circulation*, 26, 325–40
6. Shah, P.M., Gramiak, R. and Kramer, D.H. (1969). Ultrasound localization of left ventricular outflow tract obstruction in hypertrophic cardiomyopathy. *Circulation*, 40, 3–11
7. Henry, W.L., Clark, C.E., Glancy, D.L. and Epstein, S.E. (1973). Echocardiographic measurement of the ventricular outflow gradient in idiopathic hypertrophic subaortic stenosis. *N. Engl. J. Med.*, 288, 989–93
8. Pollick, C., Morgan, C.D., Gilbert, B.W., Rakowski, H. and Wigle, E.D. (1982). Muscular subaortic stenosis, the temporal relationship between systolic anterior motion of the anterior mitral leaflet and the pressure gradient. *Circulation*, 66, 1087–94
9. Pollick, C., Rakowski, H. and Wigle, E.D. (1984). Muscular subaortic stenosis: the quantitative relationship between systolic anterior motion and the pressure gradient. *Circulation*, 69, 43–9
10. Gauer, O.H. (1950). Evidence in circulatory shock of an isometric phase following ejection (Abstr.). *Fed. Proc.* 9, 47
11. Gauer, O.H. and Henry, J.P. (1964). Negative (−GZ) acceleration in relation to arterial oxygen saturation, subendocardial hemorrhage and venous pressure in the forehead. *Aerospace Med.*, 35, 533–44

12. Hernandez, R.R., Greenfield, J.C. Jr. and McCall, B.W. (1964). Pressure-flow studies in hypertrophic subaortic stenosis. *J. Clin. Invest.*, **43**, 401–7

13. Braunwald, E., Lambrew, C.T., Morrow, A.G., Pierce, G.E., Rockoff, S.D. and Ross, J. Jr. (1964). Idiopathic hypertrophic subaortic stenosis. *Circulation*, 30, IV, 1–213

14. Criley, J.M., Lewis, K.B., White, R.I. Jr. and Ross, R.S. (1965). Pressure gradients without obstruction. *Circulation*, **32**, 881–87

15. Wilson, W.S., Criley, J.M. and Ross, R.S. (1967). Dynamics of left ventricular emptying in hypertrophic subaortic stenosis. *Am. Heart J.*, **73**, 4–16

16. Goodwin, J.F. (1982). The frontiers of cardiomyopathy. *Br. Heart J.*, **48**, 1–18

17. Shabetai, R. (1984). Cardiomyopathy: How far have we come in twenty five years, how far yet to go? *J. Am. Coll. Cardiol.*, 1, 252–63

18. White, R.I. Jr., Criley, J.M., Lewis, K.B. and Ross, R.S. (1967). Experimental production of intracavitary pressure differences. Possible significance in the interpretation of human hemodynamic studies. *Am. J. Cardiol.*, **19**, 806–17

19. McLaughlin, J.S., Morrow, A.G. and Buckley, M.J. (1964). The experimental production of hypertrophic subaortic stenosis. *J. Thorac. Cardiovasc. Surg.*, **48**, 695–703

20. Burford, T.H., Hartman, A.F. Jr., Ferguson, T.P. and Ferrier, R.W. (1967). The production of muscular subaortic stenosis in dogs. *J. Thorac. Cardiovasc. Surg.*, **54**, 639–48

21. Blaufuss, A.H., Garner, D. and Criley, J.M. (1977). Experimental hypertrophy and hyperfunction of the left ventricle in conscious dogs produced by chronic sub-hypertensive norepinephrine infusion. *Clin. Res.*, **25**, 141A

22. Grose, R., Maskin, C., Spindola-Franco, H. and Yipintsoi, T. (1981). Production of left ventricular cavitary obliteration in normal man. *Circulation*, **64**, 448–55

23. Ross, J. Jr., Braunwald, E., Gault, J.H., Mason, D.T. and Morrow, A.G. (1966). The mechanism of the intraventricular pressure gradient in idiopathic hypertrophic subaortic stenosis. *Circulation*, **34**, 558–78

24. Simon, A.I., Ross, J. Jr. and Gault, J.H. (1967). Angiographic anatomy of the left ventricle and mitral valve in idiopathic hypertrophic subaortic stenosis. *Circulation*, **36**, 852–67

25. Adelman, A.G., McLoughlin, M.J., Marquis, Y., Auger, P. and Wigle, E.D. (1969). Left ventricular cineangiographic observations in muscular subaortic stenosis. *Am. J. Cardiol.*, **24**, 689–97

26. Wigle, E.D., Auger, P. and Marquis, Y. (1966). Muscular subaortic stenosis: the initial left ventricular inflow tract pressure as evidence of outflow tract obstruction. *Can. Med. Assoc. J.*, **95**, 793–7

27. Wigle, E.D., Marquis, Y. and Auger, P. (1967). Muscular subaortic stenosis initial left ventricular inflow tract pressure in the assessment of intraventricular pressure differences in man. *Circulation*, **35**, 1100–16

28. Davies, H. (1970). Hypertrophic subaortic stenosis as a complication of fixed obstruction to left ventricular outflow. *Guy's Hosp. Rep.*, **119**, 35–45

29. Thompson, R., Ahmed, M., Pridie, R. and Yacoub, M. (1980). Hypertrophic cardiomyopathy after aortic valve replacement. *Am. J. Cardiol.*, **45**, 33–41

30. Parker, D.P., Kaplan, M.A. and Connolly, J.E. (1969). Coexistent aortic valvular and functional hypertrophic subaortic stenosis. *Am. J. Cardiol.*, **24**, 307–17

31. Johnson, A.D. and Daily, P.O. (1975). Hypertrophic subaortic stenosis complicated by high degree heart block: successful treatment with an atrial synchronous ventricular pacemaker. *Chest*, **674**, 491–94

32. Brockenbrough, E.C., Braunwald, E. and Morrow, A.G. (1961). A hemodynamic technic for the detection of hypertrophic subaortic stenosis. *Circulation*, **23**, 189–94

33. Rackley, C.E., Whalen, R.E. and McIntosh, H.D. (1966). Ventricular volume studies in a patient with hypertrophic subaortic stenosis. *Circulation*, **34**, 579–84

34. Ginzton, L.E. and Criley, J.M. (1981). 'Obstructive' systolic anterior motion of the mitral valve in cavity obliteration. *Circulation*, **64**(IV), IV–30

35. Murgo, J.P., Alter, B.R., Dorethy, J.F., Altobelli, S.A. and McGranahan, G.M. Jr. (1980). Dynamics of left ventricular ejection in obstructive and nonobstructive hypertrophic cardiomyopathy. *J. Clin. Invest.*, **66**, 1369–82

36. Raizner, A.E., Chahine, R.A., Ishimori, T. and Awdeh, M. (1977). Clinical correlates of left ventricular cavity obliteration. *Am. J. Cardiol.*, **40**, 303–9

7.2
Haemodynamic, angiographic and echocardiographic evidence against impeded ejection in hypertrophic cardiomyopathy*

J.P. MURGO and J.W. MILLER

INTRODUCTION

Since the concept of a functional obstruction to left ventricular outflow was first reported by Brock nearly 30 years ago[1], the origin and physiological significance of intraventricular pressure gradients in some patients with hypertrophic cardiomyopathy (HCM) have been the source of a continuing controversy. The classic 'textbook' explanation of the mechanism for the generation of intraventricular pressure gradients invokes an abnormal anterior displacement of the mitral valve against the interventricular septum at a variable period of time during systole, resulting in an 'obstruction' against which the left ventricle is forced to eject[2-7]. Although early systolic ejection may be rapid, the later systolic left ventricular pressure gradients of patients with HCM have been invested with physiological significance similar to gradients resulting from fixed valvular aortic stenosis. This concept has led some physicians to recommend surgical therapy when gradients are 'severe', even in some asymptomatic patients.[8].

It has been difficult to demonstrate a correlation between the magnitude of the left ventricular gradients in HCM and the clinical presentation of patients with this disease. Due to the presence of rapid left ventricular emptying, high ejection fractions, cavity obliteration, and other laboratory observations inconsistent with an obstructive mechanism, other investigators have questioned the significance or presence of a mechanical, albeit dynamic, obstruction to left ventricular outflow[9-12]. With improved technological capabilities in both the non-invasive and invasive laboratory environments generating new data, this controversy has been rekindled in the last several years and has been reviewed by several recent articles and editorials[13-19].

---

* The opinions or assertions contained herein are the private views of the authors and are not to be construed as reflecting the views of the US Department of the Army or the US Department of Defense.

To some extent, this controversy has been complicated by different interpretations of the meaning of 'obstruction'. We interpret the term 'obstruction' to signify an *impediment* or *hindrance* to left ventricular ejection. In this paper, it is our purpose to present studies performed in our laboratory utilizing simultaneous pressure, flow velocity, phonocardiographic, angiographic and echocardiographic measurements of the complex dynamic events occurring from beat to beat in this intriguing disease entity. It is our belief that the results of these studies provide strong evidence against an impediment to left ventricular ejection.

STUDIES OF THE DYNAMICS OF EJECTION

Many of the early haemodynamic studies of patients with HCM arrived at conclusions regarding the dynamics of left ventricular ejection from measurements of pressure events rather than from an investigation of flow dynamics. The first published observations analysing central aortic flow in man were published by Hernandez et al.[20] in 1964. These investigators, utilizing the pressure gradient technique[21], studied ascending aortic flow in four patients with HCM and resting intraventricular gradients. They demonstrated that 80% of the stroke volume was ejected during the first half of systole, as compared with 57% in five control subjects. This was the first report of the distinctly abnormal configuration of ascending aortic flow in patients with HCM. These investigators concluded that this abnormal ejection waveform, which they observed only in patients with HCM, could have been the result of a dynamic obstruction occurring in mid-systole or, alternatively, as a result of a powerful ventricle ejecting its contents in a rapid and complete manner. In the same year, Pierce et al.[22] published a classic study in which an electromagnetic flow probe was placed around the root of the ascending aorta in several patients about to undergo ventricular myotomy–myectomy. While these patients were under general anaesthesia with an open chest, several manipulations were performed prior to the institution of extracorporeal circulation. These authors observed ejection waveforms very similar to those reported by Hernandez et al.[20], but the results of their study led them to conclude that a dynamic, mechanical obstruction existed in the outflow tract of the left ventricle and was the cause of the late systolic diminution of aortic flow in the four HCM patients they studied.

The concept of obstruction was soon challenged by Criley and coworkers[9], who believed that the ability of the left ventricle to rapidly achieve extremely low end-systolic volumes (cavity obliteration) provided an alternative explanation to the generation of high left ventricular pressure gradients during mid- and late-systole. This non-obstructive interpretation of ejection in HCM is described in detail by Criley and Siegel in Chapter 7.1. Using frame-by-frame left ventricular cineangiography, these investigators later demonstrated that left ventricular emptying in HCM occurred more rapidly than in a group of control subjects or in a group of patients with fixed obstruction, i.e. valvular aortic stenosis[10].

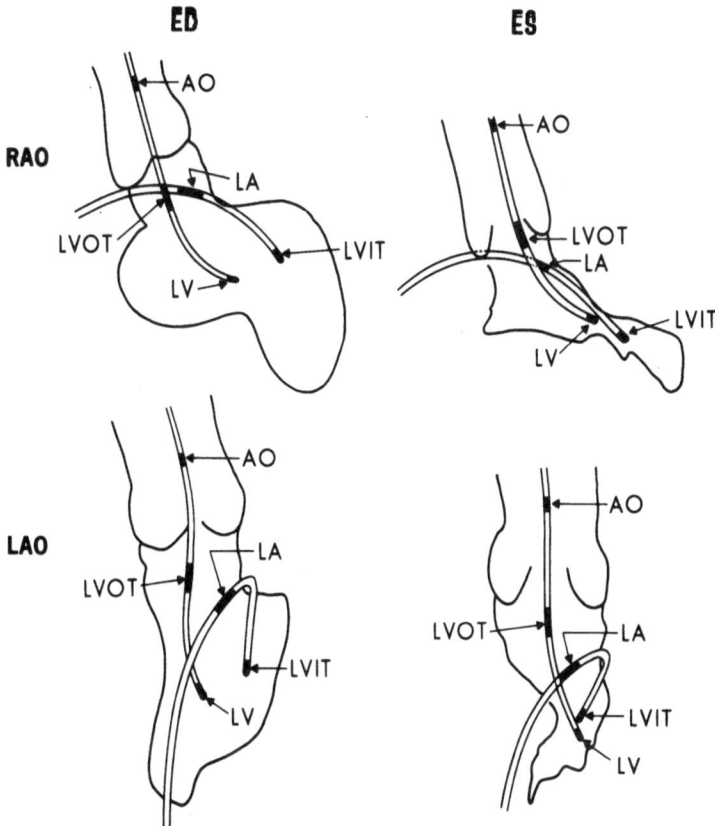

Figure 7.2.1 Simultaneous retrograde and transseptal multisensor catheterization of the left ventricle in a patient with HCM. Illustrated are end-diastolic and end-systolic silhouettes derived from an actual cineangiogram in the 30° RAO and 60° LAO projections. The locations of the micromanometers during haemodynamic measurements are shown in the left ventricular inflow tract (LVIT) and left atrium (LA) via the transseptal catheter; left ventricular cavity (LV), left ventricular outflow tract (LVOT) and aorta (Ao) via the retrograde catheter. An electromagnetic flow velocity probe was also mounted at the LVOT site shown in these diagrams. With partial withdrawal of the retrograde catheter, the LVOT pressure sensor and associated flow velocity probe could be withdrawn into the ascending aortic root

In the 10 years between 1970 and 1980, improved technology in radiographic equipment and the advent of echocardiography led to the observation that an abnormal displacement of the mitral valve apparatus against the interventricular septum occurred during systole[5,6,23]. The temporal coincidence of an intraventricular pressure gradient and systolic anterior motion of the mitral valve (SAM) led to wide acceptance of the mitral valve as the 'obstructing' structure in HCM.

In the mid and late 1970s, new techniques utilizing multisensor catheters[24] developed in our laboratory provided an ability to measure multiple, simultaneous high frequency pressure and flow events for the first time in the history of human cardiac catheterization. Figure 7.2.1 illustrates

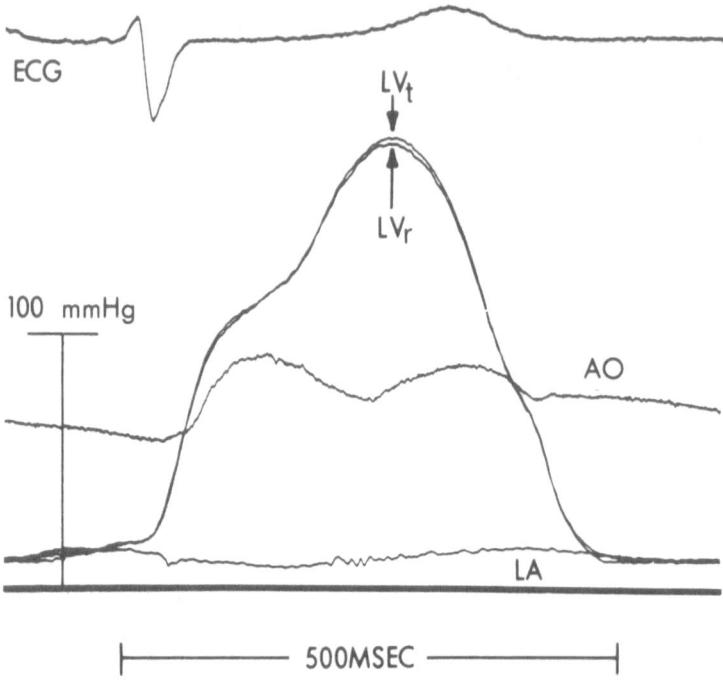

Figure 7.2.2 Selected pressure signals derived from the techniques described in Figure 7.2.1. Abbreviations as in Figure 7.2.1. Left ventricular pressure from transseptal catheter (LV_t), left ventricular pressure from retrograde catheter (LV_r). Note that the left ventricular pressures obtained from the micromanometers mounted at the tips of the transseptal and retrograde catheters are identical

the current techniques used in our laboratory to study the haemodynamics of HCM. A multisensor catheter utilizing three solid-state Millar micro-manometers is retrogradely introduced into the left ventricle and positioned to measure high frequency pressure signals in the body of the left ventricle, the left ventricular outflow tract (LVOT), and the ascending aortic root. An electromagnetic flow probe is situated at the same level as the middle pressure sensor so that LVOT flow velocity can be measured or, with partial withdrawal of the catheter, ascending aortic flow velocity may be obtained. Another multisensor catheter is placed in the left ventricular inflow tract through a sheath introduced into the left heart utilizing transseptal techniques[25]. This catheter is instrumented with Millar micromanometers at the tip to measure left ventricular inflow tract pressure and, 5 cm away, to measure left atrial pressure.

An example of the signals obtained utilizing such a technique is shown in Figure 7.2.2. Two left ventricular pressures are shown in conjunction with the aortic and left atrial pressure signals. The LVOT pressure has been eliminated from this figure for the sake of clarity. Note that both left ventricular pressures are superimposed to such a degree that the transseptal signal is barely discernible from the retrograde signal.

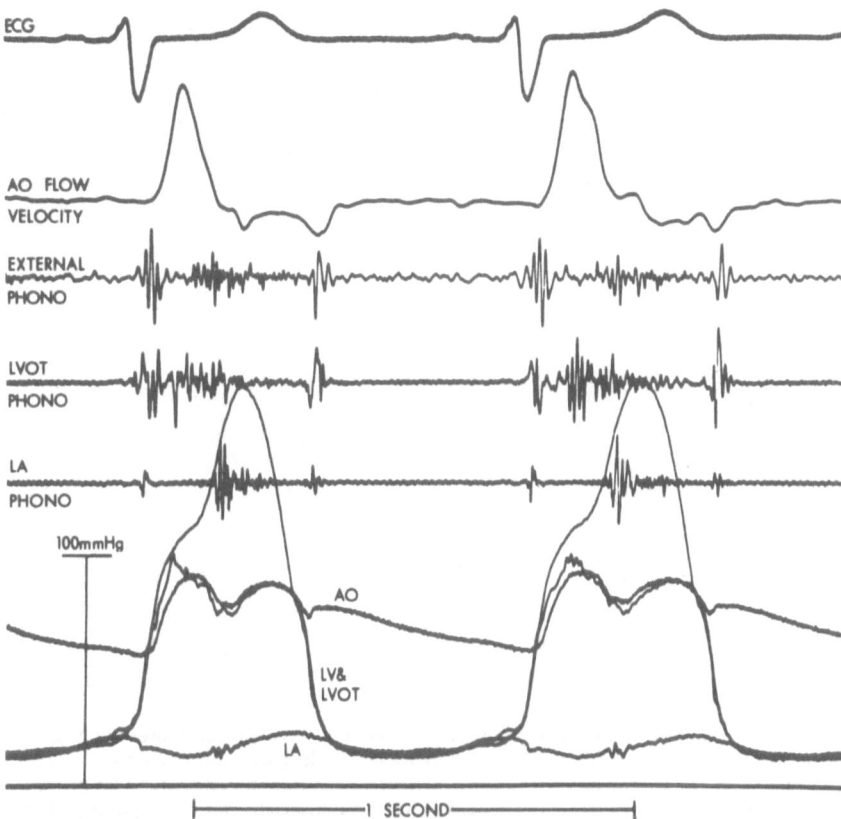

Figure 7.2.3 Multisensor catheter signals. Abbreviations as in Figure 7.2.1. Illustrates pressures from the LV, LVOT, LA and aorta with aortic flow velocity and intracardiac phonocardiograms from the LVOT and LA. Also shown is an external phonocardiogram. See text for details

Figure 7.2.3 demonstrates the full capabilities of such an approach. Micromanometer pressures are shown from the transseptal catheter in the left ventricle and left atrium and from the retrograde catheter in the LVOT and aorta; an aortic flow velocity signal is shown from the electromagnetic flow velocity probe situated in the ascending aorta just above the aortic valve, and two intracardiac phonocardiograms are shown derived from the LVOT and left atrial pressure sensors by appropriate high pass filtration. In the ascending aorta, it has been shown previously that aortic flow velocity signals may be used to represent instantaneous volumetric flow[11,26]. In this patient with a gradient of 90 mmHg, aortic flow is confined primarily to the first half of the systolic ejection period. This abnormal waveform is very similar to those reported by Hernandez *et al.*[20], and Pierce *et al.*[22], using different techniques. A separate external phonocardiogram from a lower left sternal border microphone is also shown in conjunction with the electrocar-

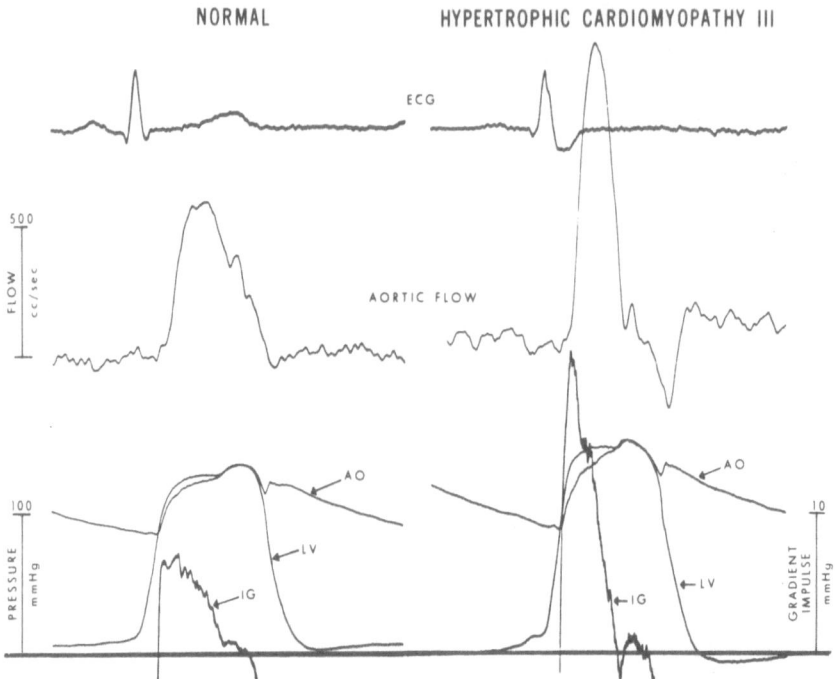

Figure 7.2.4 Impulse gradients in HCM. IG = impulse gradient; other abbreviations as in Figure 7.2.1. The instantaneous pressure difference across the aortic valve (not the LVOT) is derived by electrical subtraction of the aortic pressure signal from the left ventricular pressure signal. In the left panel, a normal flow velocity waveform is associated with an impulse gradient as shown in a control subject. In contrast, an abbreviated high velocity waveform in an HCM patient without intraventricular pressure gradients (HCM Subgroup III[11]) generates an impulse gradient with much higher amplitude and briefer duration. See text for discussion

diographic signal. These techniques provide a powerful tool to investigate instantaneous pressure-flow haemodynamics in man.

In 1980, our laboratory challenged the concept of obstruction as an impediment to left ventricular ejection by reporting the results of a study of ejection dynamics in HCM patients with and without pressure gradients[11]. An example of the results of this study is shown in Figure 7.2.4. In the left panel, a patient from the control group with normal ejection dynamics is shown with micromanometric-derived left ventricular and aortic pressures and an aortic flow velocity signal. Left ventricular ejection occurs throughout the available systolic ejection period. In contrast, the right panel demonstrates an HCM patient without intraventricular pressure gradients. Note that the aortic flow velocity signal has a distinctly different waveform from the normal control subject. As demonstrated in the patient in Figure 7.2.3, ejection occurs predominantly in the first half of systole with much higher flow rates than those encountered in the control subject. Using these techniques to examine 30 patients with HCM and 29 control subjects, we demonstrated that the abnormal ejection waveforms, which previously had been attributed to an obstruction to left ventricular outflow, were also seen in HCM patients who demonstrated no abnormal pressure gradients.

We concluded that the abnormal waveforms were the result of rapid and early ejection rather than obstruction. However, to assess instantaneous volumetric flow, we assumed that the velocity profile in the aorta was blunt[27]. To test the validity of this assumption in HCM, we employed a second, independent technique to measure ejection dynamics. Utilizing frame-by-frame cineventriculography, we studied the same group of patients and demonstrated the same results, i.e. that ventricular emptying in HCM patients was rapid, early and virtually complete, with 90% of the angiographic stroke volume ejected in the first half of systole, whether or not pressure gradients were present[11].

Recently, Gardin *et al.*[28] and Maron *et al.*[29] reported studies of aortic flow velocity utilizing pulsed Doppler techniques in HCM. Both groups reported a difference in ejection waveforms between 'obstructive' and 'non-obstructive' HCM. We believe that significant limitations exist with Doppler studies as a result of the difficulty encountered in placing a stationary sample volume in a spatial flow velocity field that moves secondary to aortic and cardiac motion. This may be a particular problem in HCM due to the hyperdynamic ejection characteristics present in this disease. In addition, data regarding criteria for diagnosing the patients with 'non-obstructive' HCM were not clear from the abstracts published, and details regarding medications were not available. In contrast, Kinoshita *et al.*[30] reported results similar to ours using transcutaneous pulsed Doppler techniques from the suprasternal notch in patients with and without pressure gradients. Sugrue and co-workers[31], utilizing nuclear scintigraphic techniques, also examined the ejection characteristics of HCM patients with and without pressure gradients, and compared the results to a group of control subjects. Their findings were consistent with the results of our invasive investigation and conclusions that the abnormal ejection waveforms present in HCM were a result of rapid ventricular emptying rather than obstructed outflow.

However, stimulated by the pulsed Doppler studies which reported results different from ours, we have studied an additional 33 patients since 1980 to yield a total of 63 patients with HCM and 29 control subjects. The similarity in ejection characteristics between HCM patients with and without pressure gradients that we reported previously has been confirmed with these additional studies.

Our laboratory has also analysed an indirect index of dynamic pulsatile flow through the aortic valve with a third and independent technique. This involves the measurement of an instantaneous difference between pressures just above and below the aortic valve, defined as the impulse gradient[32,33]. This parameter is shown in Figure 7.2.4 as an electrically derived pressure difference between the left ventricle and aorta in the normal control subject in the left panel, and in the HCM patient without intraventricular gradients in the right panel. Despite the absence of an intraventricular gradient, the amplitude and duration of the impulse gradient signal in the HCM patient is

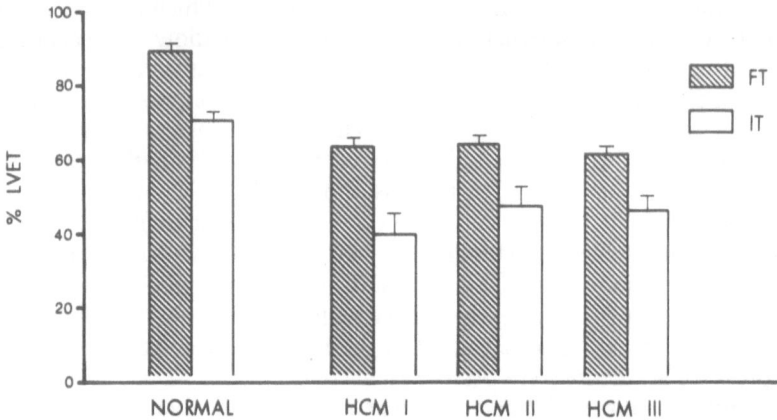

Figure 7.2.5 Flow time (FT) vs. impulse time (IT). The duration of forward aortic flow velocity (flow time) and associated impulse gradients (impulse time) are shown for a group of control subjects ($n = 29$) in the left side of this graph. The same data are illustrated for the three HCM subgroups as previously defined by our laboratory[11]. HCM Group I = patients with resting gradients ($n = 9$); HCM Group II = patients with provokable gradients ($n = 12$); HCM Group III = patients without resting or provokable gradients ($n = 9$). See text for discussion

significantly different from the control subject. These patients were chosen to illustrate this point because of similar stroke volumes. As a result, the areas circumscribed by each of the flow velocity signals in Figure 7.2.4 are identical. However, due to the stroke volume of the HCM patient being compressed into the first half of systole, a much higher flow rate is achieved and the instantaneous gradient generated across the aortic valve as the result of blood inertia is similarly higher in amplitude and shorter in duration. Figure 7.2.5 illustrates impulse gradient duration (impulse time) in the same group of patients reported earlier by our laboratory[11]. Note that there is a significant difference between the control group and all three subgroups as previously defined. All three HCM subgroups reveal significantly shorter impulse gradient durations associated with the previously shown abbreviated flow signals. Thus, whether or not *intraventricular* pressure gradients are present, the measurement of physiological flow-related *impulse gradients* across the aortic valve demonstrates no difference in ejection characteristics in HCM patients[34].

In the study of Maron *et al.*[29], a late systolic secondary rise in aortic flow velocity was identified in some of the patients they classified as 'obstructive'. They interpreted these observations as signifying a continued ejection of blood into the aorta in late systole against a significant obstruction. Our laboratory has not demonstrated late secondary systolic peaks in aortic flow using computer-averaged blood-flow velocity measurements over multiple cardiac cycles, or by deriving flow from dynamic frame-by-frame analysis of ventricular emptying. It is also noteworthy that a secondary systolic peak in aortic flow was not reported by Hernandez *et al.*[20] or Pierce *et al.*[22].

However, secondary peaks in flow velocity are more commonly seen in the LVOT when the catheter is advanced such that the flow velocity probe is introduced into the LVOT. We believe that these secondary peaks in LVOT velocity do not represent volumetrically significant flow. This conclusion is derived from observations such as those illustrated in Figure 7.2.6. In the left panel, aortic flow velocity is shown with the catheter partially withdrawn, so that the flow velocity probe is in the aorta. The deep left ventricular pressure was not recorded as a result of the catheter position, but was identical to that shown in the right panel prior to the change in catheter position. Note the short, abbreviated flow which ends just after SAM–septal contact, demonstrated on a simultaneous M-mode echocardiogram. However, in the right panel of Figure 7.2.6, when the catheter was advanced deeper into the left ventricle, a secondary peak in LVOT flow velocity occurs in late systole. While SAM–septal contact is maintained (between the two vertical lines), an initial *decrease* in velocity is associated with an *increasing* gradient, and a later *increase* in velocity is associated with a *decreasing* gradient. These changes are opposite to those predicted by fluid dynamic principles if, as suggested by the echo of the mitral valve, the LVOT dimensions remain unchanged from the onset of SAM-septal contact to its termination. These observations lead us to believe that the prominent late systolic pressure gradients in HCM *may* be dissociated from any residual late systolic flow through the LVOT. More recent studies by Yock *et al.*[30] reveal increases in LVOT velocity just prior to SAM-septal contact following which a more rapid increase in velocity occurs. However, these increases in LVOT velocity are associated with marked drops in signal amplitude *implying* that insignificant amounts of volumetric flow occur after SAM–septal contact.

SIMULTANEOUS HAEMODYNAMIC AND ECHOCARDIOGRAPHIC STUDIES

Despite the evidence that ejection dynamics are similar in HCM patients with and without pressure gradients as described above, recent studies of the temporal relationships of SAM and pressure events reported by Pollick *et al.*[36,37] have challenged the conclusions of our studies. They emphasized the following three points: the onset of the pressure gradient was virtually simultaneous with the timing of SAM–septal contact; the larger the pressure gradient, the earlier the SAM–septal contact occurred in systole; and the larger the pressure gradients, the longer was the duration of SAM–septal contact. These authors concluded that SAM was the cause of the abnormal pressure gradient seen in HCM. Furthermore, they claim that the ejection characteristics reported for Group I (patients with gradients) in our study[11] were basically derived from patients without 'significant obstruction' because the peak-to-peak pressure gradients we reported in this group averaged only 51 mmHg. Using linear regression equations derived from their studies, Pollick and co-workers claimed that by studying patients with milder gradients, virtually all of the left ventricular stroke volume was

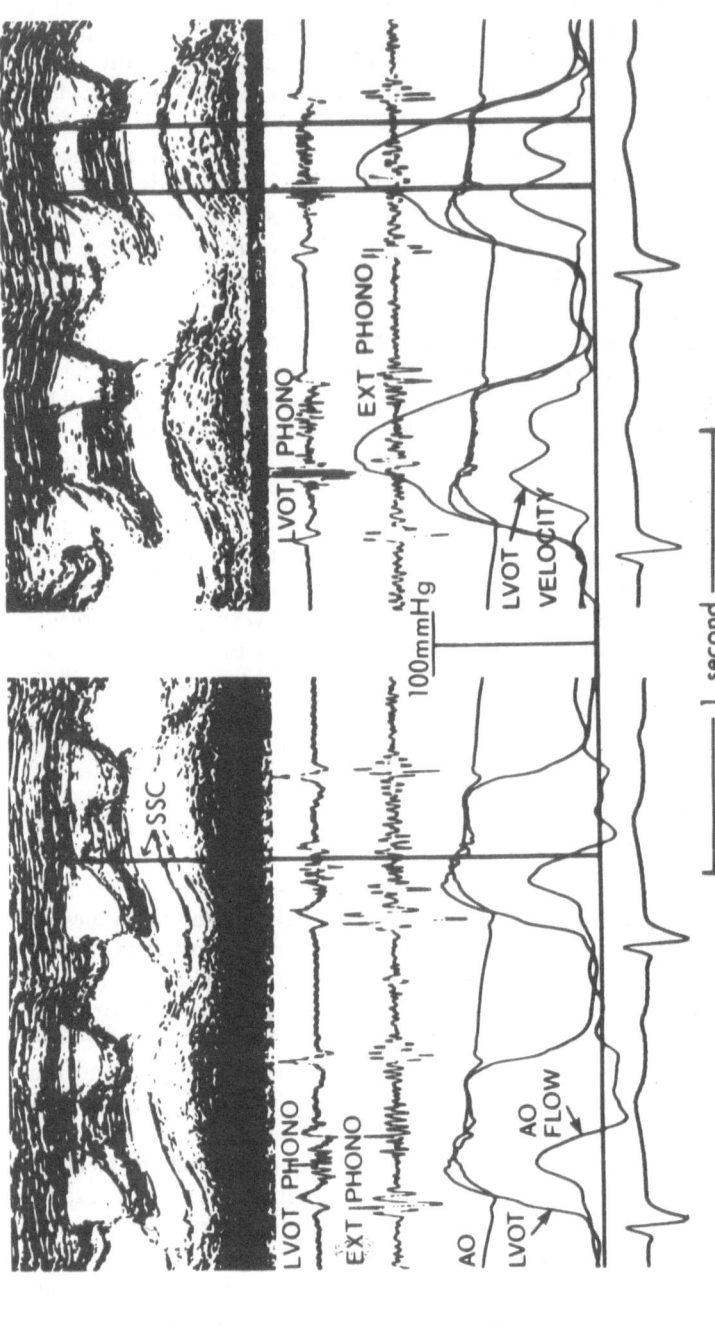

Figure 7.2.6 Simultaneous echocardiogram of SAM, phonocardiograms, pressure and flow velocity signals. Abbreviations as in Figure 7.2.1. In the left panel, the deep LV pressure was not recorded in order to obtain aortic flow velocity by partial withdrawal of the catheter. However, a pressure gradient of identical magnitude as shown in the right panel was present. The aortic flow velocity signals ends just after SAM–septal contact (vertical line). In the right panel, the catheter was remanipulated into the ventricle in order to obtain LVOT flow velocity signals. Note that a secondary rise in LV flow velocity occurs while SAM–septal contact is maintained (two vertical lines). However, no change in the LVOT or downstream aortic pressures is seen. See text for discussion

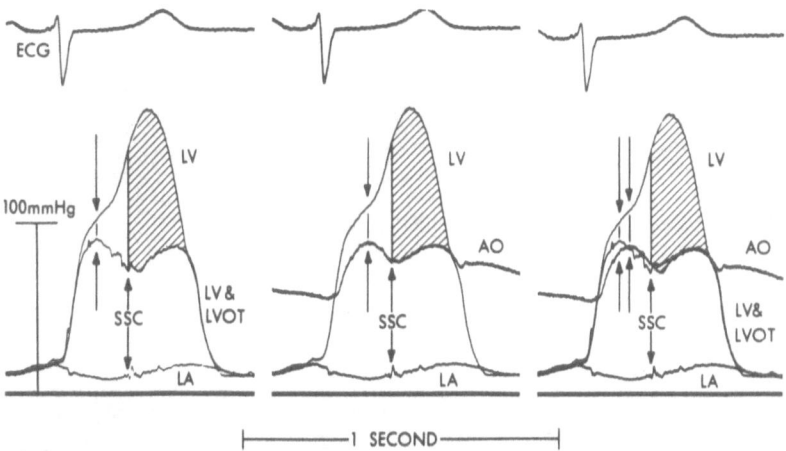

Figure 7.2.7 Definition of pressure gradient onset. **SSC** = SAM–septal contact. Hatched area highlights pressure gradient after echocardiographically identified SAM–septal contact. Abbreviations otherwise as in Figure 7.2.1. *Left panel:* Using simultaneous left ventricular and left ventricular outflow tract pressures, the onset of an 'abnormal' pressure gradient in HCM is defined as the initial divergence of these pressures after the impulse gradient. *Middle panel:* Identification of the onset of pressure gradient using deep LV and aortic pressure. *Right panel:* A difference of 45 ms results by identifying the onset of the pressure gradient using aortic pressure instead of LVOT pressure. See text for discussion

ejected in our patients prior to the onset of 'obstruction', as defined by the time at which SAM–septal contact occurred. They further claimed that, if we had studied patients with larger gradients, a significant portion of the stroke volume would have been ejected in the presence of an abnormal pressure gradient, and thereby our data would be consistent with an obstructive mechanism.

We believe that several methodological problems exist in Pollick's studies. First, the investigators utilized fluid-filled catheter systems to measure their pressure gradients and thus introduced errors in timing of all pressure events. Secondly, the authors defined the onset of the abnormal pressure gradient by the peak of the aortic 'percussion wave' just before the divergence of left ventricular inflow tract pressure and aortic pressure. However, since the abnormal gradient occurs in the left ventricular *outflow* tract, a more proper definition of the timing of the onset of this gradient requires the measurement to be accomplished utilizing the left ventricular outflow tract pressure. This is illustrated in Figure 7.2.7. In the left panel, left ventricular outflow tract (LVOT) and left ventricular inflow tract pressures are recorded simultaneously. The peak of the 'percussion wave' in the LVOT pressure is shown by the converging vertical arrows, and corresponds in time with the onset of the divergence of these two pressures which we define as the onset of the 'abnormal' pressure gradient seen in HCM. The remaining two panels of Figure 7.2.7 illustrate the problems generated when one defines the onset of such a pressure gradient by utilizing the aortic pressure waveform. Even though this signal was recorded using a

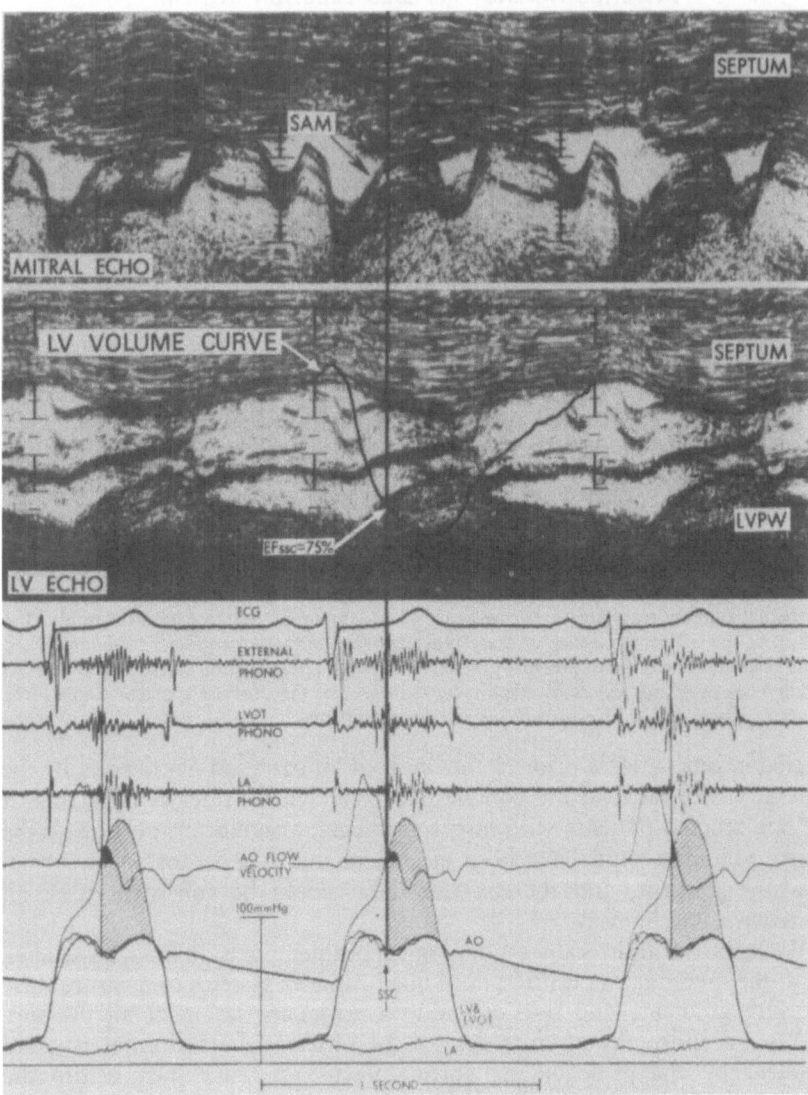

Figure 7.2.8 Haemodynamic–Echocardiographic correlates. Abbreviations: SAM = systolic anterior motion of the mitral valve; LVPW = left ventricular posterior wall. Abbreviations otherwise as in Figure 7.2.1. Shown in the top portion of this figure is an M-mode echocardiogram of the mitral valve demonstrating SAM. This echo was performed simultaneously with the haemodynamic data shown in the bottom portion of this figure. Transseptal and retrograde pressure signals are shown with aortic flow velocity, left atrial and LVOT intracardiac phonocardiograms, an external phonocardiogram and an electrocardiographic signal. Just above the haemodynamic signals is a second M-mode echocardiogram of the left ventricular internal dimensions recorded immediately after the echo of the mitral valve was obtained. An identical R–R interval preceding the middle beat was chosen, and all other haemodynamic parameters were identical. The vertical line in the middle cardiac cycle represents the onset of SAM–septal contact. Note that the majority of aortic flow velocity is completed by this time. A continuous ventricular volume curve was constructed from the digitized dimensions of the middle cardiac cycle. An ejection fraction (EF SSC) of 75% is achieved by the time SAM–septal contact occurs. See text for further discussion

198

micromanometer just above the aortic cusps, the timing of the early peak aortic pressure occurs later than that of the LVOT pressure. In this particular example, this difference is 45 ms, as shown in the right panel of Figure 7.2.7. If one adds the delays intrinsic to fluid-filled catheter manometer systems, it is clear that significant errors can be made in defining the temporal onset of this abnormal pressure gradient.

We have recently completed a study of eight patients utilizing the multisensor catheterization techniques described above with *simultaneous* echocardiography in the cardiac catheterization laboratory. An example is shown in Figure 7.2.8. The echocardiogram of the mitral valve demonstrating systolic anterior motion was performed simultaneously with the pressure, flow and phonocardiographic signals shown in conjunction with this echo. In addition, an echocardiogram of the septum and posterior left ventricular wall just below the level of the mitral valve apparatus was performed immediately after the echocardiographic recording of SAM. Cardiac cycles with R–R intervals varying no more than 2% were matched to the original echocardiogram illustrating SAM and photographically mounted together as shown in Figure 7.2.8. First, it is clear that an abnormal pressure gradient is developed much earlier than SAM–septal contact. In this example, the pressure gradient already developed at SAM–septal contact is 50 mmHg. The peak-to-peak gradient associated with this beat is 80 mmHg and, more importantly from a haemodynamic standpoint, the peak instantaneous gradient developed exceeds 90 mmHg. Yet, despite what would be interpreted by others as 'significant obstruction', the aortic flow velocity signal demonstrates that greater than 90% of the forward stroke volume is completed *prior* to SAM–septal contact. Ventricular emptying was examined by digitizing the septum and the posterior wall of the left ventricular echocardiogram and, utilizing the algorithm described by Teichholz et al.[38], a ventricular volume as a function of time was computed and displayed superimposed on the left ventricular echocardiogram. By the time SAM–septal contact occurred, the left ventricle achieved an ejection fraction of 75% out of a total ejection fraction of 92%. The residual ejected volume may represent mitral regurgitation, a combination of mitral regurgitation and insignificant forward flow across the LVOT, a change in shape rather than volume, or a combination of all three mechanisms. Most importantly, no *significant* forward stroke volume is ejected 'against an obstruction', and the ventricle has achieved a normal or supernormal ejection fraction by the time SAM–septal contact occurs.

In the example given in Figure 7.2.8, left atrial and LVOT intracardiac phonocardiograms were derived from the pressure sensors and compared to an external phonocardiogram obtained from an external microphone at the lower left sternal border. All phonocardiograms utilized identical amplifiers with a band pass frequency response of 50–500 Hz. Note that in early systole, through most of the forward flow duration as demonstrated by the aortic flow velocity signal, little murmur is generated until just before SAM–septal contact when a murmur of short duration is generated in the LVOT. After SAM–septal contact, the murmur in the LVOT diminished greatly,

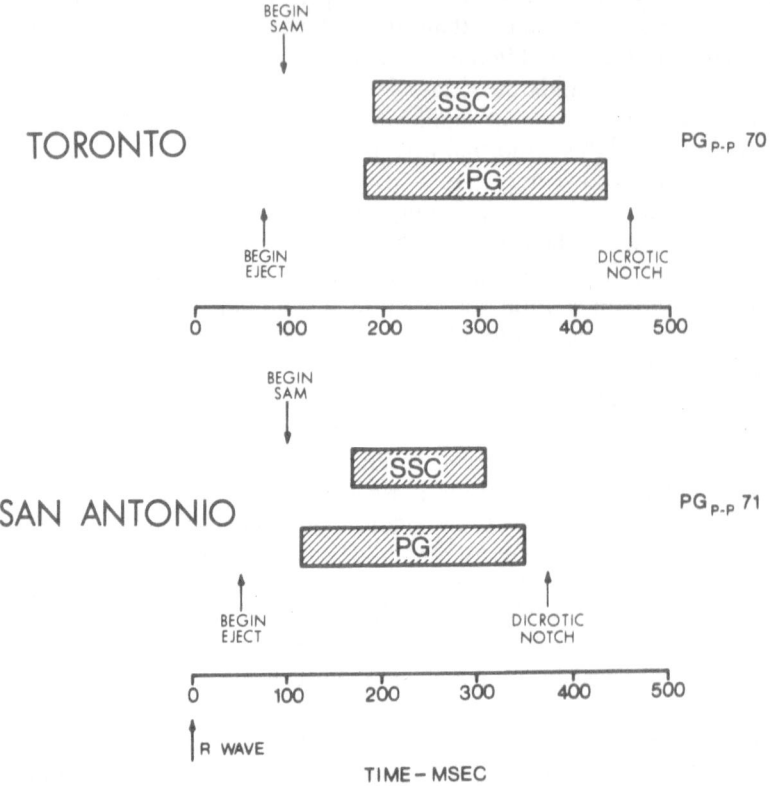

Figure 7.2.9 Temporal relationships of SAM–septal contact and the intraventricular gradient. **PG** = pressure gradient; **PG**$_{pp}$ = peak-to-peak pressure gradient. In the bottom portion of this figure, averaged data from eight patients reveals that the intraventricular pressure gradient begins well before SAM–septal contact. This is in contrast to data reported by Pollick *et al*.[35] reproduced in the top portion. See text for discussion

whereas another murmur appears in the left atrium as a result of mitral regurgitation. Accordingly, the majority of the murmur demonstrated in the external phonocardiogram may be the result of mitral regurgitation which is consistent with the findings of others[39,40]. On angiography, this patient had a trace of mitral regurgitation during normal sinus rhythm. Furthermore, the left atrial 'v' waves are normal in amplitude and the patient's left atrial size was within normal limits. Thus, the mitral regurgitation was haemodynamically insignificant, even though the majority of the murmur recorded on the external phonocardiogram appears to be due to mitral regurgitation.

The preceding methods were utilized to examine the relationship between pressure gradient and stroke volume in all eight patients, who represent a group with substantial intraventricular pressure gradients. The average peak-to-peak gradient was 71 mmHg, and the average peak instantaneous gradient was 85 mmHg. The gradients in this group of patients matched the average gradients in the cases reported by Pollick *et al.*[36]. The lower portion of Figure 7.2.9 illustrates the results obtained in these eight patients. The timing obtained for the onset of SAM, SAM–septal contact, and the duration of SAM was compared to the onset of the pressure gradient as defined above, and the duration of the pressure gradient. These parameters are temporally plotted in relationship to the peak of the R wave, the onset of ejection, and the aortic dicrotic notch. These results were purposely displayed in a format identical to that published by Pollick *et al.*[36] in order to compare our data with those published from their laboratory. Reproduced above our results are those obtained from the six patients they studied at the time of cardiac catheterization. The most significant difference between these two studies is the temporal relationship between the onset of the pressure gradient and SAM–septal contact. While Pollick *et al.* concluded that the pressure gradient began virtually simultaneously with SAM–septal contact, our study reveals that an abnormal pressure gradient begins well before SAM–septal contact. For the group, the instantaneous pressure gradient already developed at SAM–septal contact averaged 68 mmHg. Note that in the studies from both institutions, SAM–septal contact also ends considerably before the termination of the pressure gradient. The fact that the onset and termination of SAM–septal contact is not coincident with the onset and termination of the pressure gradient makes a direct cause-and-effect relationship between these two parameters more difficult to substantiate. While left ventricular internal dimensions shorten somewhat after SAM–septal contact, the volume change between SAM–septal contact and the end of systole is small. Furthermore, any residual ejection by the ventricle in this portion of systole is divided by some undetermined ratio between flow through the outflow tract and regurgitant flow into the left atrium. Indeed, mitral regurgitation may provide an 'escape' mechanism, so that only a negligible, if any, amount of residual volume left in the ventricle is ejected through the LVOT.

SIMULTANEOUS HAEMODYNAMIC AND ANGIOGRAPHIC STUDIES

A similar investigation of the relationships between pressure, flow, ventricular dimensions and mitral valve motion was made on four of the eight patients, utilizing simultaneous biplane ventriculography with multisensor pressure and flow signals. After the echocardiographic studies described above were completed, the transseptal multisensor catheter was removed and replaced with an angiographic catheter. However, the retrograde catheter remained in place in order to measure pressures in the left ventricular cavity, LVOT and ascending aorta. This approach also allowed for the measurement of ascending aortic flow velocity and selected phonocardiograms during the angiography. In order to best delineate the shape, size and dynamics of ventricular emptying, new angulations of the X-ray gantry system were utilized. In the transverse planes, a standard 30° RAO and 60° LAO projection was first obtained. This was then combined with a

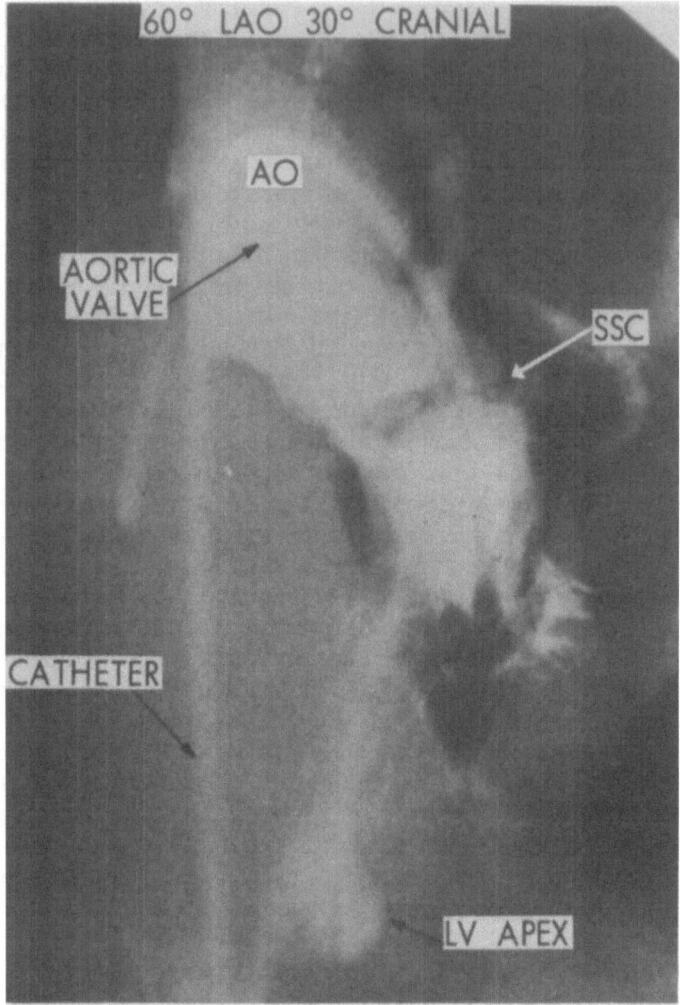

Figure 7.2.10 Angiocardiographic identification of SAM–septal contact. A 30° left anterior oblique projection with 30° of cranial-caudal angulation was utilized for angiographic visualization of SAM. Utilizing this view facilitated the tracking of SAM from its onset to SAM–septal contact. Abbreviations as in Figures 7.2.1 and 7.2.7. See text for discussion

cranial-caudal angulation of 30–35° in the LAO position, and a caudal-cranial angulation of 30–35° in the RAO position. These angulations provided significant advantages in elongating the left ventricle in the LAO view, and also provided greatly improved resolution and visualization of the mitral valve apparatus and its associated SAM during left ventriculography. Figure 7.2.10 illustrates a selected frame from a left anterior oblique projection with 30° cranial-caudal angulation at the time of SAM–septal contact.

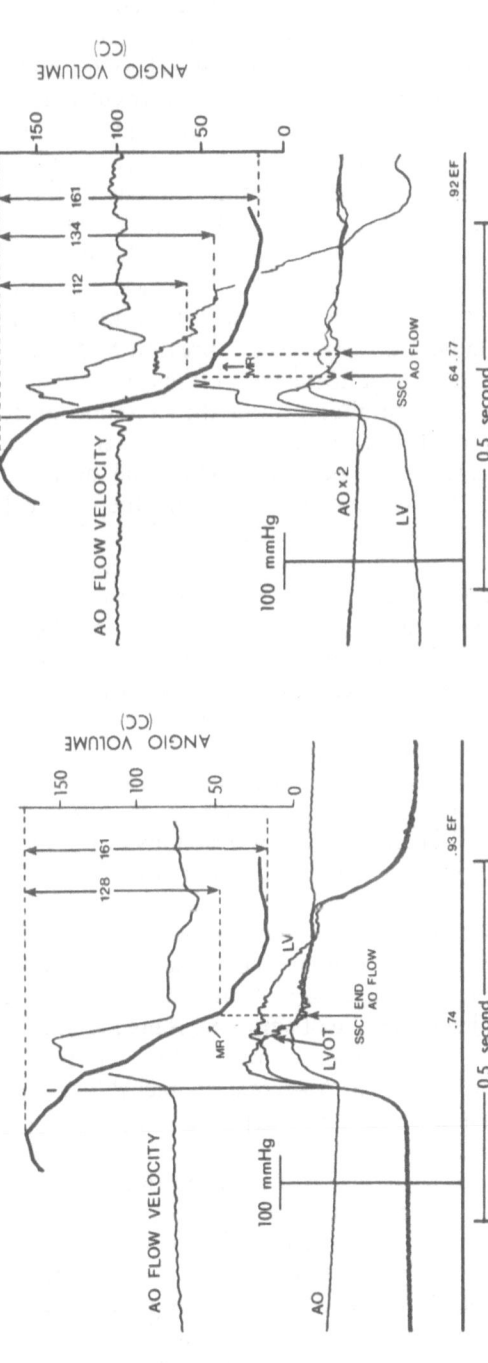

Figure 7.2.11 Simultaneous haemodynamic data obtained during ventriculography. MR = mitral regurgitation. Other abbreviations as in Figure 7.2.1. The left panel demonstrates a cardiac cycle with a maximum gradient of only 20 mmHg. After isoproterenol infusion, a gradient of 90 mmHg was generated, as shown in the right panel. Angiographic emptying curves were obtained for each of these beats by analysis of frame-by-frame angiography. See text for discussion

Using these techniques, dynamic emptying of the left ventricle was analysed while simultaneously obtaining pressure-flow data in four patients. Figure 7.2.11 illustrates data selected from the patient with the lowest resting intraventricular gradient (left panel), who underwent isoproterenol infusion to stimulate a larger intraventricular gradient (right panel). Left ventricular pressure, LVOT pressure and aortic pressure are shown in conjunction with ascending aortic flow velocity and the dynamic emptying curve derived from frame-by-frame analysis of the angiogram. Identified in each beat are the times of SAM–septal contact, the onset of mitral regurgitation, and the cessation of aortic flow. In addition, the stroke volumes at the time of SAM–septal contact, cessation of aortic flow, and end-systole are shown. In the non-provoked beat in the left panel, a maximum pressure gradient of 20 mmHg is present. SAM–septal contact occurs 100 ms after the onset of aortic ejection and is virtually coincident with the onset of mitral regurgitation and the cessation of aortic flow. However, by this time, the ventricle has already achieved an ejection fraction of 74%, similar to the echocardiographic value shown in a different patient in Figure 7.2.8. In the remainder of systole, the ventricular volume decreases by approximately another 30 cc. In the right panel, during isoproterenol infusion, a peak instantaneous gradient of 90 mmHg is generated. SAM–septal contact occurs 52 ms after the onset of systole, closely followed by the onset of mitral regurgitation and the cessation of aortic flow. The ventricular volume at the time of SAM–septal contact, onset of mitral regurgitation and cessation of aortic flow is nearly identical to that of the non-provoked beat. Both beats had identical left ventricular ejection times since the non-provoked beat was at a slower heart rate and the provoked beat was a post-PVC beat during isoproterenol infusion. Despite a much larger gradient and an earlier appearance of SAM–septal contact in the provoked beat, the ejection fractions at the time of SAM–septal contact in these two beats are both within or above accepted normal end-systolic values.

Figure 7.2.12 superimposes the two emptying curves. End-diastolic and end-systolic volumes in both beats are nearly identical, with both beats achieving overall ejection fractions of 92% and 93%. Yet, in the beat with the large pressure gradient, the rate of emptying is greater and, even though SAM–septal contact occurs earlier in the systolic ejection period, the amount ejected by the time of SAM–septal contact differs only by a few millilitres. While a residual volume of approximately 30 cc was yet to be ejected after SAM–septal contact in both beats, the beat with the larger pressure gradient did not result in a greater proportion of the stroke volume ejected after SAM–septal contact. These observations provide another argument against larger pressure gradients signifying 'more severe obstruction'. The data independently derived in the laboratory of Criley and Siegel, and presented in Chapter 7.1, reveal similar angiographic findings between beats with small pressure gradients and beats with large pressure gradients. The paradox is that a larger pressure gradient is associated within more *rapid* emptying rather than *slower* emptying.

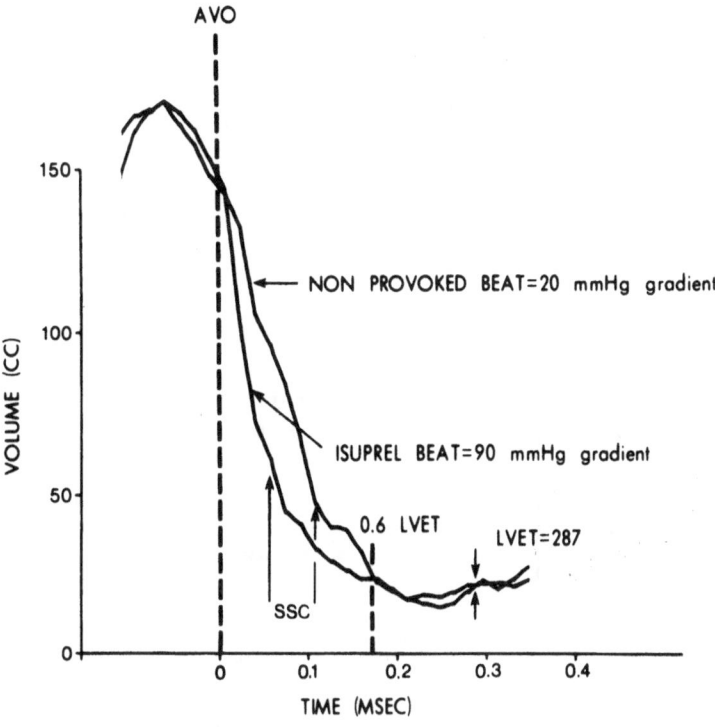

Figure 7.2.12 Superimposed angiographic emptying curves from the two cardiac cycles shown in Figure 7.2.11. AVO = aortic valve opening. The angiographic emptying curve in the beat with the 90 mmHg gradient reveals faster emptying than the beat with a 20 mmHg gradient. See text for discussion

Combining data obtained from aortic flow velocity with ventricular emptying characteristics obtained from both echocardiography and angiography, Figure 7.2.13 illustrates the relationships between the magnitude of pressure gradients generated within the left ventricle and the percentage of stroke volume that is ejected at the time of SAM–septal contact. The data shown are derived from all three techniques. Some small gradients were chosen purposefully to allow a comparison to larger gradients. An average of 80% of the forward stroke volume is ejected prior to SAM–septal contact in these patients, no matter what the magnitude of the pressure gradient. Similar results (not shown) were obtained when analysing the average ejection fraction at the time of SAM–septal contact, which equalled or exceeded the accepted norm for end-systolic values in patients without HCM[41]. These data are critical to an understanding of the relationship of ejection characteristics in HCM ventricles with respect to the magnitude of pressure gradients. This is in marked contrast to what was speculated by Pollick *et al.*[37] Since those investigators did not measure flow or derive any index of ventricular emptying from echocardiographic or angiographic data, they erroneously speculated that increased pressure gradients would cause a greater percentage of the forward stroke volume to

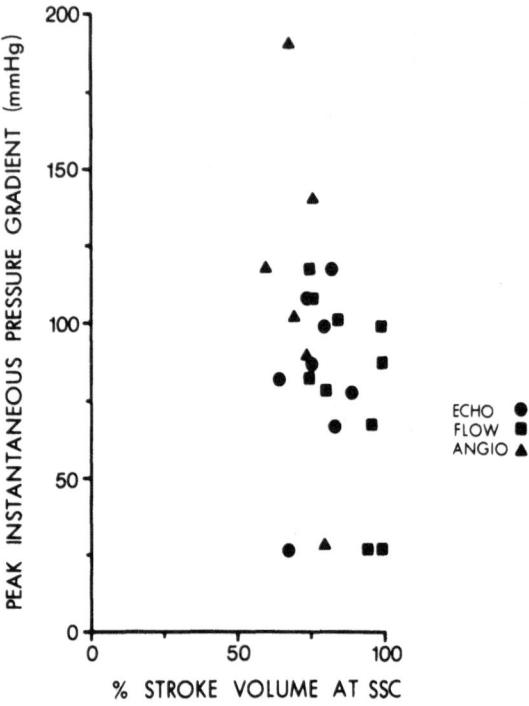

Figure 7.2.13 Relationship between pressure gradient and the per cent stroke volume ejected by SAM–septal contact (**SSC**). Data obtained from echocardiographic (circles), flow velocity (squares), and angiographic (triangles) techniques reveal an average of 80 ± 12% of the stroke volume is ejected independent of the magnitude of the developed intraventricular pressure gradient by the time SAM–septal contact occurs. See text for discussion

occur after SAM–septal contact. Our results demonstrate that this does not occur. These points are further emphasized in the final figure examining the haemodynamic effects of a premature ventricular contraction in HCM.

PVC HAEMODYNAMICS

In Figure 7.2.14, the effects of a premature ventricular contraction on simultaneous pressure, flow velocity and phonocardiographic events are shown. In the pre-PVC beat, a stroke volume of 88 cc is ejected and associated with an aortic pulse pressure of 35 mmHg. This beat would ordinarily be considered to represent a significant 'obstruction' since the instantaneous gradient exceeds 100 mmHg. Yet, the stroke volume is ejected prior to SAM–septal contact, highlighted by the vertical straight line. SAM–septal contact was determined from a simultaneous echocardiogram but, while not shown in Figure 7.2.14, is indirectly confirmed by its 'landmarks' on the left atrial pressure, LVOT pressure, and the coincident onset of mitral regurgitation in the left atrial phonocardiogram. After the premature ventricular contraction, an augmented sinus beat develops a peak instantaneous gradient of approximately 175 mmHg. SAM–septal contact

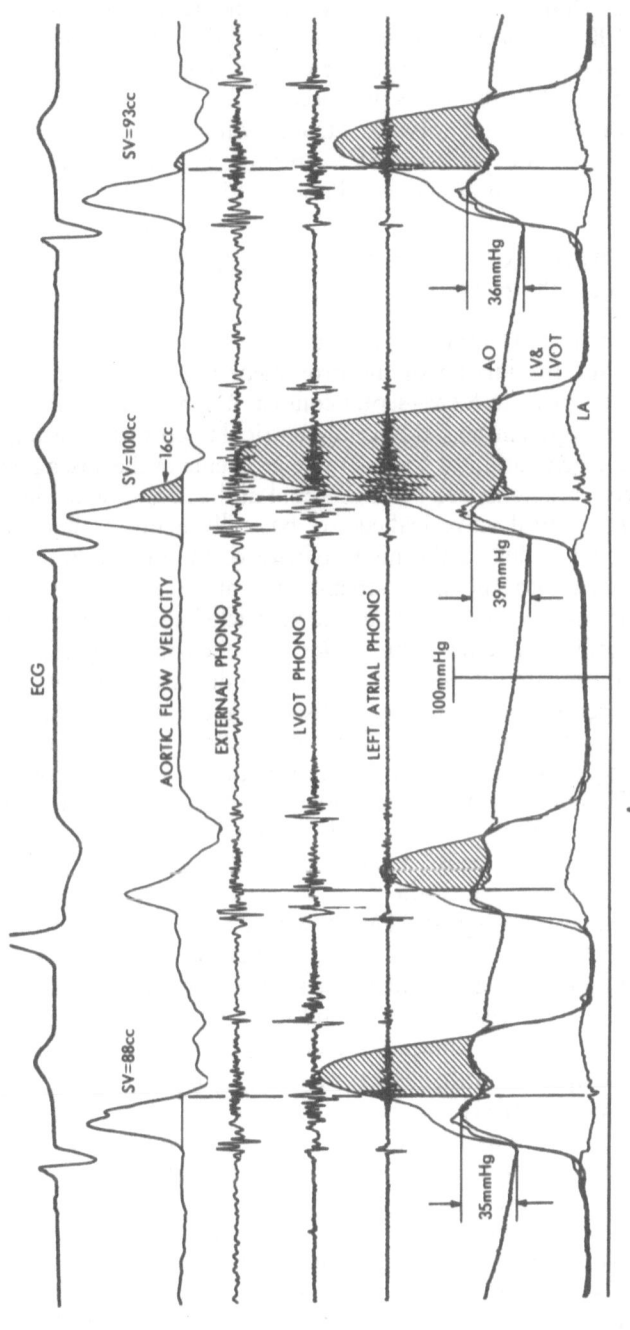

Figure 7.2.14 Effects of a premature ventricular contraction on haemodynamics in HCM. SV=stroke volume. Other abbreviations as in Figure 7.2.1. The second cardiac cycle in this illustration is a premature ventricular contraction following a sinus beat with a stroke volume of 88cc and an aortic pulse pressure of 35mmHg. The augmented sinus beat following the PVC generates a stroke volume of 100cc and associated aortic pulse of 39mmHg. This stroke volume is greater than the pre-PVC or post-augmented beat stroke volume, despite the presence of an intraventricular gradient of 175mmHg. See text for discussion

occurs earlier in the systolic ejection period and a greatly augmented murmur appears externally, in the outflow tract and in the left atrial phonocardiograms. Despite the marked increase in pressure gradient, a stroke volume of 100 cc is ejected and is associated with a pulse pressure of 39 mmHg. This observation is not consistent with the concept of increased obstruction during post-PVC beats, as proposed by Brockenbrough et al.[42]. While a small portion of the forward stroke volume is ejected after SAM–septal contact in the presence of a pressure gradient, this small portion is only 16% of the total stroke volume in this example.

POTENTIAL MECHANISMS FOR THE GENERATION OF PRESSURE GRADIENTS IN HCM

Given the evidence provided by these studies, two separate mechanisms may be responsible for the production of the prominent intraventricular gradients in HCM. First, prior to SAM–septal contact, a combination of high ejection velocity development and abnormal ventricular geometry peculiar to HCM leads to the generation of considerable gradients in the absence of an obstruction; these gradients are due to inertial and convective acceleration factors[43,44]. The mitral valve leaflets are basically neutrally buoyant structures and, probably due to the high velocity of blood flow in early systole, are entrained into the flow stream and move anteriorly until SAM–septal contact occurs. At this point, the ventricle has already ejected the majority of its contents and has achieved low systolic volumes no matter what magnitude of pressure gradient develops. Secondly, after SAM–septal contact occurs, the ventricle almost becomes 'isovolumic' and a *dissociation* of pressure and flow appears to occur. That is, the late systolic gradient which arises after SAM–septal contact may not be due to residual ejection through the LVOT, since mitral regurgitation may be responsible for the small changes in volume occurring in late systole. While small, insignificant amounts of forward flow may exist, as demonstrated by residual turbulent fluctuations in the LVOT phonocardiogram, observations of simultaneous *changes* in flow velocity through the LVOT with *changes* in the pressure gradient across the LVOT after SAM–septal contact do not seem to be consistent with an 'unchanging obstruction' suggested by the M-mode display of the mitral valve between the onset and termination of SAM–septal contact. However, M-mode techniques do not reveal what is happening in three-dimensional space and this aspect of LVOT geometry, along with measurements of LVOT flow velocity, is needed to further clarify this issue. The doppler techniques used by Yock et al.[30] to assess LV and LVOT velocities during systole may reveal that there is an *association* of the late systolic pressure gradients to increases in LVOT velocity but, as mentioned above, these studies also reveal decreases in overall signal amplitude consistent with decreases in volumetric flow. Thus, the presence of a large pressure gradient after SAM–septal contact is not associated with the movement of a significant amount of volume through the LVOT.

While high late systolic *pressures* within the left ventricle may be metabolically detrimental, to equate the presence of large intraventricular pressure *gradients* with a hindrance to left ventricular ejection is not supported by the data and observations presented here.

CONCLUSIONS

In this chapter, we have summarized the data we believe represent evidence against obstruction to left ventricular ejection in HCM. First, indices of ejection dynamics derived from flow velocity signals, angiographic and echocardiographic ventricular emptying data, and instantaneous impulse gradients across the aortic valve all reveal that ejection in HCM is early, rapid and similar in patients with and without intraventricular pressure gradients. Secondly, a detailed analysis of the timing of SAM yields several important observations inconsistent with an impediment to ejection: the HCM ventricle ejects the majority of its stroke volume and achieves a normal or supernormal ejection fraction by the time SAM–septal contact occurs, independent of the timing of SAM–septal contact and the magnitude of the gradient. Thus, we have shown that the pressure gradients present in HCM do not reflect an impediment or hindrance to left ventricular ejection.

Acknowledgements

The authors would like to acknowledge the invaluable assistance of various members of the Cardiology Service at Brooke Army Medical Center for their assistance in the complex technological studies reported in this chapter: The staff and fellow physicians of the Cardiology Service who, over several years, co-operated in referring patients to this study; Mr Ray Tamez and the technicians of the cardiac catheterization laboratory; Dr Stephen Hoadley for his assistance in performing the echocardiograms at the time of catheterization; Bernard Rubal, PhD, SFC Deo Phillip, SSG Noel Diaz, SP6 Vicki Perez, and SFC Manuel Alamo for their assistance in data processing, photography and graphics; and Ms Bettye Jo Hairston for her typing and editorial assistance. We would also like to express our gratitude to Dr J. Michael Criley, Los Angeles, California, and Dr Charles Mullins, Houston, Texas, for assisting in those catheterizations utilizing transseptal techniques. Finally, our appreciation to Ares Pasipoularides, MD, PhD, for his review and assistance in the theoretical and fluid dynamic aspects of this work.

References

1. Brock, R.C. (1959). Functional obstruction of the left ventricle (acquired aortic subvalvular stenosis). *Guy's Hosp. Rep.*, 106, 221–39
2. Braunwald, E., Morrow, A.G., Cornell, W.P., Aygen, M.M. and Hilbish, T.F. (1960). Idiopathic hypertrophic subaortic stenosis: clinical, hemodynamic and angiographic manifestations. *Am. J. Med.*, 29, 924–35
3. Wigle, E.D., Auger, P. and Marquis, Y. (1966). Muscular subaortic stenosis. The initial left ventricular inflow tract pressure as evidence of outflow trace obstruction. *Can. Med. Assoc. J.*, 95, 793–7

4. Ross, J. Jr., Braunwald, E., Gault, J.H., Mason, D.T. and Morrow, A.G. (1966). The mechanism of the intraventricular pressure gradient in idiopathic hypertrophic subaortic stenosis. *Circulation*, **34**, 558–78

5. Shah, P.M., Gramiak, C.E. and Kramer, D.H. (1969). Ultrasound localization of left ventricular outflow obstruction in hypertrophic obstructive cardiomyopathy. *Circulation*, **40**, 3–11

6. Henry, W.L., Clark, C.E., Griffith, J.M. and Epstein, S.E. (1975). Mechanism of left ventricular outflow obstruction in patients with obstructive asymmetric septal hypertrophy (idiopathic hypertrophic subaortic stenosis). *Am. J. Cardiol.*, **35**, 337–45

7. Frank, S. and Braunwald, E. (1968). Idiopathic hypertrophic subaortic stenosis. Clinical analysis of 126 patients with emphasis on the natural history. *Circulation*, **37**, 759–88

8. Reis, R.L., Hannah, H., Carley, J.E. and Pugh, D.M. (1977). Surgical treatment of idiopathic hypertrophic subaortic stenosis (IHSS). *Circulation*, **56** (Suppl. II), II–128–32

9. Criley, J.M., Lewis, K.B., White, R.I. Jr. and Ross, R.S. (1965). Pressure gradients without obstruction. A new concept of 'hypertrophic subaortic stenosis'. *Circulation*, **32**, 881–7

10. Wilson, W.S., Criley, J.M. and Ross, R.S. (1967). Dynamics of left ventricular emptying in hypertrophic subaortic stenosis: a cineangiographic and hemodynamic study. *Am. Heart J.*, **73**, 4–16

11. Murgo, J.P., Alter, B.R., Dorethy, J.F., Altobelli, S.A. and McGranahan, G.M. Jr. (1980). Dynamics of left ventricular ejection in obstructive and nonobstructive hypertrophic cardiomyopathy. *J. Clin. Invest.*, **66**, 1369–82

12. Goodwin, J.F. The frontiers of cardiomyopathy. *Br. Heart J.*, **48**, 1–18

13. Criley, J.M., Lennon, P.A., Abbasi, A.S. and Blaufuss, A.H. (1976). Hypertrophic cardiomyopathy. Clinical cardiovascular physiology. In Levine, H.J. (ed.) *Clinical Cardiovascular Physiology*. pp. 771–828. (New York: Grune and Stratton)

14. Bulkley, B.H. (1977). Idiopathic hypertrophic subaortic stenosis afflicted: idols of the cave and the marketplace. *Am. J. Cardiol.*, **40**, 476–9

15. Goodwin, J.F. (1980). Hypertrophic cardiomyopathy: a disease in search of its own identity. *Am. J. Cardiol.*, **45**, 177–80

16. Goodwin, J.F. (1980). An appreciation of hypertrophic cardiomyopathy. *Am. J. Med.*, **68**, 797–800

17. Canedo, J.I. and Frank, M.J. (1981). Therapy of hypertrophic cardiomyopathy: medical or surgical? Clinical and pathophysiologic considerations. *Am. J. Cardiol.*, **48**, 383–8

18. Murgo, J.P. (1982). Does outflow obstruction exist in hypertrophic cardiomyopathy? *N. Engl. J. Med.*, **307**, 1008–9

19. Shabetai, R. (1983). Cardiomyopathy: How far have we come in 25 years, how far yet to go? *J. Am. Coll. Cardiol.*, **1**, 253–63

20. Hernandez, R.R., Greenfield, J.R. Jr. and McCall, B.W. (1964). Pressure-flow studies in hypertrophic subaortic stenosis. *J. Clin. Invest.*, **34**, 401

21. Dry, D.L. (1959). The measurement of pulsatile blood flow by the computed pressure gradient technique. *Instit. Radio Engineers, Trans. Med. Electronics*, ME–6, **259**, 264

22. Pierce, G.E., Morrow, A.G. and Braunwald, E. (1964). Idiopathic hypertrophic subaortic stenosis III. *Circulation* **30** (Suppl. 4), 152–74

23. Simon, A.L., Ross, J. Jr. and Gault, J.H. (1967). Angiographic anatomy of the left ventricle and mitral valve in idiopathic hypertrophic subaortic stenosis. *Circulation*, **36**, 852–67

24. Murgo, J.P. (1975). New techniques in cardiac catheterization: the advantages of multisensor catheters. In *Proceedings of the International Conference on Biomedical Transducers*, Paris, France, 41–6. Comité d'Organisation du Collogne de Paris (Nov 1975)

25. Neches, W.H., Mullins, C.E., Williams, R.L., Vargo, T.A. and McNamara, D.G. (1972). Percutaneous sheath cardiac catheterization. *Am. J. Cardiol.*, **30**, 378–84

26. Nichols, W.W., Pepine, C.J., Conti, C.R., Christie, L.G. and Feldman, R.L. (1980). Evaluation of a new catheter-mounted electromagnetic velocity sensor during cardiac catheterization. *Catheter. Cardiovasc. Diagn.*, **6**, 97–113

27. Seed, W.A. and Wood, N.B. (1971). Velocity patterns in the aorta. *Cardiovasc. Res.*, **5**, 318–30

28. Gardin, J.M., Dabestani, A., Glasgow, G.A., Butman, S., Hughes, C., Burn, C. and

Henry, W.L. (1982). Doppler aortic blood flow studies in obstructive and non-obstructive hypertrophic cardiomyopathy. *Circulation*, 66 (Suppl. II), II–267 (Abstr.)

29. Maron, B.J., Gottdiener, J.S., Arce, J., Wesley, Y.E. and Epstein, S.E. (1984). Pulsed doppler aortic flow-velocity and echocardiographic findings in obstructive and non-obstructive hypertrophic cardiomyopathy: evidence of true subaortic obstruction. *J. Am. Coll. Cardiol.*, 3, 619 (Abstr.)

30. Yock, P. Hatle, L., Popp, R. (1985). Patterns and timing of doppler-detected intracavitary and aortic flow in hypertrophic obstructive cardiomyopathy. *J. Am. Coll. Cardiol.*, 5, 395 *(Abstr.)*

31. Kinoshita, N., Nimura, Y., Miyatake, K., Nagata, S., Sakakibara, H., Hayaski, T., Asao, M., Terao, Y. and Matsuo, H. (1978). Studies on flow patterns in the aortic arch in cases with hypertrophic cardiomyopathy using pulsed ultrasonic doppler technique. *J. Cardiogr. (Japan)*, 8, 325–32

32. Sugrue, D.D., McKenna, W.J., Dickie, S., Myers, M.J., Lavender, J.P., Oakley, C.M. and Goodwin, J.F. (1984). Relation of left ventricular gradient and relative stroke volume ejected in early and late systole in HCM: assessment with radionuclide cineangiography. *Br. Heart J.*, 52, 602–609

33. Spencer, J.P. and Greiss, F.C. (1962). Dynamics of ventricular ejection. *Circ. Res.*, 10, 274

34. Murgo, J.P., Altobelli, S.A., Dorethy, J.F., Logsdon, J.R. and McGranahan, G.M. (1975). Normal ventricular ejection dynamics in man during rest and exercise. *Am. Heart Assoc. Monogr.*, 46, 92–101

35. Murgo, J.P., Alter, B.R., Dorethy, J.F. and McGranahan, G.M. (1979). Dynamic aortic valve gradients in hypertrophic cardiomyopathy (HCM). *Circulation*, 60 (Suppl. II), II–604 (Abstr.)

36. Pollick, C., Morgan, C.D., Gilbert, B.W., Rakowski, H. and Wigle, E.D. (1982). Muscular subaortic stenosis: the temporal relationship between systolic anterior motion of the anterior mitral leaflet and the pressure gradient. *Circulation*, 66, 1087–94

37. Pollick, C., Rakowski, H. and Wigle, E.D. (1984). Muscular subaortic stenosis: the quantitative relationship between systolic anterior motion and the pressure gradient. *Circulation*, 69, 43–9

38. Teichholz, L.E., Kreulen, T., Herman, M.V. and Gorlin, R. (1976). Problems in echocardiographic correlations in the presence or absence of asynergy. *Am. J. Cardiol.*, 37, 7–11

39. Harris, A., Donmoyer, T. and Leatham, A. (1969). Physical signs in differential diagnosis of left ventricular obstructive cardiomyopathy. *Br. Heart J.*, 31, 501–10

40. Lindgren, K.M. and Epstein, S.E. (1972). Idiopathic hypertrophic subaortic stenosis with and without mitral regurgitation: phonocardiographic differentiation from rheumatic mitral regurgitation. *Br. Heart J.*, 34, 191–7

41. Miller, J.W., Murgo, J.P., Rubal, B.J., Damore, S. and Duster, M.C. (1984). Integration of the divergent views of obstruction and early systolic ejection in hypertrophic cardiomyopathy (HCM): Hemodynamic (H), Echocardiographic (E) and Angiographic (A) correlates. *Circulation*, 70 (Suppl II), II–17 (Abstr.)

42. Brockenbrough, E.C., Braunwald, E. and Morrow, A.G. (1961). Hemodynamic technic for the detection of hypertrophic subaortic stenosis. *Circulation*, 23, 189–94

43. Pasipoularides, A., Murgo, J.P., Bird, J.J. and Craig, W.E. (1984). Fluid dynamics of aortic stenosis. Mechanisms for the presence of subvalvular pressure gradients. *Am. J. Physiol.*, 246, H542–50

44. Pasipoularides, A., Miller, J., Rubal, B.J. and Murgo, J.P. (1984). Left ventricular (LV) ejection pressure gradients in normal man are determined by geometry, wall kinematics and velocity patterns. *Circulation*, 70 (Suppl II), II–354

7.3
Evidence for the importance of obstruction in hypertrophic cardiomyopathy

H. KUHN

The vast majority of publications on hypertrophic cardiomyopathies make no clearcut distinction between the obstructive (HOCM) and non-obstructive (HNCM) form of hypertrophic cardiomyopathies. This is because many authors believe that there are no definite differences. However, this opinion cannot be maintained any longer in view of fundamental findings and unresolved problems as reported in recent publications. These concern the genetic basis, the pathology, the pathophysiology, the diagnosis, the treatment and the prognosis of the diseases in both subsets. The importance of obstruction in hypertrophic cardiomyopathies is based on the fact that the primary distinction between patients with and without left ventricular systolic pressure difference leads to two different myocardial disease entities.

1. THE GENETIC BASIS

Both forms may be genetically transmitted. However, apparently the prevalence of relatives presenting the full clinical picture of the disease or presenting only echocardiographic changes (asymmetric septal hypertrophy) is significantly higher in patients with HOCM[1]. In addition, in our experience, both forms have not occurred together in one family with hypertrophic cardiomyopathy and, according to other authors, only very rarely[2,3]. The same holds true for the clinical course, which shows a change from one form to the other only in rare instances, and never in our own experience[4-6].

2. PATHOLOGY AND VENTRICULOGRAPHIC PATTERNS

Whereas the disarray of myofibres predominantly occurs in the intra-ventricular septum in HOCM, the free wall of the ventricles seems to be affected in addition in HNCM[7]. It should also be noted that concentric left ventricular hypertrophy (absence of asymmetric septal hypertrophy) may be found sometimes, but only in the non-obstructive type, whereas in the

213

obstructive type asymmetric septal hypertrophy is always seen[1,2,9]. This is true at least for the typical subaortic type of HOCM. The situation may be somewhat different in atypical midventricular HOCM[4].

At the gross anatomical level, the shape of the left ventricle may be different in the two types of hypertrophic cardiomyopathy. This may be concluded from ventriculographic studies (though, no gross anatomical or ventriculographic postmortem correlations have been performed[8]) which reveal a completely different left ventricular shape in more than 90% of patients with HNCM compared to that observed in HOCM. A so-called 'funnel' or 'spade-like' shape of the left ventricle in diastole, with apical obliteration of the left ventricular cavity, is seen only in HNCM[2,4,9].

3. PATHOPHYSIOLOGY

In both forms of hypertrophic cardiomyopathy, reduced ventricular compliance (distensibility) plays an important pathophysiological role. However, in some patients (because of selection criteria) a left ventricular outflow tract pressure difference (synonym: obstruction) at rest or after provocation is found in patients with HOCM, leading to increased afterload. This is not the case in HNCM, in which no pressure difference is present at rest, or on provocation. Recently, Murgo et al. investigated ejection dynamics in HOCM and HNCM and found nearly identical flow patterns and ejection characteristics (in particular ejection time was nearly identical)[10]. Therefore they concluded that obstruction plays no pathophysiological role and that no distinction should be made between the obstructive and the non-obstructive form. Furthermore, because of these conclusions, they have not referred any patient to the surgeon for myectomy[11]. In the meantime, these results have not been confirmed by other authors using different investigative techniques[12,13]. It should also be emphasized that identical experimental findings (e.g. ejection times) in both forms of hypertrophic cardiomyopathy as described by Murgo and co-workers may not imply the same aetiological origin of the findings.

4. THE DIAGNOSIS

As with the haemodynamic and ventriculographic observations so the results from echocardiographic, electrocardiographic and morphological studies in HOCM and HNCM have very different diagnostic profiles.

Besides the absence of systolic intraventricular pressure difference and the characteristic ventricular shape (funnel or spade-like deformation of the apical part of the left ventricle in diastole and systole (see pathology)[2,9] the diagnostic criteria of HNCM as compared to HOCM include a high incidence of syncope, a loud systolic murmur at rest or after exercise, a high incidence of abnormal symmetric negative T—waves in the ECG, the absence of a spike and dome form of the carotid pulse tracing and, in rare cases, concentric left ventricular hypertrophy[4]. Because the ventriculographic and echocardiographic picture of HNCM is also found in patients with myocardial storage disease (Fabry's disease, amyloid heart disease) endomyocardial catheter biopsy seems to be necessary for the definitive diagnosis of HNCM to exclude concealed myocardial storage disease (prevalence about 15%)[4].

5. TREATMENT AND PROGNOSIS

In patients with typical subaortic HOCM, both medical and surgical therapy and the evaluation of prognosis are based on fairly well established data[6,11,14-21]. However, therapeutic and prognostic knowledge of HNCM is rather scanty[2,5,6,14]. Insufficient data are available to prove the efficacy of any therapeutic approach (administration of beta-blockers, verapamil or antiarrhythmics) in this subset of hypertrophic cardiomyopathies and the same is true for the atypical midventricular HOCM.

6. CONCLUSION

From these comparative findings it may be concluded that a clear distinction must be made between the obstructive and the non-obstructive form of hypertrophic cardiomyopathy.

References

1. Köhler, E., Thurow, J., Kuhn, H., Neuhaus, C.H., Bluschke, V. and Bosilj, M. (1979). Klinische und echokardiographische Untersuchungen zur familiären Verbreitung der hypertrophisch obstruktiven (HOCM) und hypertrophisch nicht obstruktiven (HNCM) Kardiomyopathie. Z. Kardiol., 68, 511
2. Kuhn, H., Thelen, U., Köhler, E. and Lösse, B. (1980). Die hypertrophische nicht obstruktive Kardiomyopathie (HNCM) – klinische, hämodynamische, elektro-, echo- und angiokardiographische Untersuchungen. Z. Kardiol., 69, 457–69
3. Yamaguchi, H., Nishijama, S., Naganishi, S. and Nishimura, S. (1983). Electrocardiographic, echocardiographic and ventriculographic characterization of hypertrophic non obstructive cardiomyopathy. Eur. Heart J., 4, Suppl F, 105–19
4. Kuhn, H., Mercier, J., Köhler, E., Frenzel, H., Hort, W. and Loogen, F. (1983). Differential diagnosis of hypertrophic cardiomyopathies: Typical (subaortic) hypertrophic obstructive cardiomyopathy, atypical (mid-ventricular) hypertrophic obstructive cardiomyopathy and hypertrophic non obstructive cardiomyopathy. Eur. Heart J., 4, Suppl F, 93–104
5. Kawai, C., Sakurai, T., Fujiwara, H., Matsumori, A., and Yui, I. (1983). Hypertrophic obstructive and non-obstructive cardiomyopathy in Japan. Diagnosis of the disease with special reference to endomyocardial catheter biopsy. Eur. Heart J., 4, Suppl F, 121–5
6. Kogan, Y., Itaya, K. and Toshima, H. (1984). Prognosis in hypertrophic cardiomyopathy. Am. Heart J., 108, 351–59
7. Maron, B.J., Ferrans, V.J., Henry, W.L., Clark, C.E., Redwood, D.R., Roberts, W.C., Morrow, A.G. and Epstein, S.E. (1974). Differences in distribution of myocardial abnormalities in patients with obstructive and non obstructive asymmetric septal hypertrophy (ASH): Light- and electronmicroscopic findings. Circulation, 50, 436
8. Olsen, E.G.J. (1983). Anatomic and lightmicroscopic characterization of hypertrophic and non-obstructive cardiomyopathy. Eur. Heart J., 4, Suppl F, 1–8
9. Yamaguchi, H., Ishimura, T., Nishijama, S., Nasasaki, F., Naganishi, S., Tagatsu, F., Nishijo, T., Umeda, T. and Machii, K. (1979). Hypertrophic non obstructive cardiomyopathy with giant negative T waves (apical hypertrophy) Ventriculographic and echocardiographic features in 30 patients. Am. J. Cardiol., 44, 401

10. Murgo, J.P., Alter, B.R., Dorethy, J.F., Altobelli, S. A. and McGranahan, G.M. Jr. (1980). Dynamics of left ventricular ejection in obstructive and non obstructive hypertrophic cardiomyopathy. *J. Clin. Invest.*, 66, 1369–82

11. Binet, J.P., David, P.H. and Piot, J.D. (1983). Surgical treatment of hypertrophic obstructive cardiomyopathies. *Eur. Heart J.*, 4, Suppl F, 191–5

12. Gardin, J.M., Dabestani, A., Glasgow, G.A., Butman, S., Hughes, C., Burn, C. and Henry, W.L. (1982). Doppler aortic bloodflow studies in obstructive and non-obstructive hypertrophic cardiomyopathy. *Circulation*, 66, II/267

13. Jenni, R., Ruffmann, K., Vieli, A., Anliker, M. and Krayenbühl, H.P. (1984). Aortic flow in hypertrophic cardiomyopathy. *Eur. Heart J.*, 5, Suppl I, 232

14. Loogen, F., Kuhn, H., Gietzen, F., Lösse, B., Schulte, H.D. and Bircks, W. (1983). Clinical course and prognosis of patients with typical and atypical hypertrophic obstructive and with hypertrophic non-obstructive cardiomyopathy. *Eur. Heart J.*, 4, Suppl F, 145–53

15. Kober, E., Schmidt-Moritz, A., Hopf, R. and Kaltenbach, M. (1983). Long term treatment of hypertrophic obstructive cardiomyopathy – usefulness of Verapamil. *Eur. Heart J.*, 4, Suppl F, 165–74

16. Maron, B.J., Epstein, S.E. and Morrow, A.G. (1983). Symptomatic status and prognosis of patients after operation for hypertrophic obstructive cardiomyopathy: Efficacy of ventricular septal myotomy and myectomy. *Eur. Heart J.*, 4, Suppl F, 175–85

17. Frank, M.J., Abdulla, A.M., Watkins, L.O., Prisant, L. and Stefaduros, M.A. (1983). Long term medical management of hypertrophic cardiomyopathy: Usefulness of Propranolol. *Eur. Heart J.*, 4, Suppl F, 155–64

18. Lösse, B., Kuhn, H., Loogen, F. and Schulte, H.D. (1983). Exercise performance in hypertrophic cardiomyopathies. *Eur. Heart J.*, 4, Suppl F, 197–208

19. Goodwin, J.F. and Oakley, C.M. (1983) Medical and surgical treatment of hypertrophic cardiomyopathy. *Eur. Heart J.*, 4, Suppl F, 209–14

20. Rothlin, M.E., Gobet, D., Haberer, T., Krayenbühl, H.P., Turina, M. and Senning, A. (1983). Surgical treatment versus medical treatment in hypertrophic obstructive cardiomyopathy. *Eur. Heart J.*, 4, Suppl F, 215–23

21. McKenna, W.J. (1983). Arrhythmia and prognosis in hypertrophic cardiomyopathy. *Eur. Heart J.*, 4, Suppl F, 225–34

7.4
Muscular subaortic stenosis (hypertrophic obstructive cardiomyopathy): the evidence for obstruction to left ventricular outflow

E.D. WIGLE, M. HENDERSON, Z. SASSON, C. POLLICK and
H. RAKOWSKI

INTRODUCTION

Types of hypertrophic cardiomyopathy

Hypertrophic cardiomyopathy is an idiopathic form of cardiac hypertrophy, that is usually associated with myocardial fibre disarray, and may involve either the left and/or the right ventricle. In this discussion, we will concern ourselves only with left ventricular involvement. The hypertrophic process in the left ventricle may be asymmetric or symmetric (concentric) as shown in Table 7.4.1, which also indicate the approximate incidence of the

Table 7.4.1   Types of hypertrophic cardiomyopathy

	Approximate incidence
1. Teare's disease (ventricular septal hypertrophy – 50% cases also have anterolateral wall involvement)	95%
2. Asymmetric apical hypertrophy	<3%
3. Midventricular hypertrophy	<1%
4. Posteroseptal and/or lateral wall hypertrophy	<1%
5. Concentric hypertrophy	<1%

various forms of hypertrophic cardiomyopathy in our experience of some 400 cases. It is quite evident that the vast majority of our experience has to do with that variety of hypertrophic cardiomyopathy described by Teare as 'asymmetrical hypertrophy of the heart'[1]. We will deal only with this form of the disease in this discussion, as apical, midventricular, and posteroseptal or lateral wall hypertrophy do not cause outflow tract obstruction and concentric hypertrophy does so only rarely.

217

Nomenclature

In dealing with left ventricular outflow tract obstruction in hypertrophic cardiomyopathy, many terms have been used: functional obstruction of the left ventricle[2], idiopathic hypertrophic subaortic stenosis[3], obstructive cardiomyopathy simulating aortic stenosis[4], hypertrophic obstructive cardiomyopathy[5], and muscular subaortic stenosis[6], to name a few. We take all of these terms to be synonymous and in this discussion will use the term we have favoured in the past, 'muscular subaortic stenosis'.

Haemodynamic subgroups

In hypertrophic cardiomyopathy, there are a number of haemodynamic subgroups (Table 7.4.2). Muscular subaortic stenosis at rest is defined as a

Table 7.4.2 Haemodynamic classification of hypertrophic cardiomyopathy

1. Resting muscular subaortic stenosis
2. Labile muscular subaortic stenosis
3. Latent muscular subaortic stenosis
4. Midventricular obstruction
5. Non-obstructive hypertrophic cardiomyopathy

patient who consistently has a pressure gradient across the left ventricular outflow tract, under resting conditions. It should be understood that, in our hands, such a pressure gradient begins at the time of mitral leaflet – ventricular septal contact[7,8] and the pressure drop occurs in the left ventricular outflow tract. Labile muscular subaortic stenosis is a relatively rare form of the condition in our experience in which the pressure gradient appears to come and go apparently for no reason. In some cases, this lability may be attributed to the act of inspiration[9]. We also believe, however, that much of the lability of pressure gradients reported in the literature in muscular subaortic stenosis is related to the inadvertent movements of the retrograde left heart catheter from high to low pressure areas of the left ventricle and vice versa. Latent muscular subaortic stenosis is defined as no pressure gradient at rest, but upon appropriate provocation, a pressure gradient, due to mitral leaflet–septal contact, develops in the left ventricular outflow tract. Midventricular obstruction is due to massive midventricular hypertrophy where the obstruction occurs at the level of the papillary muscles. This type of obstruction is not due to mitral leaflet–septal contact and the pressure gradient occurs at the midventricular level, not in the left ventricular outflow tract[10]. Non-obstructive hypertrophic cardiomyopathy is defined as there being no pressure gradient at rest or on provocation.

In discussing the evidence in favour of true outflow tract obstruction in muscular subaortic stenosis, we will deal principally with information derived from the study of our own cases with muscular subaortic stenosis at rest in whom the obstructive pressure gradient (1) begins with mitral leaflet–septal contact, (2) peaks in late systole, (3) is located in the left ventricular outflow tract and (4) is associated with prolongation of the left ventricular ejection time as is the case with other forms of outflow tract obstruction. Other types of intraventricular pressure differences and gradients will be discussed later in this chapter.

HISTORICAL BACKGROUND

Brock first drew attention to left ventricular outflow obstruction in hypertrophied hearts when he described 'functional obstruction to the left ventricle' in 1957[2]. Subsequently, workers in the United States[3], England[4,5], Canada[6], and elsewhere, accepted the fact that the pressure gradients recorded within the left ventricle in hypertrophic cardiomyopathy were indicative of obstruction to left ventricular outflow. As no medical therapy was available for muscular subaortic stenosis at that time, patients who presented with symptoms of angina, syncope and dyspnoea, a loud apical systolic murmur and a high outflow tract pressure gradient were operated upon by means of the ventriculomyotomy/myectomy procedure with gratifying abolition of the symptoms, the murmur and the pressure gradient[11,12]. Such was the state of affairs when, in 1965, Criley and associates reported their concept of 'pressure gradients without obstruction'[13]. This work pointed out that patients with hypertrophic cardiomyopathy often had supranormal ejection fractions on angiography and demonstrated the phenomenon of cavity obliteration at end-systole[13]. These authors drew attention to the fact that apically placed catheters became 'enfolded'[13] or 'engulfed'[13] by the myocardium in areas of left ventricular cavity obliteration with resultant generation of high intraventricular pressures. It was suggested that cavity obliteration and not left ventricular outflow tract obstruction was responsible for the intraventricular pressure differences recorded in patients with muscular subaortic stenosis. Furthermore, it was suggested that surgery was inappropriate for such patients in that there was no obstruction to operate upon or remove. Needless to say, this non-obstructive concept startled the cardiological world at the time, but more importantly it stimulated a number of investigators, including ourselves, to further investigate the nature of intraventricular pressure differences in patients with hypertrophic cardiomyopathy. It should be remembered that in the mid-1960s there was no echocardiography, nuclear cardiology or Doppler ultrasound, and cineangiography was in its infancy. Thus, the reinvestigation of the nature of intraventricular pressure gradients in hypertrophic cardiomyopathy was principally haemodynamic and to a lesser extent cineangiographic[14-17].

NATURE AND HAEMODYNAMIC SIGNIFICANCE OF THE INTRAVENTRICULAR PRESSURE DIFFERENCES IN HYPERTROPHIC CARDIOMYOPATHY

The initial left ventricular inflow tract pressure concept

As the result of this controversy about the nature of intraventricular pressure differences in hypertrophic cardiomyopathy, we[14,15] and others[16]

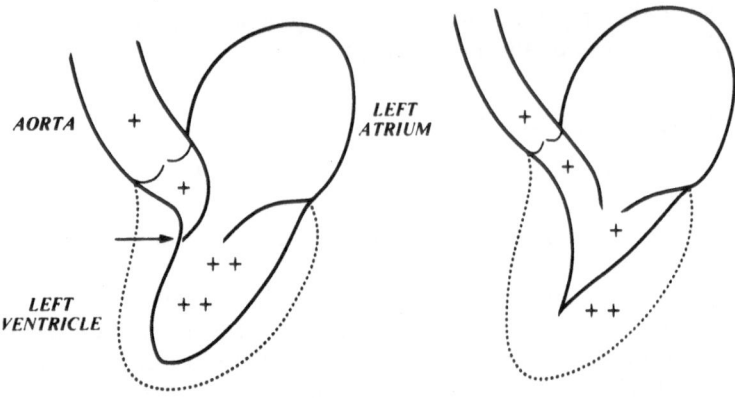

INTRAVENTRICULAR PRESSURE GRADIENT DUE TO MUSCULAR SUBAORTIC STENOSIS

INTRAVENTRICULAR PRESSURE DIFFERENCE DUE TO CAVITY OBLITERATION

Figure 7.4.1 *left*, In muscular subaortic stenosis, because the obstruction to left ventrivular outflow (arrow) is caused by anterior mitral leaflet–ventricular septal apposition, the intraventricular pressure distal to the stenosis (and proximal to the aortic valve) is low (+), whereas all ventricular pressures proximal to the stenosis, including the one just inside the mitral valve (the inflow tract pressure) are elevated (++). *Right*, When an intraventricular pressure difference is recorded, due to catheter entrapment by the myocardium as the result of cavity obliteration, the elevated ventricular pressure is recorded only in the area of cavity obliteration (++). The intraventricular systolic pressure in all other areas of the left ventricular cavity, including that in the inflow tract, just inside the mitral valve, is low (+) and equal to the aortic systolic pressure. *Note* that in cavity obliteration, there is an intraventricular pressure difference between the apex and the inflow tract and also the outflow tract. In muscular subaortic stenosis there is no intraventricular pressure difference between the apex and the inflow tract as they are both elevated above the outflow tract pressure. The three areas of the left ventricle represented by the + signs in each of these diagrams are, from above downward, the outflow tract just below the aortic valve (subaortic region), the inflow tract just inside the mitral valve, and the left ventricular apex

---

Figure 7.4.2 *(facing)* Catheter placement and corresponding intracardiac pressures in a patient with muscular subaortic stenosis who subsequently underwent successful ventriculomyotomy–myectomy surgery. The left panel indicates the position of the transseptal catheter, just proximal to the mitral valve, when recording left atrial pressure. The position of the aortic catheter is also shown. The centre panel indicates the position of the transseptal catheter when recording the elevated left ventricular inflow tract pressure, just inside the mitral valve. The right panel shows that advancing the transseptal catheter further into the left ventricular cavity did not alter the elevated left ventricular pressure. The transseptal cather could be moved freely in the left ventricular cavity without altering the elevated left ventricular systolic pressure. Note in the centre and right panels that the left ventricular pressure falls at the time of the dicrotic notch in the aortic pressure tracing. With the distal tip of the transseptal catheter sitting in the left ventricular inflow tract as in the centre and right panels, when the proximal end of the transseptal catheter was opened, blood could be withdrawn in systole and diastole and indeed 'shot out' in systole, indicating that the distal tip of the catheter was in a high-pressure, blood-filled area of the left ventricle, i.e. the left ventricular inflow tract. The catheters in this and subsequent catheter placement pictures had been outlined with dashed lines for clarity of illustration. (From Wigle *et al.* (1967). *Circulation*, **35**, 1100, by permission of the American Heart Association, Inc.)

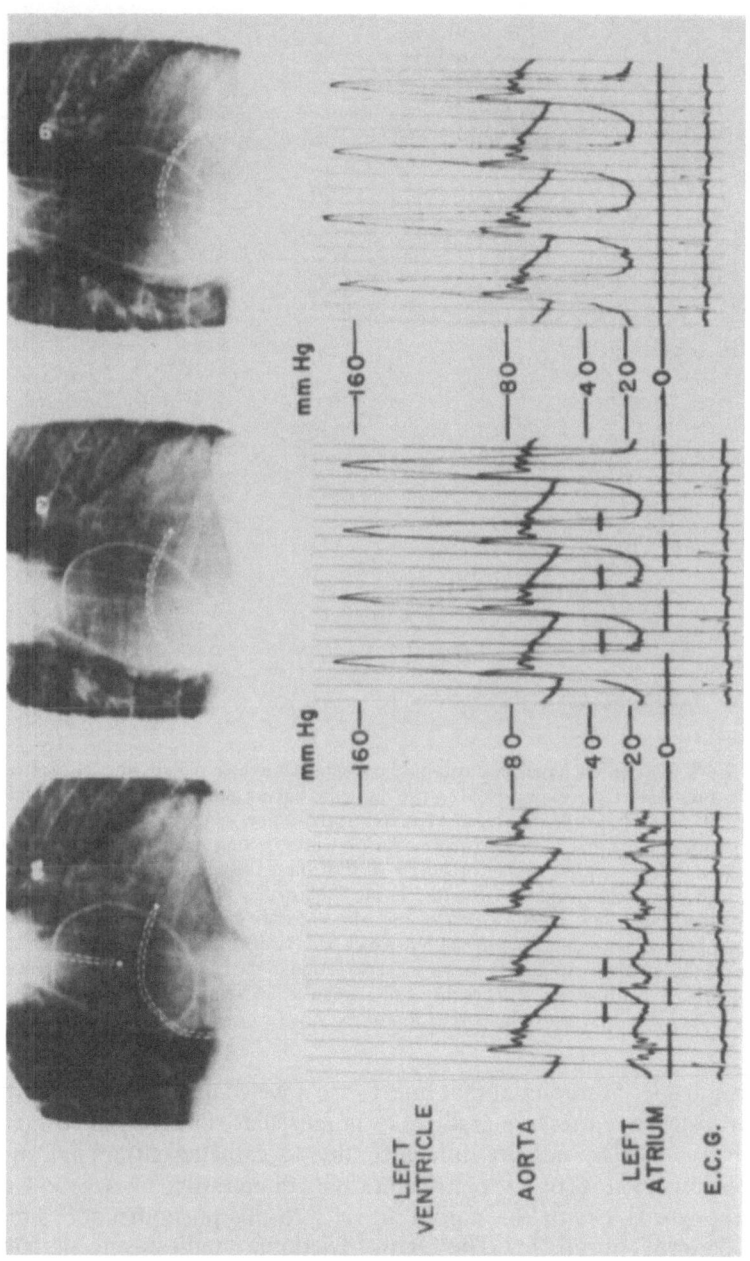

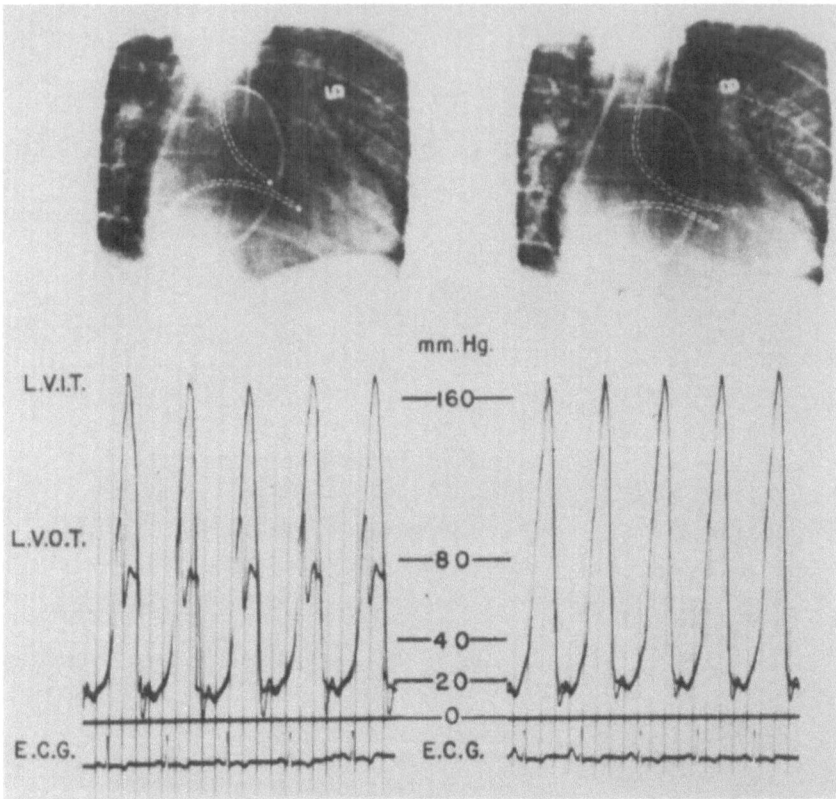

Figure 7.4.3 In the left panel, the end-hole retrograde catheter records the left ventricular outflow tract (LVOT) pressure, distal to the muscular subaortic stenosis, while the end-hole transseptal catheter records the elevated left ventricular inflow tract (LVIT) pressure proximal to the stenosis. Note that these two ventricular pressures decline simultaneously. In the right panel the inflow tract pressures recorded via each of these catheters were precisely superimposed, providing strong evidence that the elevated ventricular pressures were being recorded from a blood-filled high pressure area of the left ventricle. The systolic pressure difference measured between two catheters in the left panel or between the position of the retrograde catheter in the left and right panels, locate the obstruction to the area of the outflow tract of the left ventricle. Recordings made from the same patient as in Figure 7.4.2. (From Wigle *et al.* (1967). *Circulation*, 35, 1100, by permission of the American Heart Association, Inc.)

undertook special studies at that time to see if we could distinguish between a true obstructive pressure gradient as in muscular subaortic stenosis from an intraventricular pressure difference, due to catheter entrapment in the myocardium in areas of left ventricular cavity obliteration[14,15]. (*Note:* Criley used the words 'engulf' or 'enfold' to refer to this phenomenon[13] and we used the term 'entrap'[14,15]. The Oxford Dictionary indicates no significant difference in the meaning of these three words.) The studies we then undertook led to the development of the initial left ventricular inflow tract pressure concept, as a means to distinguish these two types of intraventricu-

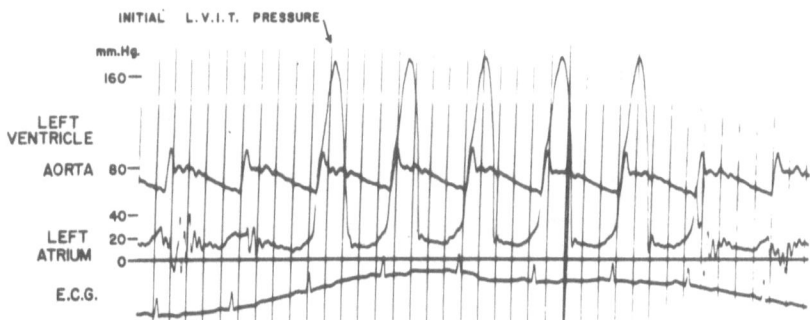

Figure 7.4.4 Pressure recordings from the case of muscular subaortic stenosis illustrated in Figures 7.4.2 and 7.4.3. The aortic pressure recording was continuous, while the end-hole transseptal catheter was introduced into, and then withdrawn from, the left ventricle, via the mitral valve. On passing the catheter from the left atrium to left ventricle, and vice versa, the first ventricular pressure on entering the left ventricle, (the initial inflow tract pressure) and the last ventricular pressure on withdrawal from the left ventricle were elevated above the aortic systolic pressure

lar pressure difference[14,15]. The initial inflow tract pressure is defined as the first left ventricular systolic pressure recorded as an end-hole-only transseptal catheter is introduced through the mitral valve, into the left ventricle[14,15]. This concept, as initially hypothesized and then proven, is depicted in Figure 7.4.1. In muscular subaortic stenosis (Figure 7.4.1, *left*), all intraventricular pressures proximal to the outflow tract obstruction (due to mitral leaflet–septal contact), including the initial inflow tract pressure, are elevated above the outflow tract or aortic pressures. In cases with catheter entrapment by the myocardium due to cavity obliteration, on the other hand, the high intraventricular pressure occurred only in obliterated areas of the ventricle, and the initial inflow tract pressure was low and equal to the outflow tract and aortic pressures[14-16] (Figure 7.4.1, *right*). In our cineangiographic studies and those of Ross *et al.*[16], the area of the left ventricular inflow tract did not become angiographically obliterated during systole. Thus, it would be difficult for catheters in this location to become entrapped by the myocardium. Figures 7.4.2–7.4.5 amplify this concept by demonstrating an elevated inflow tract pressure in muscular subaortic stenosis and a low inflow tract pressure in cavity obliteration. Additional means to distinguish between these two types of intraventricular pressure difference, were developed during these studies[14,15]. Thus, in muscular subaortic stenosis, it was shown that when blood was withdrawn from the proximal end of the transseptal catheter recording the high left ventricular inflow tract pressure, it could be freely withdrawn in systole and diastole and indeed 'shot-out' in systole, thus demonstrating that the distal tip of the catheter in the left ventricular inflow tract was in a high-pressure, blood-filled area of the ventricle. Catheters in this location could be moved without altering the high pressures recorded(Figure 7.4.2), and indeed multiple catheters could be placed in the left ventricular inflow tract and all recorded identically elevated systolic pressures (Figure 7.4.3)[14-16]. In contrast, when blood was

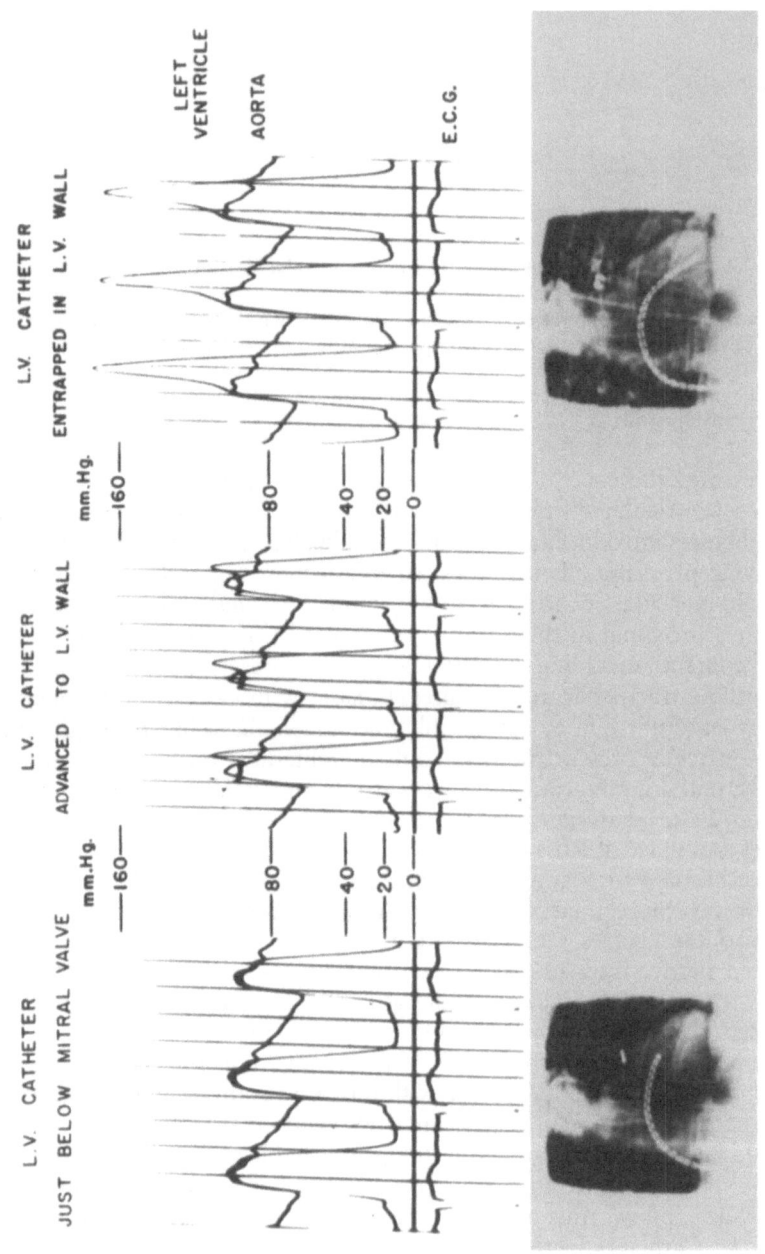

withdrawn from the proximal end of a catheter, recording a high intraventricular pressure due to the entrapment of the catheter tip in an
obliterated area of the ventricle, it could only be withdrawn in diastole
because of the entrapment in systole. Moving such a catheter changed the
configuration of the high ventricular pressure. In muscular subaortic
stenosis, left ventricular pressure fell at the time of the aortic dicrotic notch
(Figure 7.4.2), whereas in catheter entrapment, due to cavity obliteration,
the left ventricular pressure frequently fell after the aortic dicrotic notch
(Figure 7.4.5).

Importantly, the pressure gradient in muscular subaortic stenosis was
clearly located in the left ventricular outflow tract (Figures 7.4.1–7.4.3),
whereas in cavity obliteration the pressure drop occurred between the
entrapped catheter at the cardiac apex, recording the high pressure, and any
other area of the left ventricle that was blood filled and not obliterated
(Figures 7.4.1 and 7.4.5). Thus, in cavity obliteration, there was a pressure
difference between the apex of the left ventricle and the left ventricular
inflow tract (Figures 7.4.1 and 7.4.5), whereas this never occurred in
muscular subaortic stenosis (Figures 7.4.1 and 7.4.3).

Another interesting difference between these two types of intraventricular
pressure difference was the fact that the act of inspiration had the opposite
effect on the intraventricular pressure difference (Figure 7.4.6). Thus, in
muscular subaortic stenosis, inspiration lessened the obstructive pressure
gradient, presumably by afterloading the left ventricle[9], whereas the intraventricular pressure difference of cavity obliteration with catheter entrapment was increased by inspiration (Figure 7.4.6). This latter effect could be
explained by inspiration acting to displace the catheter towards the left
ventricular apex and/or decreasing left heart venous return, either of which
would favour further catheter entrapment and thus a higher systolic
pressure.

Figure 7.4.5 Catheter placement pictures and corresponding pressure recordings from a
patient with hypertrophic non-obstructive cardiomyopathy in whom cineangiography demonstrated marked systolic emptying of the apex of the left ventricle with cavity obliteration. In the
left panel with the transseptal catheter in the inflow tract, just inside the mitral valve, there was
no systolic pressure difference between the left ventricle (LV) and aorta, i.e. the left ventricular
inflow tract pressure was not elevated. Contrast the normal aortic pressure contour, in this case
of non-obstructive hypertrophic cardiomyopathy versus the spike and dome contour seen in
muscular subaortic stenosis in Figure 7.4.2 and 7.4.4. In the centre panel with the transseptal
catheter advanced further into the left ventricle there was a small late systolic pressure
difference between the left ventricle and the aorta. In the right panel, the transseptal catheter
had been advanced towards the left ventricular apex into the area of cavity obliteration. In this
loction, a large left ventricular-aortic systolic pressure difference is recorded due to entrapment
of the transseptal catheter in the area of cavity obliteration. Note that left ventricular pressure
declined after the dicrotic notch in aortic pressure in the presence of an intraventricular
pressure difference due to cavity obliteration. With the tip of the transseptal catheter located at
the left ventricular apex, when the proximal end of the catheter was opened, blood did not
shoot out in systole and when an attempt was made to withdraw blood from the proximal end
of the catheter, this was possible in diastole, but not in systole, due to the entrapment of the
distal tip of the catheter. (From Wigle et al. (1967). Circulation, 35, 1100, by permission of the
American Heart Association, Inc.)

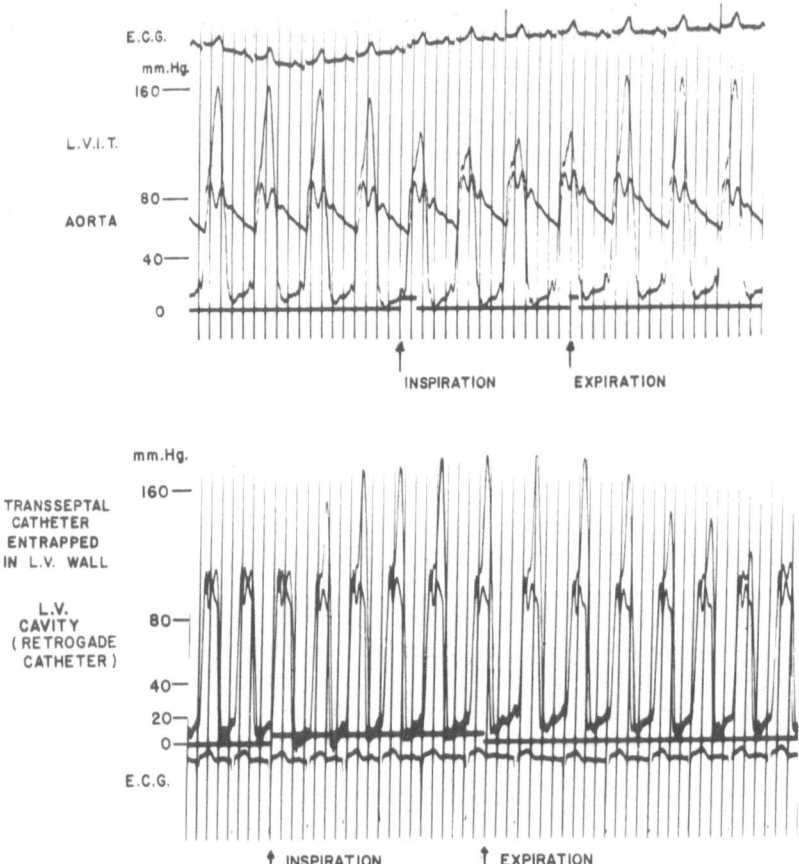

Figure 7.4.6 The effect of inspiration on the pressure gradient in muscular subaortic stenosis (*top*) contrasted with the effect of inspiration on the intraventricular pressure difference due to catheter entrapment from cavity obliteration (*bottom*). Inspiration decreases the pressure gradient in muscular subaortic stenosis and increases the intraventricular pressure difference in cavity obliteration (*see* text). Abbreviations as in previous figure legends

Left ventricular ejection time in muscular subaortic stenosis

In addition to these detailed catheter studies at that time we demonstrated that left ventricular ejection time in muscular subaortic stenosis was prolonged in direct relation to the magnitude of the pressure gradient, as is true with other types of left ventricular outflow tract obstruction (Figure 7.4.7)[17]. In contrast, left ventricular ejection time was not prolonged in the presence of an intraventricular pressure difference due to cavity obliteration[17]. Indeed, in cavity obliteration, the greater the pressure difference the shorter the ejection time, which of course is the absolute reverse of the relationship seen in muscular subaortic stenosis (Figure 7.4.8). Manoeuvres which abolished the pressure gradient in muscular subaortic

MUSCULAR SUBAORTIC STENOSIS

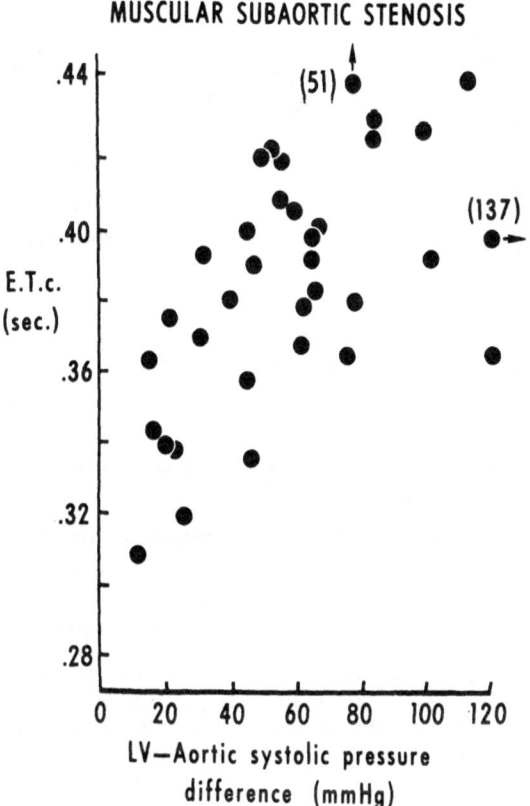

Figure 7.4.7 The relation between left ventricular ejection time corrected for heart rate (ETc) and the left ventricular (LV)–aortic systolic pressure gradient in 35 cases of muscular subaortic stenosis. With increasing magnitude of the pressure gradient there is progressive prolongation of the ejection time as would be expected with an obstruction to left ventricular outflow. (From Wigle *et al.* (1967). *Circulation*, **36**, 36, by permission of the American Heart Association, Inc.)

stenosis (angiotensin, norepinephrine, successful surgery) also shortened the left ventricular ejection time as would be expected with the relief of outflow tract obstruction (Figure 7.4.9)[17]. Pharmacological agents which increased the gradient in muscular subaortic stenosis (amyl nitrite, iso-proterenol) also prolonged the ejection time[17]. Prolongation of left ventricular ejection time in muscular subaortic stenosis has also been demonstrated by a number of groups by clinical[3,12], haemodynamic[7,8], phono-cardiographic[18] and echocardiographic[19] as well as Doppler flow techniques[19].

Some authors who do not believe that the pressure gradient in muscular subaortic stenosis represents true obstruction to left ventricular outflow have nevertheless demonstrated a prolongation of left ventricular ejection time in their own studies[20]. They have attempted to explain the prolonged ejection time on abnormalities of left ventricular relaxation[20]. To our knowledge, there is no scientific basis for such a suggestion. Indeed, in the

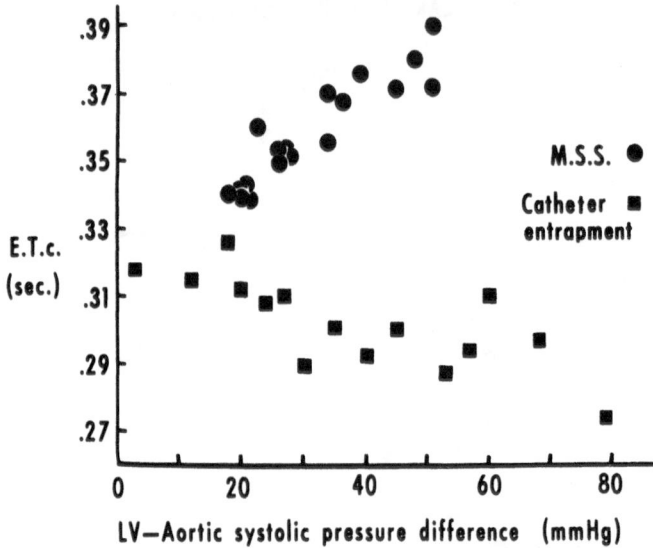

Figure 7.4.8 The relationship between corrected left ventricular ejection time (ETc) and left ventricular (LV)–aortic systolic pressure gradient in a patient with muscular subaortic stenosis (MSS, ●) and in a patient in whom there was an intraventricular pressure difference, due to catheter entrapment from cavity obliteration (■). In both patients, the pressure difference varied spontaneously with respiration. With increasing magnitude of the pressure gradient in muscular subaortic stenosis, there was progressive prolongation of the ejection time (a direct relationship), whereas when the pressure difference due to cavity obliteration with catheter entrapment increased, there was a shortening of the ejection time (an inverse relationship) (*see* text and Figure 7.4.6). (From Wigle *et al.* (1967). *Circulation*, 36, 36, by permission of the American Heart Association, Inc.)

isolated muscle preparation experiments of Brutsaert *et al.*[21,22] application of a load in the first one third to one half of systole (contraction loading) also results in prolonged contraction and delay in the *onset* of relaxation. One could in fact look upon muscular subaortic stenosis as the human counterpart of Brutsaert's isolated muscle experiments, in that a load is applied during the first half of contraction in both, and in each, contraction (systole) is prolonged. This prolongation of left ventricular ejection time in muscular subaortic stenosis is all the more dramatic evidence of obstruction to left ventricular outflow in that all cases with resting obstruction also have mitral regurgitation, which tends to reduce left ventricular ejection time[23-26]. This direct relationship between the magnitude of the pressure gradient and left ventricular ejection time in muscular subaortic stenosis holds true today[7,8] just as it did in the 1960s[17].

As the result of these studies involving the initial left ventricular inflow tract pressure concept and the relation of the pressure gradient to the left ventricular ejection time, and their importance in distinguishing the two types of intraventricular pressure difference, we have continued to employ combined transseptal and retrograde left heart catheterization in the investigation of patients with hypertrophic cardiomyopathy, in order to be

MUSCULAR SUBAORTIC STENOSIS

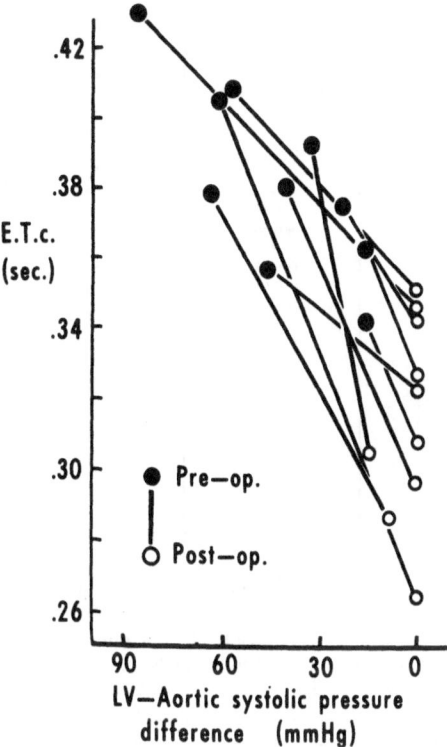

Figure 7.4.9 The relationship between corrected left ventricular ejection time (ETc) and left ventricular (LV)–aortic systolic pressure gradient (increasing from right to left on the abscissa) in ten patients with muscular subaortic stenosis before (●) and after (○) undergoing the ventriculomyotomy operation. When the pressure gradient was reduced or abolished surgically, there was a concomitant reduction in left ventricular ejection time as one would expect with relief of outflow tract obstruction (*see* text). (From Wigle *et al.* (1967). *Circulation*, **36**, 36, by permission of the American Heart Association, Inc.)

certain of whether we are dealing with true outflow tract obstruction or not. We feel that the use of these haemodynamic techniques has permitted us to make accurate correlations with non-invasive techniques of investigation that have subsequently become available for use in these patients.

NON-SIMULTANEOUS HAEMODYNAMIC– ECHOCARDIOGRAPHIC CORRELATIONS IN HYPERTROPHIC CARDIOMYOPATHY

In these studies we performed detailed one-dimensional echocardiographic examinations on 70 patients with hypertrophic cardiomyopathy[27], who previously had been haemodynamically classified into haemodynamic subgroups by the techniques described[14,15,17]. Fifteen patients had non-

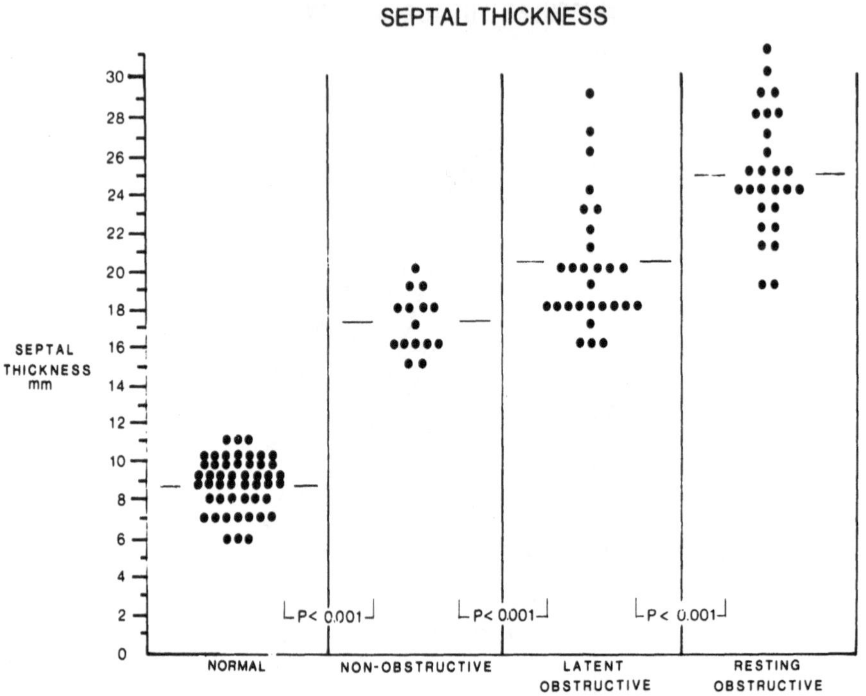

SEPTAL THICKNESS

Figure 7.4.10 Ventricular septal thickness measured by one-dimensional echocardiography at the level of the mitral leaflet tips in 50 normal individuals and 70 patients with hypertrophic cardiomyopathy, haemodynamically classified as having no outflow obstruction, latent obstruction or resting obstruction (*see* text). In all cases of hypertrophic cardiomyopathy, the ventricular septum was at least 15 mm thick. Note the highly significant increasing septal thickness from the non-obstructive to the latent obstructive group, then from the latent obstructive group to the resting obstructive group. (From Gilbert *et al.* (1980). *Am. J. Cardiol.*, **45**, 861, by permission)

obstructive hypertrophic cardiomyopathy, 28 had latent muscular subaortic stenosis, and 27 had muscular subaortic stenosis at rest. The thickness of the ventricular septum measured at the tips of the mitral leaflets was 15 mm or more in all cases, and was significantly thicker in those with resting muscular subaortic stenosis than in those with latent muscular subaortic stenosis, which in turn had thicker septa than those with hypertrophic non-obstructive cardiomyopathy ($p < 0.001$) (Figure 7.4.10). Concomitantly, the left ventricular outflow tract diameter at the onset of systole was narrowest in those with resting muscular subaortic stenosis and widest in those with hypertrophic non-obstructive cardiomyopathy, while in latent muscular subaortic stenosis, this diameter was intermediate between the other groups[27] (Figure 7.4.11). It is worthwhile noting here that, although patients with latent muscular subaortic stenosis have significantly thicker septa by one dimensional echocardiography than those with hypertrophic non-obstructive cardiomyopathy, the extent of the hypertrophy determined by two-dimensional echocardiography in latent muscular subaortic stenosis

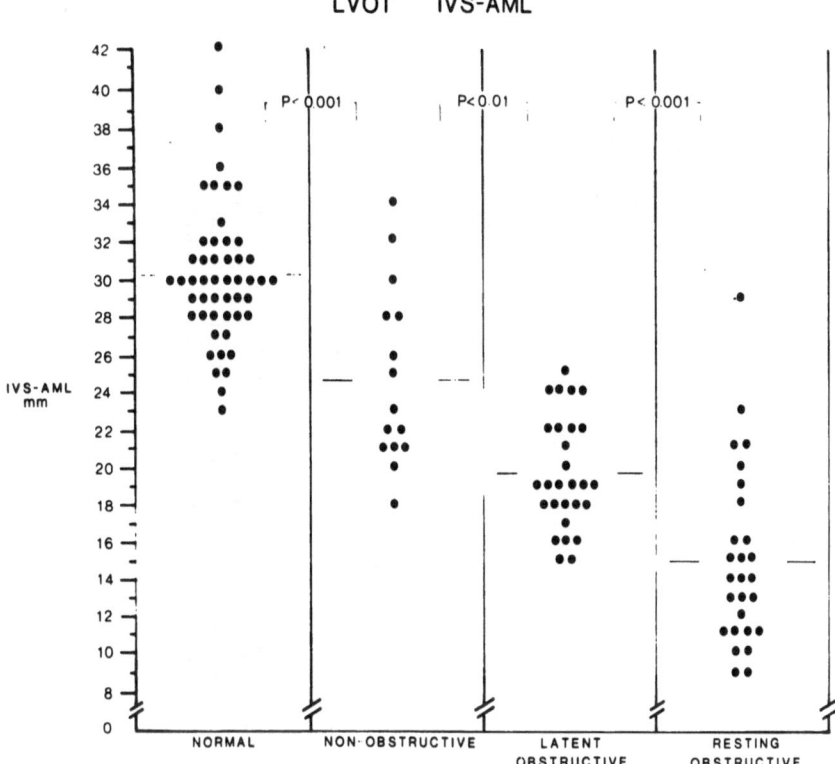

Figure 7.4.11 The left ventricular outflow tract (**LVOT**) width measured as the interventricular septal (**IVS**)–anterior mitral leaflet (**AML**) distance at the onset of systole determined by one-dimensional echocardiography in 50 normal individuals and 70 haemodynamically categorized patients with hypertrophic cardiomyopathy (*see* text). There is progressive and significant narrowing of the left ventricular outflow tract at the onset of systole from normals to non-obstructive patients, from non-obstructive patients to latent obstructive patients, and from latent obstructive patients to patients with resting outflow tract obstruction. (From Gilbert *et al.* (1980). *Am. J. Cardiol.*, **45**, 861, by permission)

is usually quite limited. Thus, in 80% of cases of latent muscular subaortic stenosis, the septal hypertrophy by two-dimensional echocardiography involved only the upper one third to two thirds of the septum, whereas in resting muscular subaortic stenosis, and hypertrophic non-obstructive cardiomyopathy, the hypertrophy usually involved the whole length of the septum, down to the apex, as well as extending into the anterolateral wall[28] (Figure 7.4.12). These differences in the two-dimensional echocardiographic extent of hypertrophy in the different haemodynamic subgroups may well be responsible for the usully normal left ventricular end-diastolic pressure in latent muscular subaortic stenosis, with limited hypertrophy, and the elevation of this pressure in the other haemodynamic subgroups with more extensive hypertrophy[28].

In order to grade the severity of the systolic anterior motion (SAM) of the anterior mitral leaflet in the 70 haemodynamically classified cases of

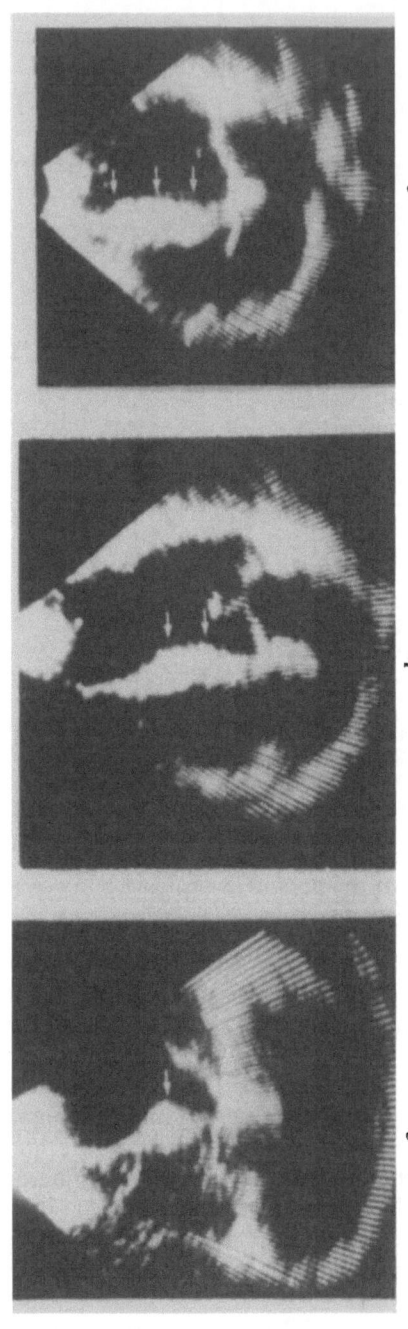

Figure 7.4.12 Two-dimensional echocardiograms (apical four-chamber view) in three different patients with hypertrophic cardiomyopathy defined by a septal–posterior wall ratio of 1.5 or greater by one-dimensional echocardiography. **a**, only the upper one third of the ventricular septum is thickened, as indicated by the arrow; **b** the upper two thirds of the ventricular septum is thickened, as indicated by the two arrows, **c**, the ventricular septum is thickened from base to apex, as indicated by the three arrows. It can be seen that patients who have the one-dimensional echocardiographic criteria for hypertrophic cardiomyopathy, Teare's disease, may have a tremendously variable extent of hypertrophy (*see* text)

Table 7.4.3   Degree of systolic anterior motion of the anterior mitral leaflet in the haemodynamic subgroups of hypertrophic cardiomyopathy

	Cases (n)	Absent	Mild	Moderate	Severe
Non-obstructive hypertrophic cardiomyopathy	15	13	2	—	—
Latent muscular subaortic stenosis	28	2	9	17	—
Muscular subaortic stenosis at rest	27	—	—	—	27

See text regarding quantification of mild, moderate, and severe systolic anterior motion

hypertrophic cardiomyopathy, we defined mild SAM as not coming within 10 mm of the septum, moderate SAM as coming within 10 mm of the septum, or establishing brief septal contact, and severe SAM as that in which anterior mitral leaflet–septal contact existed for greter than 30% of echocardiographic systole (Figure 7.4.13). Table 7.4.3 shows the degree of SAM in each of the haemodynamic subgroups. Resting obstruction was always associated with severe SAM (with early and prolonged septal contact), while the non-obstructive cases usually had no SAM, or at most, a mild degree. Latent muscular subaortic stenosis was associated with moderate SAM twice as frequently as mild SAM and rarely with no SAM. These striking differences in the degree of systolic anterior motion in the different haemodynamic subgroups of hypertrophic cardiomyopathy is strong supportive evidence that the cause of the left ventricular outflow tract obstruction in muscular subaortic stenosis is early and prolonged mitral leaflet–septal contact.

Aortic valve notching occurred in all 25 cases of muscular subaortic stenosis at rest, in which this parameter could be assessed, in only three of 28 cases with latent muscular subaortic stenosis and never in non-obstructive hypertrophic cardiomyopathy. Left atrial enlargement occurred in 25 of 27 cases with muscular subaortic stenosis at rest, but in only four of 28 cases with latent muscular subaortic stenosis and two of 15 cases with hypertrophic non-obstructive cardiomyopathy. Since all cases with resting obstruction have mitral regurgitation[23-26] we would interpret the left atrial enlargement in this haemodynamic subset to be due, at least in part, to the mitral leak.

Two-dimensional echocardiography has helped to further elucidate the mitral valve structures involved in mild, moderate and severe SAM[28]. Thus, in severe SAM by one-dimensional echocardiography, the distal one third to one half of the anterior mitral leaflet can be seen by two-dimensional echocardiography to move anteriorly during left ventricular systole and to establish prolonged contact with the interventricular septum (Figure 7.4.14). Mild to moderate degrees of SAM by one-dimensional echocardiography are shown by two-dimensional echocardiography to involve the anterior movement of the anterior mitral leaflet tip and/or its attached chordae tendineae. In cases of latent muscular subaortic stenosis, following provocation, the mild to moderate degree of SAM by one-dimensional

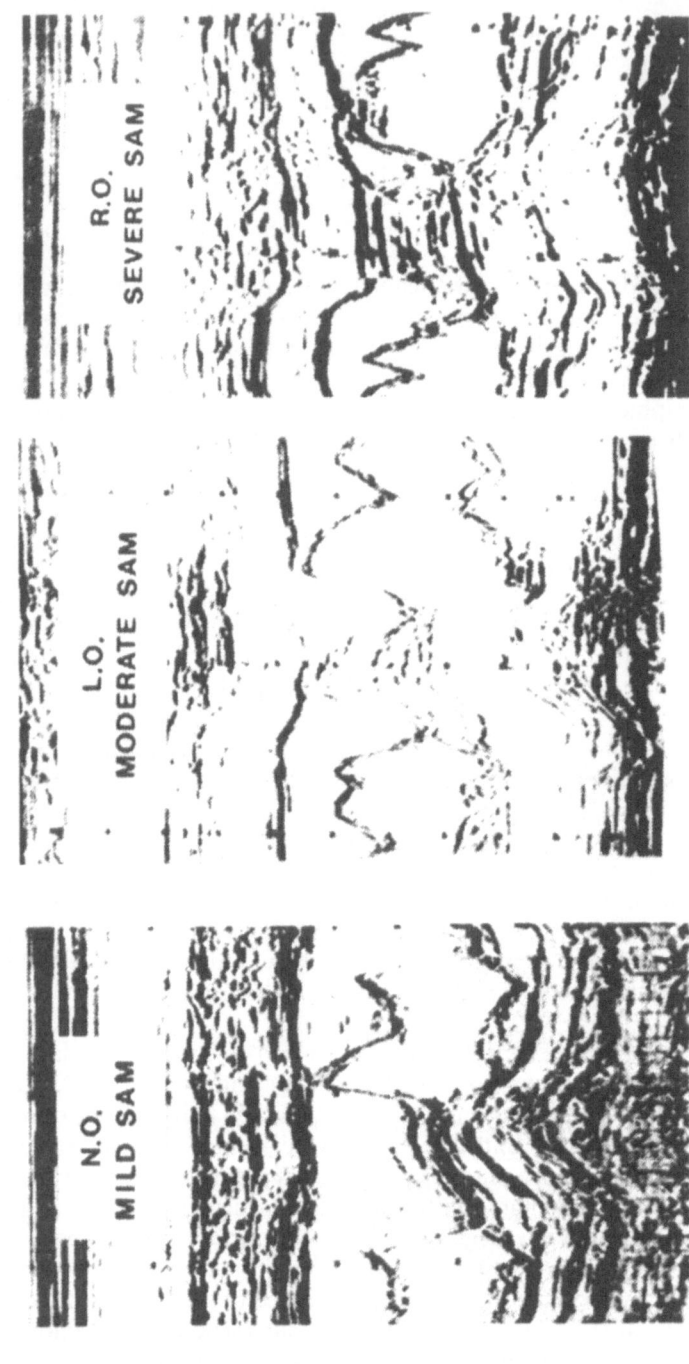

Figure 7.4.13 One-dimensional echocardiograms from: *left*, a patient with no outflow tract obstruction (NO), and mild systolic anterior motion of the anterior mitral leaflet (SAM); *centre*, a patient with latent obstruction (LO) with moderate SAM (centre); and *right*, patient with resting outflow tract obstruction and severe SAM. (*See* text for the criteria for quantitating SAM.) (From Gilbert *et al.* (1980). *Am. J. Cardiol.*, 45, 861, by permission)

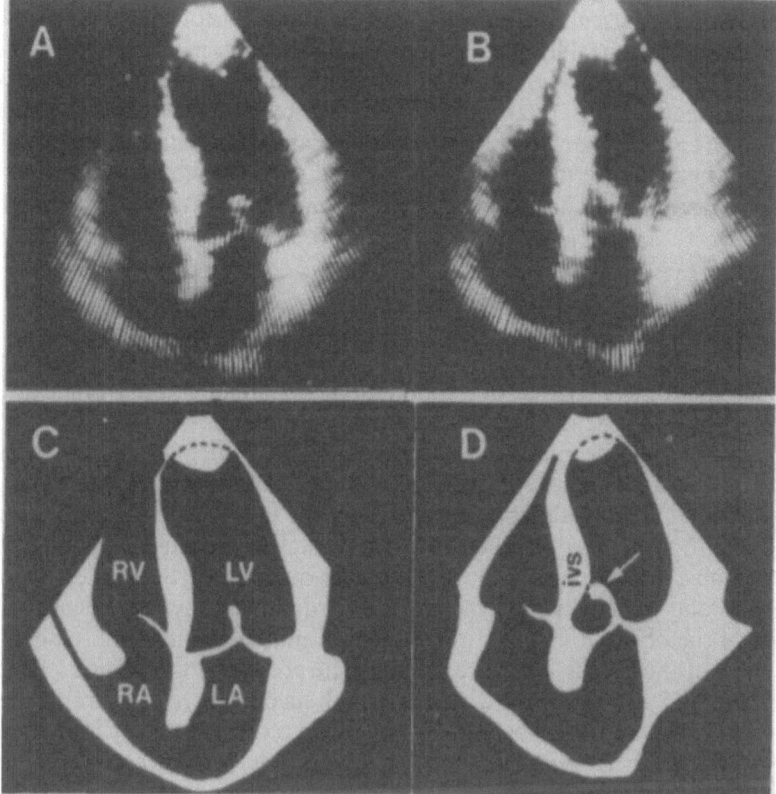

Figure 7.4.14 Two-dimensional echocardiogram (apical four-chamber view) from a patient with muscular subaortic stenosis. A and B are the echocardiograms in diastole and systole respectively. C and D are lined diagrams of A and B respectively. Note that the distal one half of the anterior mitral leaflet (arrow) comes into contact with the interventricular septum (IVS) early in systole at a time when the left ventricular (LV) cavity is not greatly reduced in size (no cavity obliteration) (*see* text). RV = right ventricle; RA = right atrium; LA = left atrium

echocardiography becomes severe and by two-dimensional echocardiography the leaflet tip SAM comes to involve the distal one third to one half of the anterior mitral leaflet. Mild degrees of SAM, due to anterior chordal motion, have been identified by both one- and two-dimensional echocardiographic studies in a number of clinical situations[27,29]. With provocation, this type of SAM does not increase in severity[29]. Pseudo-SAM refers to anterior movement of the whole mitral apparatus in late systole and is due to posterior wall contraction. Once recognized, it should not be confused with mitral leaflet SAM, that is responsible for outflow tract obstruction. On several occasions we have seen a vegetation due to infective endocarditis, attached to the ventricular surface of the anterior mitral leaflet, give rise to apparent SAM on one-dimensional echocardiography. Two-dimensional echocardiography quickly establishes the problem in such cases.

Two-dimensional echocardiography has been solely responsible for the recognition of muscular subaortic stenosis, due to systolic anterior motion of the posterior mitral leaflet[30]. Normally, the anterior mitral leaflet extends into the left ventricle further than does the posterior leaflet. In cases of posterior leaflet SAM, it appears that the posterior leaflet extends further into the ventricle than is normal, either because the leaflet is abnormally long, or because the mitral annulus is tilted such that the posterior leaflet extends further than normal into the left ventricular cavity.

SIMULTANEOUS HAEMODYNAMIC–ECHOCARDIOGRAPHIC CORRELATIONS IN MUSCULAR SUBAORTIC STENOSIS

Recently, we have carried out simultaneous one-dimensional echocardiographic–haemodynamic correlative studies in muscular subaortic stenosis, to ascertain the time relationships between mitral leaflet–septal contact and the pressure gradient[7,8]. All pressure gradients were measured between an unentrapped transseptal catheter placed in the left ventricular inflow tract and a retrograde aortic catheter with its distal tip, located just above the aortic valve[14,15]. Because impulse gradients occur in early systole, both in normals and patients with hypertrophic cardiomyopathy[31], we defined the onset of the obstructive pressure gradient in muscular subaortic stenosis as the peak of the percussion wave in the aortic pressure trace (Figure 7.4.15). Figure 7.4.15 illustrates the virtually simultaneous onset of mitral leaflet–septal contact and the obstructive pressure gradient onset defined as the peak of the aortic percussion wave. Figure 7.4.16 illustrates the highly significant correlation between these two systolic events in muscular subaortic stenosis. Figures 7.4.17 and 7.4.18 demonstrate that the magnitude of the pressure gradient in muscular subaortic stenosis is strongly correlated to the time of onset and duration of mitral leaflet–septal contact[7,8]. Thus, a large obstructive pressure gradient is associated with early and prolonged mitral leaflet–septal contact, whereas a small pressure gradient is associated with late onset and short duration of mitral leaflet–septal contact (Figure 7.4.19). In Figure 7.4.17, it is worth noting that when mitral leaflet–septal contact occurs after 55% of the left ventricular ejection time, no pressure gradient develops. This finding, together with the information that mitral leaflet–septal contact ceases at approximately 75% of the left ventricular ejection period[7], is very much in keeping with our earlier studies to the effect that mitral leaflet–septal contact must be present for approximately 30% of left ventricular systole in order for there to be an obstructive pressure gradient of any significance[27].

In these simultaneous one-dimensional echocardiographic–haemodynamic studies, we utilized fluid filled catheter systems. Thus, it is possible that the timing of the peak of the aortic percussion wave (onset of pressure gradient), might have been delayed by up to 10 ms. If this were true, it would merely mean that the obstructive pressure gradient began immediately prior to mitral leaflet–septal contact rather than simultaneously with

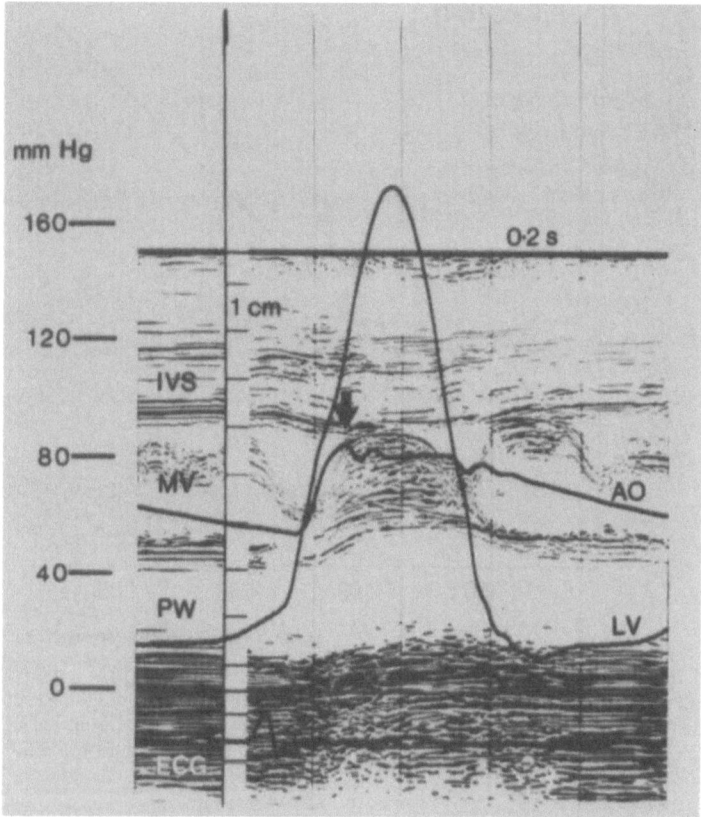

Figure 7.4.15 Simultaneous haemodynamic and echocardiographic recordings in a patient with muscular subaortic stenosis (gradient 86 mmHg). Arrow indicates onset of mitral leaflet–septal contact and onset of the pressure gradient (defined as the peak of the aortic percussion wave), which are virtually simultaneous. Note how early in systole onset of mitral leaflet–septal contact and pressure gradient occur in patients with severe outflow tract obstruction. IVS = interventricular septum; MV = mitral valve; PW = posterior wall; AO = central aortic pressure; LV = left ventricular pressure. (From Pollick *et al.* (1982). *Circulation*, **66**, 1087, by permission of the American Heart Association, Inc.)

it. Such a change would not alter the significant correlations between these two systolic events in muscular subaortic stenosis.

MITRAL REGURGITATION IN MUSCULAR SUBAORTIC STENOSIS

Mitral regurgitation has been recognized to be a potentially important part of the pathophysiology of muscular subaortic stenosis, from the time of the early indicator dilution[23–26] and angiographic studies[32–34] of this condition. Angiographic evidence of mitral regurgitation is only present in about two thirds of cases of muscular subaortic stenosis[34].

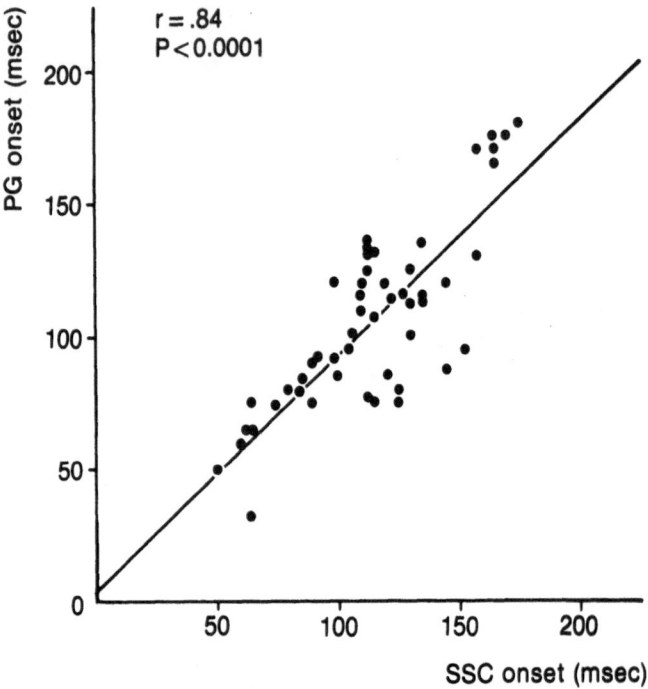

Figure 7.4.16 Correlation between pressure gradient (PG) onset and SAM–septal contact (SSC) onset in a series of patients with muscular subaortic stenosis, in whom the haemodynamic and echocardiographic investigation was carried out simultaneously. (From Pollick *et al.* (1982). *Circulation*, **66**, 1087, by permission of the American Heart Association, Inc.)

Beginning in the early 1960s, we have investigated the mitral regurgitation in muscular subaortic stenosis by means of an indicator dilution technique that provides a semiquantitative estimation of the mitral leak[23–26]. In these studies, one retrograde catheter was placed in the ascending aorta, another in the high pressure area of the left ventricle, while a transseptal catheter was placed in the left atrium. Indocyanine green dye was injected over several cardiac cycles into the left ventricle while blood was continually withdrawn from the left atrium, through the transseptal catheter. Mitral regurgitation was detected by the early appearance of green dye in the left atrium and depending on the amount of the early appearing dye, compared with the recirculation peak, an estimate of the degree of mitral regurgitation was obtained. This technique had the advantage of there being no catheter across the mitral valve, extrasystoles could be avoided and the pressure gradient was ascertained virtually simultaneously with the estimation of the degree of mitral regurgitation. Additionally, pharmacological agents could be administered and the effect on the pressure gradient and the degree of mitral regurgitation ascertained (Figures 7.4.20 and 7.4.21). Results of these studies throw an important light on the pathophysiology of muscular subaortic stenosis.

In 100 consecutive cases of muscular subaortic stenosis with a gradient at

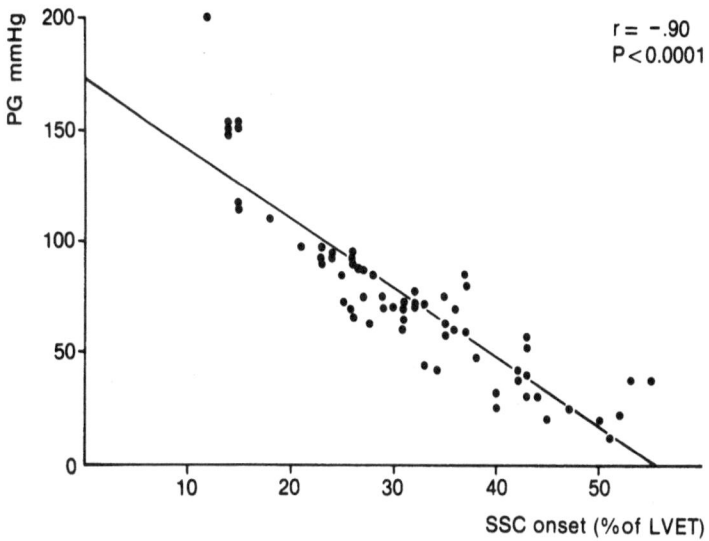

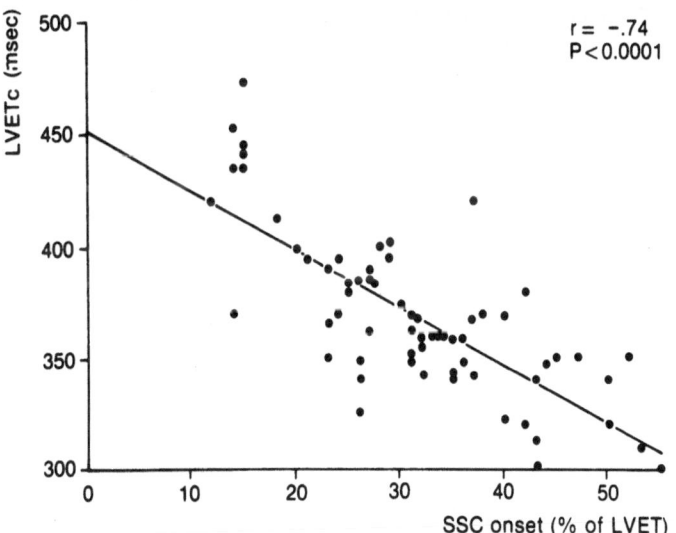

Figure 7.4.17 Correlation between the percentage of systolic ejection period that SAM–septal contact (SSC) first occurs and the magnitude of the pressure gradient (*top*) and left ventricular ejection time corrected for heart rate (LVETc) (*bottom*) in a series of patients with muscular subaortic stenosis in whom the echocardiographic and haemodynamic investigations were carried out simultaneously. (From Pollick *et al.* (1984). *Circulation*, **69**, 43, by permission of the American Heart Association Inc.)

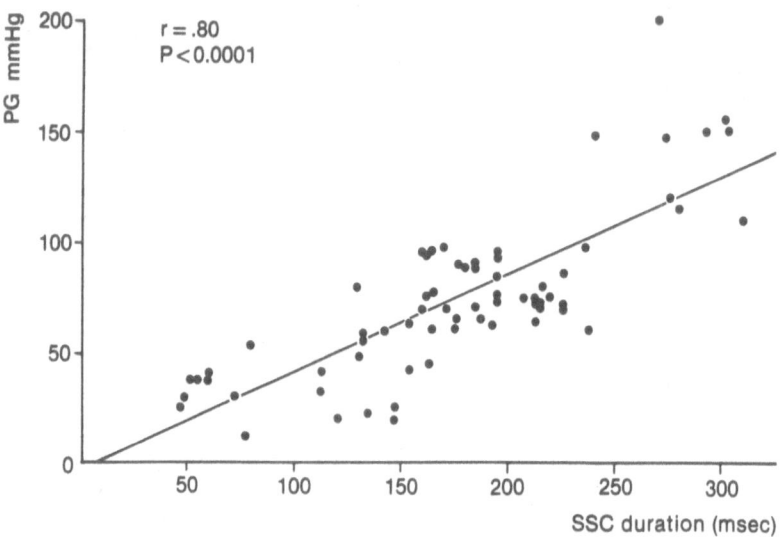

Figure 7.4.18 Correlation between the magnitude of the pressure gradient and the duration of SAM–septal contact (SSC) in a series of patients with muscular subaortic stenosis, undergoing simultaneous haemodynamic and echocardiographic investigation. (From Pollick *et al.* (1984). *Circulation*, **69**, 43, by permission of the American Heart Association, Inc.)

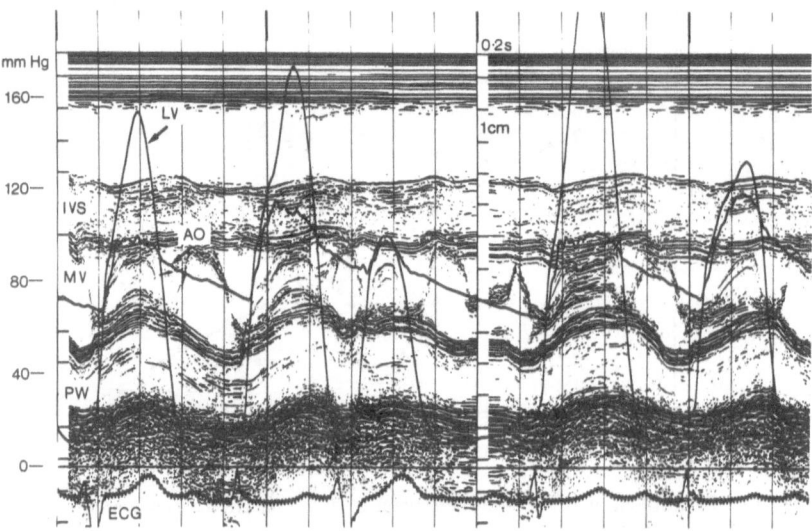

Figure 7.4.19 Simultaneous left ventricular (LV) inflow tract and aortic (AO) pressure tracings and one-dimensional echocardiogram in a case of muscular subaortic stenosis demonstrating that the variation in the severity of SAM determines the magnitude of the obstructive pressure gradient. Note that SAM–septal contact occurs earlier in systole and lasts longer in the postextrasystolic beat (beat 4) with the highest pressure gradient, than it does in beat 2 with a moderate pressure gradient. In beat 5, SAM–septal contact occurs late and its duration is relatively brief, resulting in small pressure gradient. In beat 3, note that SAM does not make contact with the septum and there is no pressure gradient. IVS = interventricular septum; MV = mitral valve; PW = posterior wall

240

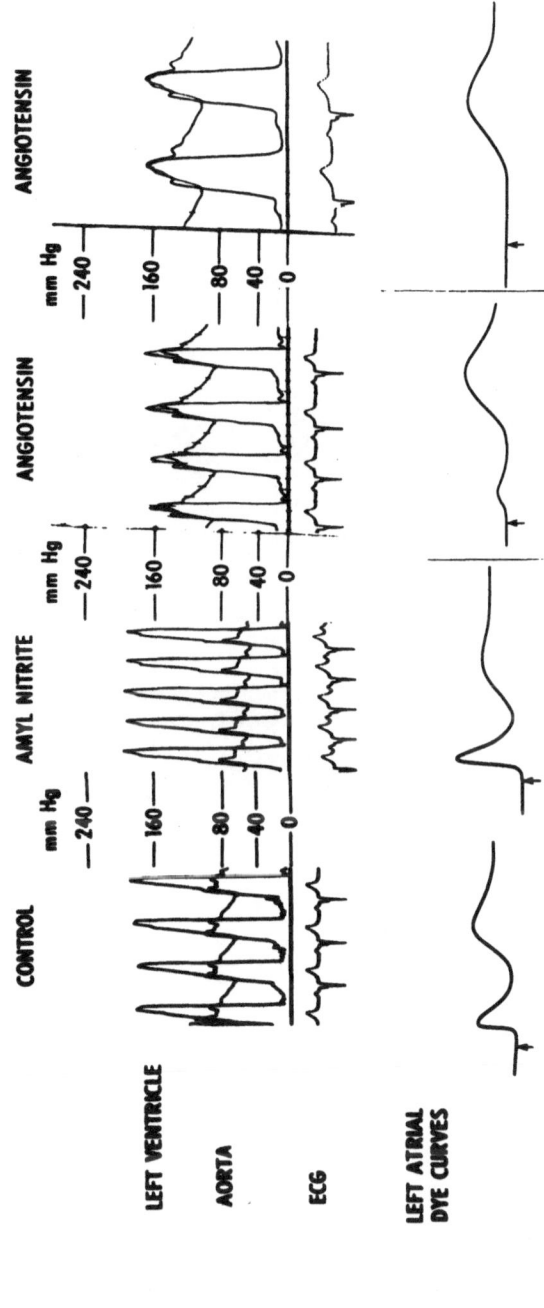

Figure 7.4.20 Simultaneous left ventricular and aortic pressure recordings (*top*) and left atrial dye dilution curves (*bottom*), inscribed from left to right, after left ventricular injection of 2 ml of indocyanine green dye in a patient with muscular subaortic stenosis, in control conditions (first panel), after amyl nitrite inhalation (second panel), and during angiotensin infusion (third and fourth panels). The amount of dye leaking back into the left atrium is indicated by the upward deflection of the dye curve that occurs immediately to the right of the arrow, which indicates the time of left ventricular injection of the dye. To the right of this regurgitant dye deflection is the recirculation concentration. The intensification of the outflow tract obstruction, due to administration of amyl nitrite, was accompanied by an increase in the amount of regurgitant dye appearing in the left atrium (second panel). Angiotensin infusion initially reduced (third panel) and eventually abolished (fourth panel) both the outflow tract obstruction and the mitral regurgitation (*see text*) (From Wigle *et al.* (1969). *Am. J. Cardiol.*, **24**, 698, by permission)

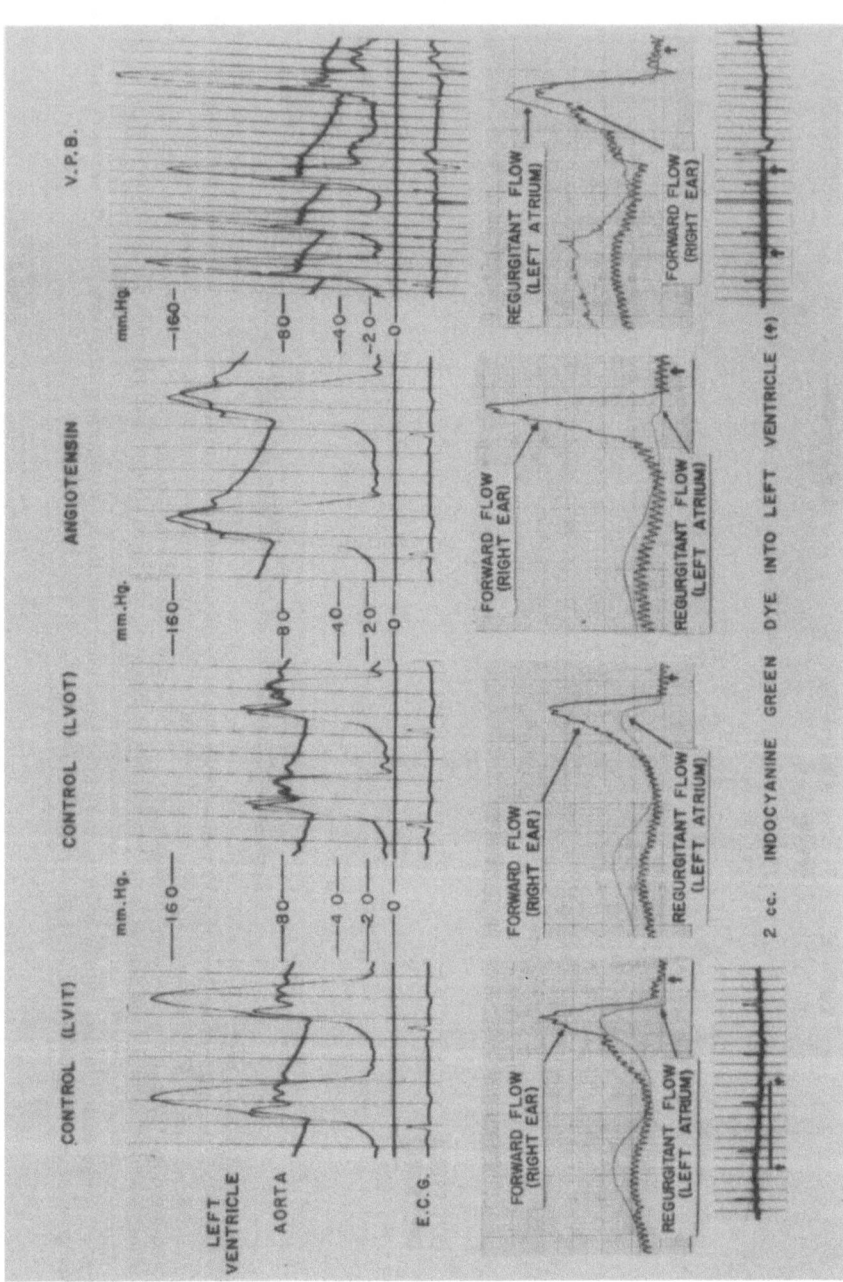

Figure 7.4.21

242

rest, mitral regurgitation was present in every case, and tended to be greatest in those cases with the highest pressure gradient[24,26]. Pharmacological manipulation of the pressure gradient in any given case also usually revealed a direct relationship between the pressure gradient and the degree of mitral regurgitation (Figures 7.4.20 and 7.4.21). Thus, amyl nitrate and isoproterenol increased the pressure gradient and the mitral regurgitation, while angiotensin usually but not always decreased the pressure gradient and the mitral regurgitation (Figure 7.4.20). Considering the fact that there is mitral leaflet–septal contact in cases of muscular subaortic stenosis with a pressure gradient at rest, it is our belief that the mitral regurgitation in muscular subaortic stenosis is related to this anterior motion of the mitral leaflet, rendering the mitral valve apparatus incompetent. Furthermore, since the pressure gradient is related to the severity of the systolic anterior motion of the anterior mitral leaflet, it is not surprising that the degree of mitral regurgitation should be related to the magnitude of the systolic anterior motion and the pressure gradient. In a few studies we have combined the haemodynamic assessment of the gradient, echocardiographic assessment of SAM and either indicator dilution or Doppler assessment of the mitral regurgitation. As SAM decreases in severity or disappears by pharmacological manipulation, both the pressure gradient and the mitral regurgitation decreases or disappears in similar fashion (unpublished observations). Studies by Marquis et al. using hydrogen ion as an indicator have demonstrated that the mitral regurgitation in muscular subaortic stenosis begins during the development of systolic anterior motion or at the time of mitral leaflet–septal contact and continues thereafter[35].

In 55 of 100 cases studied by these indicator dilution techniques, we administered angiotensin to abolish the pressure gradient in order to ascertain the effect on the mitral regurgitation[26]. In 80% of these cases, the mitral regurgitation was either greatly reduced or abolished when the pressure gradient was abolished[26]. Successful ventriculomyotomy–myectomy surgery in these cases abolished the systolic anterior motion, the pressure gradient and the mitral regurgitation[36]. In 20% of these cases, however, angiotensin did not significantly decrease the mitral regurgitation

Figure 7.4.21 Simultaneous left ventricular and aortic pressure tracings (top), and forward flow and regurgitant flow dye dilution curves (bottom) inscribed from right to left after left ventricular ejection of 2 ml of indocyanine green dye in a patient with muscular subaortic stenosis. The forward flow curve was recorded by means of an ear oximeter. The regurgitant flow curve was recorded by withdrawal of blood continuously via a transseptal catheter placed in the left atrium. In control conditions, with the dye being injected into the left ventricular inflow tract (LVIT) there is a moderate amount of regurgitant dye appearing in the left atrium and distortion of the downslope of the forward flow curve. In the second panel, the dye was injected into the left ventricular outflow tract (LVOT) and there was evidence of less mitral regurgitation both in the forward flow and regurgitant flow curves. In the third panel, during angiotensin infusion, the gradient was almost abolished as was the mitral regurgitation. In the fourth panel, the dye was injected into the inflow tract of the left ventricle, immediately prior to an extrasystole. As a result, there was a marked increase in mitral regurgitation as indicated by both the regurgitant flow curve as well as the forward flow curve. The vertical arrows indicate the time of injection of the dye into the left ventricle (see text)

when the pressure gradient was abolished. Successful surgery in these cases abolished the systolic anterior motion and the pressure gradient, but not the mitral regurgitation. Pathology of the mitral valves in some of these cases revealed marked fibrosis (?due to repeated mitral leaflet–septal contact), rheumatic or congenital abnormalities[24,26]. Thus, in about 20% of cases with muscular subaortic stenosis, mitral regurgitation was at least partly related to an independent abnormality of the mitral valve, while in 80% of cases, mitral regurgitation appeared to be entirely related to the systolic anterior motion of the anterior mitral leaflet.

A number of investigators have now demonstrated the occurrence of mitral regurgitation in muscular subaortic stenosis by Doppler ultrasound techniques and have confirmed that if there is systolic anterior motion and a pressure gradient, there is also mitral regurgitation, which is frequently considerable in degree[19,37]. The mitral regurgitation detected by Doppler ultrasound tends also to begin with the development of systolic anterior motion and to be greatest during the period of mitral leaflet–septal contact[19]. The degree of mitral regurgitation is significantly greater in hypertrophic cardiomyopathy patients with obstructive pressure gradients than in patients with hypertrophic non-obstructive cardiomyopathy, in whom the mitral regurgitation by Doppler ultrasound is either non-existent or very mild[37]. This confirmation of the presence of mitral regurgitation in muscular subaortic stenosis is important in that it is not always perceived on cineangiograms and yet it is one of the important factors in explaining the small end-systolic volume of the left ventricle in hypertrophic cardiomyopathy patients with outflow tract obstruction.

We have also carried out these indicator dilution studies in cases of non-obstructive hypertrophic cardiomyopathy and latent muscular sub-aortic stenosis. In non-obstructive hypertrophic cardiomyopathy, there is either no mitral regurgitation or a very mild amount[24], which is in keeping with the Doppler studies[37]. In latent muscular subaortic stenosis, where systolic anterior motion is mild or usually moderate in degree, the amount of mitral regurgitation is greater than in hypertrophic non-obstructive cardiomyopathy, but less than that seen in patients with resting outflow tract obstruction. Pharmacological provocation of latent muscular subaortic stenosis by amyl nitrite or isoproterenol resulted in the development of severe systolic anterior motion, a pressure gradient and an increased degree of mitral regurgitation[24,26].

MECHANISM OF SYSTOLIC ANTERIOR MOTION OF THE ANTERIOR MITRAL LEAFLET (AND HENCE THE PRESSURE GRADIENT AND MITRAL REGURGITATION)

A number of mechanisms have been suggested to explain systolic anterior motion (SAM) of the anterior or posterior mitral leaflet in cases of muscular subaortic stenosis. Thus, systolic tethering of the anterior mitral leaflet by chordae tendineae attached to malaligned papillary muscles has been suggested[38,39]. If this were the mechanism for SAM, one would expect that

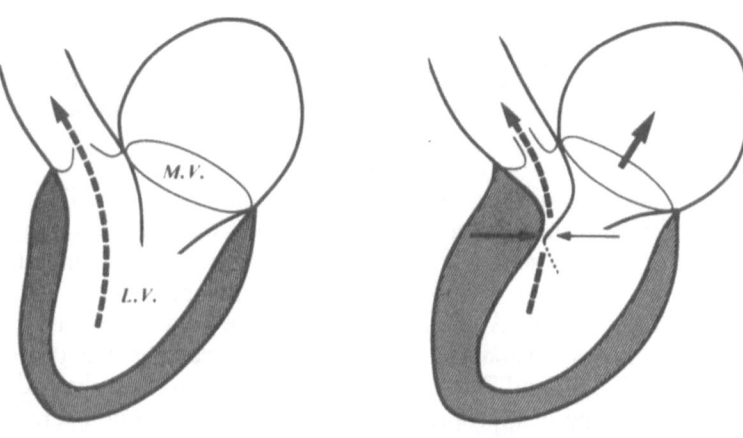

NORMAL   **MUSCULAR SUBAORTIC STENOSIS**

Figure 7.4.22   Proposed mechanism of systolic anterior motion of the anterior mitral leaflet in muscular subaortic stenosis. In normals (*left*) blood ejected from the left ventricle (dashed line) takes a relatively direct path to the aorta, through a wide open outflow tract. In muscular subaortic stenosis (*right*) the ventricular septum is thickened (left, small arrow) which narrows the outflow tract. The path of the blood being ejected from the left ventricle (LV) (dashed line) passes closer to the anterior mitral leaflet than is usual and this leaflet is drawn into the outflow tract towards the septum by a Venturi effect (right, small arrow). Mitral leaflet–septal contact results in obstruction to left ventricular outflow. Mitral regurgitation (oblique large arrow) results from the anterior mitral leaflet being out of its normal systolic position (*see* text)

anterior mitral leaflet–septal contact would be maintained until the end of papillary muscle contraction, i.e. until end-systole. Anterior mitral leaflet–septal contact, however, ceases about three quarters of the way through the systolic period[7], making this mechanism unlikely. Similarly, hyperkinetic contraction of the posterior wall, as part of cavity obliteration, has been suggested as a cause of anterior mitral leaflet motion[40]. Detailed studies have indicated that the timing and rate of development of SAM bears no relation to posterior wall motion[7].

In 1970, we first suggested that a Venturi mechanism could be the cause of systolic anterior motion of the anterior mitral leaflet[25]. Figure 7.4.22 depicts how we believe this mechanism to be operative in muscular subaortic stenosis. Over the years, we have reasoned that the thickened upper septum in cases of muscular subaortic stenosis narrows the left ventricular outflow tract and causes the path of ejection of blood to pass closer to the anterior mitral leaflet than is normal. A rapid ejection of blood from the hypertrophic ventricle, passing close to the anterior mitral leaflet, draws the latter forward toward the ventricular septum, where in cases of muscular subaortic stenosis with a resting gradient, prolonged mitral leaflet–septal contact occurs. The maintenance of mitral leaflet–septal contact could either be due to continued Venturi forces, or to haemodynamic factors such as the high ventricular pressure holding the anterior mitral leaflet against the septum[7,25,41]. The fact that anterior mitral leaflet–septal contact ceases before end-systole could be due to the diminished ejection

245

velocity (reduced Venturi effect) and/or to reduced left ventricular pressure towards the end of systole[7].

Evidence in support of a Venturi mechanism being the cause of systolic anterior motion of the anterior or posterior mitral leaflets can be summarized as follows:

(1) One- and two-dimensional echocardiographic studies indicate that the septum is thicker and the left ventricular outflow tract narrower in patients with muscular subaortic stenosis at rest than in patients with hypertrophic non-obstructive cardiomyopathy[27,41,42] (Figures 7.4.10 and 7.4.11). As might be expected, the values for patients with latent muscular subaortic stenosis fall between these two groups (Figures 7.4.10 and 7.4.11). These studies indicate that the pathological anatomy is appropriate for a Venturi effect to be operative in patients with muscular subaortic stenosis at rest.

(2) Bellhouse and Bellhouse of Oxford built a model of the left ventricle in muscular subaortic stenosis, following correspondence with ourselves. In this model, there were no papillary muscles and no posterior wall motion, but rather an ejection jet was passed close to a modelled mitral valve. The anterior mitral leaflet and sometimes the posterior leaflet as well, opened in systole when the ejection jet was rapid enough and close enough to the anterior leaflet (Bellhouse, B. and Bellhouse, T., personal communication, 1970).

(3) Any known manoeuvre that can affect the pressure gradient in muscular subaortic stenosis can be explained by the Venturi mechanism causing systolic anterior motion of the mitral leaflets. Preload, afterload, and contractility affect the stroke volume of normal man and also affect the degree of systolic anterior motion and pressure gradient magnitude in muscular subaortic stenosis. Thus, diminished afterload, or increased contractility, would increase the early ejection velocity, which in turn would increase the Venturi forces on the anterior mitral leaflet and, thus, increase SAM, the pressure gradient and the mitral regurgitation (Figure 7.4.20). Increased afterload or diminished contractility would reduce early systolic velocity and the Venturi forces on the anterior mitral leaflet, and thus would reduce or abolish SAM, the pressure gradient and the mitral regurgitation (Figure 7.4.20). Preload could affect these events by increasing or decreasing the anatomical size of the left ventricular outflow tract. It may be that ventricular volume (preload) is less important in regulating the magnitude of the pressure gradient than is either afterload or contractility, which more directly affect the ejection velocity and hence the magnitude of the Venturi forces on the anterior mitral leaflet. In the postextrasystolic beat in muscular subaortic stenosis, systolic anterior motion of the anterior mitral leaflet and hence the pressure gradient and mitral regurgitation all become more severe (Figures 7.4.19 and 7.4.21). In this beat,

contractility is increased (postextrasystolic potentiation) and after-load is decreased (lowered aortic diastolic pressure after the long pause, Figure 7.4.21), both factors acting to increase ejection velocity and hence the magnitude of the Venturi forces on the anterior mitral leaflet. Preload, on the other hand, is, if anything, increased in the postextrasystolic beat, which would tend to diminish the Venturi forces and systolic anterior motion. Obviously, afterload and con-tractility by directly affecting the Venturi mechanism predominate in the postextrasystolic beat intensification of the left ventricular out-flow tract obstruction (Figures 7.4.19 and 7.4.21).

(4) The results of surgery can readily be explained if the Venturi mechanism is the cause of systolic anterior motion of the anterior or posterior mitral leaflet and hence the pressure gradient and mitral regurgitation. Thus, either the ventriculomyotomy operation or the ventriculomyotomy–myectomy operation thins the ventricular sep-tum and hence significantly widens the left ventricular outflow tract. This surgery thus alleviates the perceived initial cause of the problem. As a result of the thinned septum and widened left ventricular outflow tract, the rapid ejection jet no longer passes so close to the anterior leaflet and as a result the Venturi forces acting on the leaflet are no longer sufficient to draw it into the left ventricular outflow tract. Thus, the obstruction to left ventricular outflow and the mitral regurgitation are abolished.

(5) Further evidence that the above explanation is valid comes from the recent cross-sectional, two-dimensional echocardiographic observa-tions where the surgical incision and myectomy have been placed a bit too far laterally[43]. In these cases, the lateral part of the systolic anterior motion has been abolished (where the septum was thinned and the outflow tract widened), but the medial part of the systolic anterior motion of the anterior mitral leaflet remained (where the septum was untouched, and the left ventricular outflow tract was as narrow as preoperatively).

(6) There have now been a number of reports of the occurrence of systolic anterior motion of the anterior mitral leaflet and a pressure gradient in patients with concentric hypertrophy of the left ventricle, or with normal hearts, particularly if left ventricular contraction is hyperkinetic or the patient is hypovolaemic[44,45]. Given the appropriate anatomy (a narrow outflow tract for whatever reason), and a high velocity ejection, passing close to the anterior mitral leaflet, a Venturi effect can equally well explain systolic anterior motion and the pressure gradient in these patients. Some cases of muscular subaortic stenosis may have an anterior mitral leaflet that is longer than normal, rendering it more susceptible to Venturi forces[46]. However, this is not a prerequisite to the development of systolic anterior motion of the anterior mitral leaflet (unpublished observations).

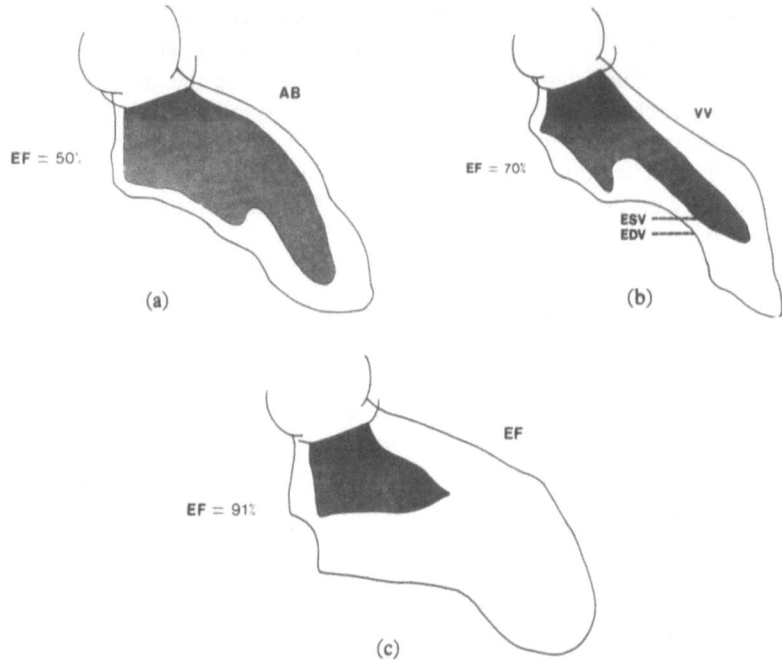

Figure 7.4.23 Line drawings outlining the end-diastolic (**EDV**) and end-systolic (**ESV**) right anterior oblique cineangiographic frames in three patients with muscular subaortic stenosis, who subsequently underwent the ventriculomyectomy operation because of disabling symptoms associated with a large obstructive pressure gradient. Note the variation in ejection fraction (**EF**) and the fact that the area of the left ventricular inflow tract did not become obliterated even with an ejection fraction of 91%. It would be difficult to envisage an intraventricular pressure difference due to cavity obliteration occurring in patient AB with an ejection fraction of 50% (*see* text)

(7) Finally, the Venturi mechanism can also explain SAM of the posterior mitral leaflet when the anatomy is appropriate, i.e., when this leaflet protrudes further into the left ventricle than is normal[30].

CINEANGIOGRAPHIC OBSERVATIONS IN MUSCULAR SUBAORTIC STENOSIS

There have been many detailed descriptions of the cineangiographic appearance of the left ventricle in hypertrophic cardiomyopathy[32-34]. Typically, the papillary muscles are prominent, trabeculation is marked, the ventricular walls are thickened and a variable degree of cavity obliteration occurs (Figure 7.4.23). In our studies, a well defined cavity has always been present in the inflow tract of the left ventricle, even when cavity obliteration is extreme (Figure 7.4.23). (This fact is important relative to the concept of left ventricular inflow tract pressure as a means of distinguishing between an obstructive pressure gradient in muscular subaortic stenosis from an

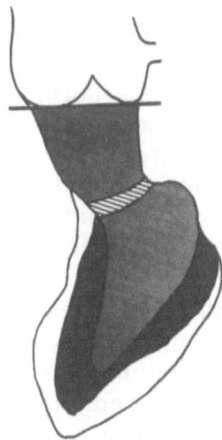

Figure 7.4.24 Line drawings of left anterior oblique, left ventricular cineangiographic frames in a patient with muscular subaortic stenosis at end-diastole (outer line) at the time of mitral leaflet–septal contact (cross-hatched area) (middle line) and at end-systole (inner line). The left ventricular area reduction before mitral–septal contact is indicated by the white area within the end-diastolic silhouette. The left ventricular area reduction after mitral–septal contact is indicated by the dark stippled area. The light stippled area represents the end-systolic area of the left ventricle. A significant portion of left ventricular emptying occurred after the development of mitral leaflet–septal contact and the pressure gradient (ref. 47)

intraventricular pressure difference in cavity obliteration.) In cases with left ventricular outflow tract obstruction, one can visualize systolic anterior motion of the anterior mitral leaflet as well as a radiolucent line, indicating mitral leaflet–septal contact (Figure 7.4.24). This is seen best in the left anterior oblique projection, but also can be seen in the right anterior oblique projection[34]. Although Doppler and indicator dilution studies indicate that the mitral regurgitation may commence just before or with the onset of mitral leaflet-septal contact[19,35], mitral regurgitation is usually best visualized cineangiographically in the last half of systole, during which time it contributes to the small end-systolic volume of the left ventricle[34]. In either the left anterior oblique or right anterior oblique projections, careful observations reveal the following sequence of events in muscular subaortic stenosis:

(1) An early rapid ejection into the ascending aorta, following opening of the aortic leaflets

(2) The development of systolic anterior motion and then mitral leaflet–septal contact (radiolucent line), associated with partial closure of the aortic leaflets and the onset of mitral regurgitation

(3) Continuation of the mitral regurgitation in the last half of systole, accompanied by an ever decreasing left ventricular systolic volume. The aortic valve leaflets reopen in the last half of systole.

This sequence is virtually identical to the eject–obstruct–leak sequence that we described some years ago[34].

More recently, we have investigated cineangiographic left ventricular emptying in a group of nine patients with muscular subaortic stenosis and a mean pressure gradient at rest of 88 mmHg[47]. We studied left anterior oblique, left ventricular cineangiograms, in order to ascertain the amount of left ventricular emptying that occurred before and after the development of the radiolucent line in the left ventricular outflow tract. In these patients, the radiolucent line was first seen at 37.5% of the end-diastolic to end-systolic angiographic interval, while in the same patients, echocardiographic mitral leaflet–septal contact occurred at 38.1% of the 'R' wave end-systolic interval[47]. This virtually simultaneous development of echocardiographic mitral leaflet–septal contact and the angiographic radiolucent line provides strong evidence that the radiolucent line indeed represents mitral leaflet–septal contact and the onset of the pressure gradient. In this group of patients, left ventricular angiographic area reduction was 34% before and 66% after the development of the radiolucent line, indicating that a significant amount of left ventricular emptying occurred in the presence of a pressure gradient[47]. Mitral regurgitation was first evidenced cineangiographically at the onset of mitral leaflet–septal contact, and continued throughout the rest of systole, during which time it appeared to significantly affect left ventricular emptying, which continued until end-systole. From these studies, we would conclude that the development of mitral leaflet–septal contact places a significant haemodynamic burden on the left ventricle, in that a major portion of left ventricular emptying occurred in the presence of a pressure gradient. In addition, the mitral regurgitation began with mitral leaflet–septal contact, and was most evident in the last half of systole. The degree of mitral regurgitation appeared to be the principal determinant of left ventricular end-systolic size[47].

Recent studies by Grose et al. add important confirmation of the above studies on muscular subaortic stenosis as well as new and very pertinent information (Grose, R.M., Strain, J.E. and Spindola-Franco, H., personal communication, 1984). Using simultaneous micromanometry and caudocranial left anterior oblique, left ventricular cineangiography, these authors demonstrated that the obstructive pressure gradient began simultaneously with angiographic mitral leaflet–septal contact (radiolucent line) (Grose et al., personal communication, 1984). Distinguishing between an obstructive and an obliterative pressure gradient by means of the left ventricular inflow tract pressure concept[14–16] (Figures 7.4.1–7.4.5), mitral leaflet–septal contact was only seen in patients with an obstructive gradient. Cavity obliteration occurred in only 50% of cases with obstructive pressure gradients and did so *after* the peak gradient and up to 220 ms, after mitral leaflet–septal contact (Grose et al., personal communication, 1984). (In our earlier simultaneous haemodynamic–echocardiographic studies, peak posterior wall motion occurred an average of 219 ms after mitral leaflet–septal contact.) In cases with cavity obliterative intraventricular pressure differences, the cavity obliteration occurred *before*, rather than after, the onset of the pressure difference (Grose et al., personal communication, 1984).

CRITIQUE OF THE NON-OBSTRUCTIVE POINT OF VIEW

In the foregoing sections we have reviewed the evidence in favour of there being haemodynamically significant obstruction to left ventricular outflow in muscular subaortic stenosis. We have provided evidence that there are very significant differences between an obstructive pressure gradient in muscular subaortic stenosis and a cavity obliterative intraventricular pressure difference[14-16] (Figures 7.4.1–7.4.9). Criteria for differentiating these intraventricular pressure differences are summarized in Table 7.4.4, which also indicates the characteristics of the impulse gradient[31] and the gradient encountered in midventricular obstruction[10]. As all four of these pressure differences may be encountered in the various types of hypertrophic

Table 7.4.4   Differentiation of intraventricular pressure differences that may be encountered in hypertrophic cardiomyopathy

	Muscular subaortic stenosis	Cavity obliteration	Impulse gradient	Midventricular obstruction
(1) *Haemodynamics:*				
Elevated LV inflow pressure	+	−	+	−
Entrapment criteria*	−	+	−	−
Time of peak systolic gradient	Late	Late	Early	Late
Spike and dome aortic pressure	+	−	−	−
Spike and plateau aortic flow	+	−	−	−
LV ejection time	Increased	Normal (or short)	Normal (or short)	Normal
(2) *Cineangiography:*				
Mitral–septal contact (Radiolucent line)	+	−	−	−
LV end-systolic volume	Variable	Small	Normal	Base Small Apex Large
Mitral regurgitation	++	±	−	−
LV cavity obliteration	± Late if +	Early	−	−
(3) *Echocardiography:*				
(a) *ID:*				
Severe SAM	+	−	−	−
Left atrium	+	−	−	±
Aortic valve notch	+	−	−	−
(b) *2D:*				
Leaflet SAM–septal contact	+	−	−	−
(4) *Clinical:*				
Apical murmur	3–4/6	0–2/6	±	?
Reversed split S$_2$	+	−	−	−

*See text

cardiomyopathy, we believe it behoves everyone working in this field to be sure what type of pressure difference they are dealing with in any given patient, at any given time. But, alas, such is not the case!

The reasons for some authors believing that there is no obstruction to left ventricular outflow vary considerably. Criley[13,40,48] has espoused the view that intraventricular pressure differences in hypertrophic cardiomyopathy patients are the result of cavity obliteration and not outflow tract obstruction, yet he has chosen never to try to distinguish between an obstructive pressure gradient and an intraventricular pressure difference due to cavity obliteration, in spite of the fact that there are so many distinguishing features[14-16] (Figures 7.4.1–7.4.9, Table 7.4.4). He claims that the left ventricular inflow tract becomes obliterated in hypertrophic cardiomyopathy, rendering the left ventricular inflow tract pressure concept less than useful. This has not been our experience in some 200–300 cineangiographically investigated patients with hypertrophic cardiomyopathy (Figure 7.4.23). We have never seen an obliterated left ventricular inflow tract in one of our cases, but have viewed some cineangiograms shown by Criley, that do suggest a degree of inflow tract obliteration. We can only conclude that this phenomenon must be extremely rare, so rare that it certainly would not invalidate the left ventricular inflow tract pressure concept[14-16] whose value has just been reaffirmed this very year (Grose et al., personal communication, 1984).

Criley has suggested that systolic anterior motion[40,48] of the anterior mitral leaflet as well as aortic valve notching are due to left ventricular cavity obliteration. Earlier, he had suggested that systolic anterior motion was due to posterior wall hyperkinesis, which is essentially the same thing as it being due to cavity obliteration[40]. There are several strong points of evidence against systolic anterior motion of the anterior mitral leaflet being caused by cavity obliteration. Firstly, the rate of systolic anterior motion of the anterior mitral leaflet towards the septum in early systole, is three times the rate of the inward movement of the posterior wall of the left ventricle during the same time period[7] (Figure 7.4.15). Secondly, peak systolic anterior motion occurs at the time of mitral leaflet–septal contact, which in our studies occurred some 219ms prior to peak posterior wall motion[7] (Figure 7.4.15). Finally, echocardiographic[19] (Figure 7.4.15), cineangiographic[47] (Figure 7.4.24), and the combination of haemodynamic–echocardiographic[7] (Figure 7.4.15), and haemodynamic–cineangiographic (Grose et al., personal communication, 1984) studies have revealed no evidence of cavity obliteration at the time of mitral leaflet–septal contact. Instead, all of these studies have indicated that a very significant proportion of left ventricular stroke volume is ejected *after* the onst of mitral leaflet–septal contact and the pressure gradient. All of these data would indicate that cavity obliteration is not present at the time of mitral leaflet–septal contact, and hence Criley's contention that it is, cannot be sustained; in fact, it can be vigorously denied!

Murgo and associates have also thrown doubt on the concept of there being haemodynamic obstruction to the left ventricular outflow in patients with hypertrophic cardiomyopathy and pressure gradients[20]. These authors base their viewpoint mainly on the fact that the velocity flow profile in the ascending aorta was apparently the same whether or not a pressure gradient was present in patients with hypertrophic cardiomyopathy. The velocity flow profile in patients with no gradient, provocable gradients, and resting gradients all demonstrated rapid early systolic flow that was completed in 61%, 63% and 69% of the systolic ejection period, respectively[20]. Normals took 90% of the systolic ejection period to complete forward flow. The fact that the hypertrophic cardiomyopathy patients finished forward ejection earlier than normals, and that there was no apparent difference in the velocity flow profile between hypertrophic cardiomyopathy patients, whether or not a pressure gradient was present, was taken as evidence against the presence of left ventricular outflow tract obstruction. Similar to Criley's reports in the 1960s, Murgo's paper published in 1980[20] has had a considerable impact on the cardiological world and has similarly stimulated renewed interest in the subject.

Recently, we had reanalysed Murgo's data in considerable detail in light of our own work on the timing of mitral leaflet–septal contact and the pressure gradient[7,8], and believe that he and his associates demonstrated some very significant differences in both forward flow time and systolic ejection period between patients with and without pressure gradients. It is important to realize that these authors studied eight patients with gradients averaging 51 mmHg and that two of these patients had gradients of less than 20 mmHg[20]. From our studies[7,8] (Figure 7.4.17), patients with a gradient of 50 mmHg would have the onset of mitral leaflet–septal contact at 40% of the left ventricular ejection period. At this precise time in Murgo's studies, the flow curve of patients with gradients crosses over the flow curve of those without gradients at a time when 80% of the stroke volume has been ejected in unobstructed fashion. Following mitral leaflet–septal contact at 40% of the systolic ejection period, a gradient of 50 mmHg develops and the last 20% of the stroke volume is ejected against the pressure gradient, representing obstruction to left ventricular outflow. In keeping with this obstruction, the patients with gradients took 32 ms (48%) longer to eject the last 20% of stroke volume than did patients without a gradient. This prolongation of flow time for the last 20% of stroke volume in the patients with gradients, accounts for the difference in the total flow time in those with gradients versus those without (69% versus 61% of the systolic ejection period). Concomitantly, the systolic ejection period was 30 ms longer in those with gradients than those without.

In the analysis of the angiographic data in this paper[20], the flow curve of patients with gradients crosses over that of the patients without gradients at 30% of the systolic ejection period, at a time when 45% of the stroke volume still had to be ejected. We presume this cross-over of the flow curves in the angiographic data has the same significance as in the velocity flow probe data, i.e. mitral leaflet–septal contact occurred at 30% of the systolic ejection period, which caused the cross-over of the flow curves and resulted in the last 45% of stroke volume being ejected in the presence of a pressure gradient of 75–80 mmHg (predicted from Figure 7.4.17). The fact that four of the six beats analysed angiographically were postextrasystolic beats[20] accounts for the earlier cross-over of the flow curves, the earlier mitral leaflet–septal contact, the higher estimated pressure gradient and the greater percentage of systole that is obstructed than was the case in the velocity flow probe data (45% versus 20%). In keeping with this greater degree of obstruction during angiographic analysis, left ventricular ejection time was prolonged by 53 ms, but forward flow time was only prolonged 17 ms, possibly because of the greater degree of mitral regurgitation in the postextrasystolic beat.

Murgo's flow data are a plot of percentage stroke volume against percentage systolic ejection period[20]. We have plotted our data relating the magnitude of the pressure gradient and the left ventricular ejection time against the time of mitral leaflet–septal contact as a percentage of the systolic ejection period (which we have called left ventricular ejection time[7,8]; Figure 7.4.17). By combining the data from the two studies[8,20] it would appear that we can relate the pressure gradient, the left ventricular ejection time (systolic ejection period), and the percentage of stroke volume that is obstructed and unobstructed to any given timing of mitral leaflet–septal contact. The latter is expressed as a percentage of the systolic ejection period. The results of such a tabulation are shown in Table 7.4.5. The

Table 7.4.5   Time of onset of mitral leaflet–septal contact as the determinant of the percentage of stroke volume obstructed, the pressure gradient and the ejection time in muscular subaortic stenosis

	Onset mitral leaflet–septal contact as % LV ejection period					
	10%	20%	30%	40%	50%	60%
Gradient	140	110	80	50	20	0
LVETc	425	400	375	350	320	300
% SV Unobstructed	8%	30%	55%	80%	90%	100%
% SV Obstructed	92%	70%	45%	20%	10%	0%

Gradient = pressure difference across left ventricular outflow tract (mmHg); LVETc = left ventricular ejection time corrected for heart rate (ms); SV = stroke volume

The values indicated in this table are based on recalculations of data provided in the work of Murgo et al.[20] and our own studies[8]. To the best of our understanding the indicated values should be approximately correct but it has to be appreciated that the two studies were not carried out simultaneously (see text)

information in this table must be taken as very tentative at this time, in that the studies from which it was derived were not carried out simultaneously[8,20]. Nevertheless, we believe it could be quite valuable in providing insight into the unique situation in muscular subaortic stenosis by drawing attention to the percentage of total stroke volume that is obstructed for any given onset of SAM–septal contact and pressure gradient (Table 7.4.5). Thus, when mitral leaflet–septal contact occurs at 20% of the systolic ejection period, the gradient would be 110 mmHg and 70% of the stroke volume would be ejected against an obstruction, resulting in the left ventricular ejection time being prolonged to 400 ms. Contrast this with what would happen when mitral leaflet–septal contact occurred at 40% of the systolic ejection period. In this instance, the pressure gradient would be 50, but only the last 20% of stroke volume ejection would be obstructed resulting in only a slight prolongation of ejection time of 350 ms. The important message is that the time of onset of mitral leaflet–septal contact during systole is *the* factor that determines the percentage of stroke volume that is obstructed as well as the magnitude of the pressure gradient and the degree of prolongation of left ventricular ejection time. For mitral leaflet–septal contact times from 10% to 40% of the systolic ejection period, each 10% change will result in a 25% difference in the amount of stroke volume that is obstructed, a 30 mmHg change in the pressure gradient and a 25 ms change in the left ventricular ejection time. We believe that the integration of Murgo's important studies and our own data lead to an important improvement in understanding the significance of obstruction in patients with muscular subaortic stenosis.

Goodwin and his associates do not believe that there is obstruction to left ventricular outflow in hypertrophic cardiomyopathy in the usual sense of the word[39,49]. Indeed, they have described the concept of obstruction to outflow as a 'myth'[39] and 'incidental'[49] to the disease, yet they advise surgery for those with significant pressure gradients and symptoms[39]! They believe that the papillary muscles rather than the mitral leaflets are the cause of SAM and speak of 'cavity elemination' rather than cavity obliteration[39]. We would regard their viewpoint as rather similar to that of Criley and associates[13,40,48], but the latter would not recommend surgery for symptomatic patients with gradients!

A number of investigators, in addition to Murgo and associates, have performed aortic flow studies in patients with muscular subaortic stenosis. Thus, Hernandez et al.[50] used the pressure differential technique, while Pierce and associates[51] studied ascending aortic flow by means of an electromagnetic flow meter at the time of surgery for muscular subaortic stenosis. Both of these authors found a sharp deceleration of aortic flow in early systole together with a lower plateau of late systolic forward flow in patients with obstructive pressure gradients[50,51]. When patients did not have pressure gradients, the pattern of ascending aortic flow resembled that seen in normals. This has also been the case with ascending aortic[19,52], carotid[53] and descending aortic [54,55] flow studies using Doppler techniques in patients with hypertrophic cardiomyopathy with and without pressure gradient. In patients with pressure gradients, all of these Doppler studies have shown a high velocity, early systolic flow, followed by rapid deceleration in the first half of systole, followed by systolic forward flow in the last half of systole. The Doppler flow profile was essentially normal in patients without gradients. It is not immediately evident why pressure differential[50], electromagnetic[51], and Doppler[19,52-55] velocity flow profile showed dramatic differences between patients with and without pressure gradients, while

Murgo's catheter mounted velocity flow probe[20] showed only minor differences. It is conceivable that these differing results are explained by the different pressure gradients in these studies. Thus, the pressure gradients in Murgo's studies[20] average 51 mmHg (only the last 20% of stroke volume would be obstructed) – whereas in the other studies[19,50-55] the pressure gradients were usually greater than 75 mmHg, where 50% or more of the stroke volume would be obstructed (Table 7.4.5). If only a small percentage of stroke volume is obstructed one would not expect much distortion of forward flow[20]. With large gradients, however, it appears that forward flow is distinctly abnormal and characterized by a sharp deceleration in the first half of systole with maintenance of a smaller volume of forward flow in the last half of systole[50-55].

The studies of Pierce et al.[51] are important from several other viewpoints, in that they measure the pressure gradient simultaneously with their flow studies. They have clearly demonstrated that, in patients with large pressure gradients, a large percentage of forward flow (67–80%) occurs in the presence of a pressure gradient. This is in keeping with the data shown in Table 7.4.5. These authors also demonstrated that the stroke volume fails to increase, or actually decreases, in the postextrasystolic beat[51]. Aortic constriction, on the other hand, increases stroke volume, by relieving the outflow tract obstruction[51]. If cavity obliteration were responsible for the pressure gradients in the cases studied, the stroke volume changes would have been in the opposite direction.

Our studies have demonstrated that the onset of mitral leaflet–septal contact and the pressure gradient (defined by the peak of the percussion waves) are virtually simultaneous[7]. The studies of Henry and associates indicate that the onset of mitral leaflet–septal contact is associated with the onset of rapid deceleration of the aortic flow in early systole[19]. Pierce's studies indicate that the onset of rapid deceleration of aortic flow is virtually simultaneous with the peak of the percussion wave in the aortic pressure tracing[51]. It would appear very feasible that the onset of mitral leaflet–septal contact causes the rapid deceleration of aortic flow, which in turn is responsible for the decline in aortic pressure after the percussion wave by Newton's second law. The familiar spike and dome aortic pressure trace is only seen in patients with obstructive gradients and virtually parallels the velocity flow profiles obtained by Doppler[19,52-55] pressure differential[50] and electromagnetic[51] methods. Aortic valve notching is also virtually only seen in patients with obstructive pressure gradients. It would appear to us that the maintained systolic flow in the last half of systole is the only means by which one could explain the dome in the aortic pressure tracing and the reopening of the aortic valve following the notch.

OTHER FEATURES OF HYPERTROPHIC CARDIOMYOPATHY

In this chapter we have been asked to express our views on the significance of the obstructive pressure gradient in muscular subaortic stenosis and we have done just that. Some authors in this field appear to assume that if one believes there is outflow tract obstruction in muscular subaortic stenosis, then, as a corollary, diastolic abnormalities are not important. Nothing could be further from the truth, in view of the fact that we were one of the first groups to draw attention to the problems of decreased compliance in this condition, when in 1962 we said 'some of these patients may be more disabled from decreased compliance in diastole than from the outflow tract obstruction in systole'[6]. Subsequently, we have all come to realize that the diastolic problems in hypertrophic cardiomyopathy are twofold – namely, abnormal relaxation as well as decreased compliance[28]. It would appear evident that the degree and site of hypertrophy in hypertrophic cardiomyopathy is a major determinant of both the systolic and diastolic abnormalities, as well as the occurrence of atrial and ventricular arrhythmias and prognosis[28]. Hypertrophic cardiomyopathy is a disease of many facets. This section deals with but one of them, the obstruction to left ventricular outflow.

CLINICAL MANIFESTATIONS OF OUTFLOW TRACT OBSTRUCTION IN HYPERTROPHIC CARDIOMYOPATHY

Many authors who do not believe in outflow tract obstruction in hypertrophic cardiomyopathy cite, as evidence against its importance, the fact that patients with and without pressure gradients have similar symptoms[20,39,40]. This is not surprising, since both the obstructive and non-obstructive patients often have extensive hypertrophy and significant arrhythmias. However, in our population of patients, those with resting outflow tract obstruction (mean gradient 70 mmHg) had significantly more angina and dyspnoea and were more disabled than were patients with non-obstructive disease. This recent information would coincide very well with the dramatic relief of symptoms that is seen following successful ventriculomyotomy–myectomy surgery[12,36].

The physical findings are also significantly different between patients with and without obstructive pressure gradients. Thus, the incidence of a grade III–IV/VI apical systolic murmur and reversed splitting of the second heart sound was significantly greater in those with obstruction than those without ($p < 0.001$). It is perhaps worth noting that the apical systolic murmur extends well into the latter part of systole in keeping with continuing mitral regurgitation and outflow tract obstruction. A murmur of this length and loudness in late systole would be rather incompatible with virtually total cavity obliteration or elimination in the early part of systole, as had been suggested to occur by some authors.

PATIENT MANAGEMENT IN HYPERTROPHIC CARDIOMYOPATHY

In the foregoing discussions, we have provided evidence to the effect that there are three principal haemodynamic subgroups of hypertrophic cardiomyopathy: (1) muscular subaortic stenosis at rest, (2) latent muscular subaortic stenosis and (3) hypertrophic non-obstructive cardiomyopathy. Patients with latent muscular subaortic stenosis have provocable left ventricular outflow tract obstruction, but because the vast majority (80%) of our patient population have a limited degree of hypertrophy, they have not suffered from diastolic function abnormalities or significant arrhythmias. Thus, therapy has been directed at preventing the provocation of left ventricular outflow obstruction. We have managed these patients for over 20 years now with modest doses of β-adrenergic blocking agents, with gratifying results. There have been no deaths in the 70 or more patients followed for up to 20 years and the relief of symptoms has been very satisfactory and at times quite spectacular. We continue to treat these patients in this manner, but recognize that ventriculomyotomy–myectomy is a therapeutic option[56]. Calcium blocking agents could be effective in preventing provocation of obstruction in these patients, by their negative inotropic effect, but the peripheral vasodilator properties of these drugs could conceivably provoke obstruction to left ventricular outflow.

The therapy of patients with hypertrophic non-obstructive cardiomyopathy today is principally calcium blocking agents, which have been demonstrated to rather dramatically improve left ventricular relaxation in the short and long term[57–61]. Some studies have suggested improvement in left ventricular compliance following long term therapy[60,61]. Propranolol, on the other hand, has been shown not to improve left ventricular relaxation and we rarely use it in these patients today[59]. Because of the extent of hypertrophy in these patients, they are prone to ventricular arrhythmias and frequently require antiarrhythmic therapy.

Patients with muscular subaortic stenosis at rest may be managed with drug therapy or surgery. Patients with mild obstruction to outflow often did well on β-adrenergic blocking therapy but we were never impressed with this form of therapy in cases with significant outflow tract obstruction[36], although others are[62]. The calcium blocking drugs, verapamil and nifedipine, benefit left ventricular relaxation and generally reduce pressure gradients in these patients, but in some the subaortic stenosis increases, and there have been some serious side-effects and deaths on this form of therapy[63].

Currently, our choice of therapy in patients with resting obstruction is either disopyramide or surgery, both of which we believe act by affecting the Venturi effect on the mitral leaflets. Disopyramide, through its negative inotropic action, decreases the ejection velocity in the outflow tract, thus lessening the Venturi forces on the anterior mitral leaflet. As a result, systolic anterior motion is lessened or abolished. Surgery acts by decreasing septal thickness and widening the left ventricular outflow tract; thus, the ejection jet does not pass as close to the anterior mitral leaflet, again lessening the Venturi forces on the leaflet and reducing or abolishing the systolic anterior motion. By acting to decrease the Venturi forces on the anterior mitral leaflet and decreasing or abolishing systolic anterior motion, the two forms of therapy have remarkably similar effects, i.e. they both decrease or abolish the pressure gradient, the mitral regurgitation, the aortic valve notching, and the aortic spike and dome flow profile and pressure pulse. Both may also lower left ventricular end-diastolic pressure, reduce the ejection time, restore normal splitting of the second heart sound and reduce or abolish the apical murmur and symptoms of left ventricular outflow tract obstruction. Successful surgery may also lessen the left atrial size in patients under 40 years of age, thereby rendering them more likely to remain in normal sinus rhythm[64].

Currently, we initially try disopyramide either during acute invasive or non-invasive studies, together with an initial trial of oral therapy. If the response is good, we continue with medical therapy, if not, we do not hesitate to advise surgery. There have been no surgical or late follow-up deaths in the last 40 cases operated upon. Successful surgery appears to have more dramatic haemodynamic and clinical effects than does any form of medical therapy including disopyramide. Arrhythmias must be sought out and appropriately managed both pre- and postoperatively.

SUMMARY AND CONCLUSIONS

Hypertrophic cardiomyopathy is characterized by variable degrees of usually asymmetric cardiac hypertrophy with resultant systolic and diastolic function and rhythm abnormalities. We have reviewed the evidence indicating that true obstruction to left ventricular outflow exists in those patients defined as having obstructive pressure gradients. We have drawn attention to the uniquely characteristic features of patients with muscular subaortic stenosis at rest, in whom the obstruction to outflow is caused by mitral leaflet–ventricular septal apposition. Evidence has been provided that a Venturi effect on the anterior mitral leaflet is responsible for the systolic anterior motion of this structure. Medical and surgical therapy is directed at lessening the Venturi forces on the mitral valve leaflets. A successful ventriculomyotomy–myectomy procedure affords the most dramatic haemodynamic and clinical benefits to patients with muscular subaortic stenosis and resting outflow tract obstruction. To deny that an obstruction to overflow exists in this condition, is to deny patients the benefit of appropriate therapy.

References

1. Teare, R.D. (1958). Asymmetrical hypertrophy of the heart in young adults. *Br. Heart J.*, **20**, 1–8
2. Brock, R.C. (1957). Functional obstruction of the left ventricle. *Guy's Hosp. Rep.*, **160**, 221–38
3. Braunwald, E., Morrow, A.G., Cornell, W.P., Aygen, M.M. and Hilbish, T.F. (1960). Idiopathic hypertrophic subaortic stenosis. *Am. J. Med.*, **29**, 924–45
4. Goodwin, J.F., Hollman, A., Cleland, W.P. and Teare, D. (1960). Obstructive cardiomyopathy simulating aortic stenosis. *Br. Heart J.*, **22**, 403
5. Cohen, J., Effat, H., Goodwin, J.F., Oakley, C.M. and Steiner, R.E. (1964). Hypertrophic obstructive cardiomyopathy. *Br. Heart J.*, **26**, 16–32

6. Wigle, E.D., Heimbecker, R.O. and Gunton, R.W. (1962). Idiopathic ventricular septal hypertrophy causing muscular subaortic stenosis. *Circulation*, **26**, 325–40
7. Pollick, C., Morgan, C.D., Gilbert, B.W., Rakowski, H. and Wigle, E.D. (1982). Muscular subaortic stenosis: the temporal relationship between systolic anterior motion of the anterior mitral leaflet and pressure gradient. *Circulation*, **66–5**, 1087–93
8. Pollick, C., Rakowski, H. and Wigle, E.D. (1984). Muscular subaortic stenosis: the quantitative relationship between systolic anterior motion and the pressure gradient. *Circulation*, **69**, 43–9
9. Buda, A.J., MacKenzie, G.W. and Wigle, E.D. (1981). Effect of negative intrathoracic pressure on left ventricular outflow tract obstruction in muscular subaortic stenosis. *Circulation*, **63**, 875–81
10. Falicov, R.E., Resnekov, L., Bharati, S. and Lev, M. (1976). A variant of obstructive cardiomyopathy: Mid-ventricular obstruction. *Am. J. Cardiol.*, **37**, 432–7
11. Morrow, A.G. and Brockenbrough, E.C. (1961). Surgical treatment of idiopathic hypertrophic subaortic stenosis: Technic and hemodynamic results of subaortic ventriculomyotomy. *Ann. Surg.*, **154**, 181–9
12. Wigle, E.D., Chrysohou, A. and Bigelow, W. (1963). Results of ventriculomyotomy in muscular subaortic stenosis. *Am. J. Cardiol.*, **11**, 572–86
13. Criley, J.M., Lewis, K.B., White, R.I. and Ross, R.S. (1965). Pressure gradients without obstruction. A new concept of 'hypertrophic subaortic stenosis'. *Circulation*, **32**, 881–7
14. Wigle, E.D., Auger, P. and Marquis, Y. (1966). Muscular subaortic stenosis: Initial left ventricular inflow tract pressure as evidence of outflow tract obstruction. *Can. Med. Assoc. J.*, **95**, 793–7
15. Wigle, E.D., Marquis, Y. and Auger, P. (1967). Muscular subaortic stenosis: Initial left ventricular inflow tract pressure in the assessment of intraventricular pressure difference in man. *Circulation*, **35**, 1100–17
16. Ross, J., Braunwald, E., Gault, J.H., Mason, D.T. and Morrow, A.G. (1966). Mechanism of the intraventricular pressure gradient in idiopathic hypertrophic subaortic stenosis. *Circulation*, **34**, 558–78
17. Wigle, E.D., Auger, P. and Marquis, Y. (1967). Muscular subaortic stenosis: the direct relation between the intraventricular pressure difference and left ventricular ejection time. *Circulation*, **36**, 36–44
18. Boiteau, G.M. and Allenstein, B.J. (1961). Hypertrophic subaortic stenosis: Clinical and hemodynamic studies with special reference to pulse contour measurement. *Am. J. Cardiol.*, **8**, 614–23
19. Glasgow, G.A., Gardin, J.M., Burn, C.S., Childs, W.J. and Henry, W.L. (1980). Echocardiographic and doppler flow observations in idiopathic hypertrophic subaortic stenosis (IHSS). *Circulation*, **62**, III, 99 (Abstr.)
20. Murgo, J.P., Alter, B.R., Dorethy, J.F., Altobelli, S.A. and McGranahan, G.M. (1980). Dynamics of left ventricular ejection in obstructive and nonobstructive hypertrophic cardiomyopathy. *J. Clin. Invest.*, **66**, 1369–82
21. Brutsaert, D.L., Housmans, P.R. and Goethals, M.A. (1980). Dual control of relaxation. Its role in the ventricular function in the mammalian heart. *Circ. Res.*, **47**, 637–52
22. Brutsaert, D.L., Rademakers, F.E. and Sys, S.U. (1984). Triple control of relaxation: implications in cardiac disease. *Circulation*, **69**, 190–6
23. Wigle, E.D., Marquis, Y. and Auger, P. (1967). Pharmacodynamics of mitral insufficiency in muscular subaortic stenosis. *Can. Med. Assoc. J.*, **97**, 299–301
24. Wigle, E.D., Adelman, A.G., Auger, P. and Marquis, Y. (1969). Mitral regurgitation in muscular subaortic stenosis. *Am. J. Cardiol.*, **24**, 698–706
25. Wigle, E.D., Adelman, A.G. and Silver, M.D. (1971). Pathophysiological considerations in muscular subaortic stenosis. In Wolstenholme, G.E.W. and O'Connor, M. (eds.) *Hypertrophic Obstructive Cardiomyopathy*. (Ciba Foundation Study Group 37) pp. 63–76. (London: Churchill)
26. Silver, M.D., Buda, A.J., MacKenzie, G.W. and Wigle, E.D. (1977). The variable nature of mitral regurgitation in muscular subaortic stenosis. *Circulation*, **56**–III, 217 (Abstr.)
27. Gilbert, B.W., Pollick, C., Adelman, A.G. and Wigle, E.D. (1980). Hypertrophic cardiomyopathy: subclassification by M-mode echocardiography. *Am. J. Cardiol.*, **45**, 861

28. Wigle, E.D., Rakowski, H., Pollick, C., Henderson, M.A. and Ruddy. T.D. (1981). Future trends in cardiomyopathy. Part II. Cardiomyopathy: Predictions for the foreseeable future. In Yu, P.N. and Goodwin, J.F. (eds) *Progress in Cardiology.* Vol. 10, pp. 185–203. (Philadelphia: Lea & Febiger)

29. Boughner, D., Rakowski, H. and Wigle, E.D. (1978). Mitral valve systolic anterior motion in the absence of hypertrophic cardiomyopathy. *Circulation,* 58–II, 235

30. Maron, B.J., Harding, A.M., Spirito, P., Roberts, W.C. and Waller, B.F. (1983). Systolic anterior motion of the posterior mitral leaflet: a previously unrecognized cause of dynamic subaortic obstruction in patients with cardiomyopathy. *Circulation,* 68–II, 282–93

31. Murgo, J.P., Altobelli, S.A., Dorethy, J.F., Logsdon, J.R. and McGranahan, G.M. (1974). Normal ventricular ejection dynamics in man during rest and exercise. *Am. Heart Assoc. Monogr.,* **46,** 92–101

32. Dinsmore, R.E., Sanders, C.A. and Harthorne, J.W. (1966). Mitral regurgitation in idiopathic hypertrophic subaortic stenosis. *N. Engl. J. Med.,* 275, 1225–8

33. Simon, A.L., Ross, J. and Gault, J.H. (1967). Angiographic anatomy of the left ventricle and mitral valve in idiopathic hypertrophic subaortic stenosis. *Circulation,* 36, 852–67

34. Adelman, A.G., McLoughlin, M.J., Marquis, Y., Auger, P. and Wigle, E.D. (1969). Left ventricular cineangiographic observations in muscular subaortic stenosis. *Am. J. Cardiol.,* **24,** 689–97

35. Marquis, Y., Gateau, P., Alsac, J. and Laurenceau, J.L. (1980). L'insufficance mitrale dans la cardiomyopathie obstructive. *Arch. Mal. Coeur,* 73, 1259–68

36. Wigle, E.D., Adelman, A.G. and Felderhof, C.H. (1974). Medical and surgical treatment of cardiomyopathies. *Circ. Res.,* 34, 196–207

37. Kinoshita, N., Nimura, Y., Okamoto, M., Miyatake, K., Nagata, S. and Sakakibara, H. (1983). Mitral regurgitation in hypertrophic cardiomyopathy. Non-invasive study by two dimensional Doppler echocardiography. *Br. Heart J.,* 49, 574–83

38. Reis, R.L., Bolton, M.R., King, J.F., Pugh, D.M., Dunn, M.I. and Mason, D.T. (1974). Anterior-superior displacement of papillary muscles producing obstruction and mitral regurgitation in idiopathic hypertrophic subaortic stenosis. *Circulation,* 49–II, 181–7

39. Goodwin, J.F. (1982). The frontiers of cardiomyopathy. *Br. Heart J.,* 48, 1–18

40. Criley, M.J., Lennon, P.A, Abbasi, A.S., Blaufuss, A.H. (1976). Hypertrophic Cardiomyopathy. In Levine, H.J. (ed.) *Clinical Cardiovascular Physiology.* pp. 771–827. (New York: Grune & Stratton)

41. Henry, W.L., Clark, C.E., Griffith, J.M. and Epstein, S.E. (1975). Mechanism of left ventricular outflow obstruction in patients with obstructive asymmetric septal hypertrophy (idiopathic hypertrophic subaortic stenosis). *Am. J. Cardiol.,* 35, 337–45

42. Spirito, P. and Maron, B.J. (1983). Significance of left ventricular outflow tract cross-sectional area in hypertrophic cardiomyopathy: a two-dimensional echocardiographic assessment. *Circulation,* 67, 1100–8

43. Pollick, C., Williams, W.G., Rakowski, H. and Wigle, E.D. (1984). Post ventriculomyectomy eccentric SAM: Further evidence for the Venturi mechanism. *J. Am. Coll. Cardiol.,* **3–III,** 492 (Abstr.)

44. Maron, B.J., Gottdiener, J.S., Roberts, W.C., Henry, W.L., Savage, D.D. and Epstein, S.E. (1978). Left ventricular outflow tract obstruction due to systolic anterior motion of the anterior mitral leaflet in patients with concentric left ventricular hypertrophy. *Circulation,* 57, 527–33

45. Come, P.C., Bulkley, B.H., Goodman, Z.D., Hutchins, G.M., Pitt, B. and Fortuin, N.J. (1977). Hypercontractile cardiac states simulating hypertrophic cardiomyopathy. *Circulation,* 55, 990–8

46. Shah, P., Taylor, R.D. and Wong, M. (1981). Abnormal mitral valve coaptation in hypertrophic obstructive cardiomyopathy: Proposed role in systolic anterior motion of mitral valve. *Am. J. Cardiol.,* 48, 258–62

47. Morgan, C.D., Pollick, C. and Wigle, E.D. (1979). Cineangiographic timing of left ventricular outflow obstruction and systolic emptying in muscular subaortic stenosis. *Circulation,* 60–II, 262 (Abstr.)

48. Criley, J.M. (1979). The bottom line syndrome, hypertrophic cardiomyopathy revisited. *West. J. Med.,* 130, 350–3

49. Goodwin, J.F. (1980). Hypertrophic cardiomyopathy: a disease in search of its own identity. *Am. J. Cardiol.*, **45**, 177–80
50. Hernandez, R.R., Greenfield, J.C. and McCall, B.W. (1964). Pressure-flow studies in hypertrophic subaortic stenosis. *J. Clin. Invest.*, **43**, 401–7
51. Pierce, G.E., Morrow, A.G. and Braunwald, E. (1964). Idiopathic hypertrophic subaortic stenosis. III. Intraoperative studies of the mechanism of obstruction and its hemodynamic consequences. *Circulation*, **30** (Suppl. 4), 152–207
52. Gardin, J.M., Dabestani, A., Glasgow, G.A., Butman, S., Hughes, C., Burn, C. and Henry, W.L. (1982). Doppler aortic blood flow studies in obstructive and nonobstructive hypertrophic cardiomyopathy. *Circulation*, **66** (Suppl. II), II–267 (Abstr.)
53. Joyner, C.R., Harrison, F.S. and Gruber, J.W. (1971). Diagnosis of hypertrophic subaortic stenosis with a Doppler velocity detector. *Ann. Intern. Med.*, **74**, 692–6
54. Boughner, D.R., Schuld, R.L. and Persaud, J.A. (1975). Hypertrophic obstructive cardiomyopathy. Assessment by echocardiographic and doppler ultrasound techniques. *Br. Heart J.*, **37**
55. Boughner, D.R., Rakowski, H. and Wigle, E.D. (1976). Idiopathic hypertrophic subaortic stenosis: Combined doppler and echocardiographic assessment. *Circulation*, **54**, II–191 (Abstr.)
56. Maron, B.J., Merrill, W.H., Frieier, P.A., Kent, K.M., Epstein, S.E. and Morrow, A.G. (1978). Long-term clinical course and symptomatic status of patients after operation for hypertrophic subaortic stenosis. *Circulation*, **57**–VI, 1205–13
57. Lorell, B.H., Paulus, W.J., Grossman, W., Wynne, J. and Cohn, P.F. (1982). Modification of abnormal left ventricular diastolic properties by Nifedipine in patients with hypertrophic cardiomyopathy. *Circulation*, **65**, 499–507
58. Bonow, R.O., Rosing, D.R. and Epstein, S.E. (1983). The acute and chronic effects of verapamil on left ventricular function in patients with hypertrophic cardiomyopathy. *Eur. Heart J.*, **4**–F, 57–65
59. Hess, O.M., Grimm, J. and Krayenbuehl, H.P. (1983). Diastolic function in hypertrophic cardiomyopathy: effects of propranolol and verapamil on diastolic stiffness. *Eur. Heart J.*, **4**–F, 47–56
60. Kaltenbach, M., Hopf, R., Kober, G., Bussmann, W.D., Keller, M. and Petersen, A.Y. (1979). Treatment of hypertrophic obstructive cardiomyopathy with verapamil. *Br. Heart J.*, **42**, 35–42
61. Chatterjee, K., Raff, G., Anderson, D. and Parmley, W.W. (1982). Hypertrophic cardiomyopathy-therapy with slow channel inhibiting agents. *Prog. Cardiovasc. Dis.*, **25**, 193–210
62. Frank, M.J., Abdulla, A.M., Watkins, L.O., Prisant, L. and Stefadouros, M.A. (1983). Long-term medical management of hypertrophic cardiomyopathy: usefulness of propranolol. *Eur. Heart J.*, **4**–F, 155–64
63. Rosing, D.R., Condit, J.R., Maron, B.J., Kent, K.M., Leon, M.B., Bonow, R.O., Lipson, L.C. and Epstein, S.E. (1981). Verapamil therapy: A new approach to the pharmacologic treatment of hypertrophic cardiomyopathy: III. Effects of long term administration. *Am. J. Cardiol.*, **48**, 545–53
64. Watson, D.C., Henry, W.L., Epstein, S.E. and Morrow, A.G. (1976). Effects of operation on left atrial size and the occurrence of atrial fibrillation in patients with hypertrophic subaortic stenosis. *Circulation*, **55**, 178–81

8.1
Dilated (congestive) cardiomyopathy – the evidence for and against a disorder of cellular immunity and infection

P.J. LOWRY and W.A. LITTLER

The cause of congestive cardiomyopathy is unknown but it has been postulated that it may be triggered by a virus infection and perpetuated by an immunological mechanism[1–3]. There has been a considerable accumulation of data concerning possible humoral mechanisms in the aetiology of congestive cardiomyopathy, and the body of evidence to date suggests that antiheart antibodies are present in congestive cardiomyopathy. Unfortunately, the relevance and true incidence of antiheart antibodies has been obscured by confused terminology and poor trial design. Many studies have not been performed in a blind manner[4–7], and some did not have control groups[8], or used the same control group for different studies while continuing to test more cardiomyopathic patients[9,10]. These studies have given rise to the erroneous impression that antiheart antibodies may have a significant aetiological role in congestive cardiomyopathy. However, studies performed with blinded, independent observers and repeated observations[11–14] have not corroborated this impression, and to date there is no evidence to suggest that antiheart antibodies are anything more than non-specific findings in heart disease whatever the underlying abnormality. Work attempting to clarify the role of cellular immune mechanisms in congestive cardiomyopathy may be open to similar errors.

Let us examine evidence for viral involvement first of all and then that for a disorder of cellular immunity.

VIRUS INFECTION AND CONGESTIVE CARDIOMYOPATHY

It is likely that a virus has caused a disease when the virus can be isolated from the affected tissue or when viral antigen can be detected in the damaged sites; where a virus can be isolated and shown to produce a similar disease in an animal model, the association is even more secure[15]. Attempts at isolation of virus or demonstration of viral antigen in congestive cardiomyopathy have not met with much success. Hibbs et al.[16]

263

found viral-like particles on electron miscroscopy in the myocardium of a patient with congestive cardiomyopathy but the virus may have been deposited during the patient's final illness rather than at the time of initial presentation of congestive cardiomyopathy several years earlier. A case report in 1982[17] documented the presence of herpes-like virus particles in a patient with congestive cardiomyopathy who had chickenpox prior to the onset of his illness; however, no virus was grown from another myocardial biopsy taken at the same time, and the varicella antibody titre was not elevated. In 1971, Kawai[18] sought the presence of viral antigen in congestive cardiomyopathy by an immunofluorescence technique and demonstrated only one positive case out of 20 studied. Cambridge et al.[19] failed to culture virus or identify virus particles on electron miscroscopy in 18 endomyocardial biopsies from patients with congestive cardiomyopathy. Thus, if virus is associated with congestive cardiomyopathy, it must be present early and all trace gone before clinical presentation.

One may attribute the cause of a disease to a viral aetiology when the disease is associated with isolation of the virus from the pharynx or the faeces, or when a fourfold rise in specific viral antibody titre can be demonstrated in paired sera[20]. Cambridge et al.[19] demonstrated that patients with congestive cardiomyopathy have high antibody titres to Coxsackie B viruses especially when the duration of illness prior to study was less than 1 year and where it began with fever. Kawai[18] also reported significantly higher antibody titres to Coxsackie B viruses in congestive cardiomyopathy compared with controls. In contrast, Fletcher et al.[21] and Sanders[22] were unable to demonstrate elevated viral titres in congestive cardiomyopathy; Grist and Bell[20] could obtain no serological evidence of recent Coxsackie infection in 'chronic heart disease'. A different study in 1978[23] failed to isolate virus from myocardial biopsies or demonstrate changing serological viral titres even in patients with an acute onset suggestive of an influenza-like illness.

In our own laboratory, we have failed to show that patients with congestive cardiomyopathy have been infected with Coxsackie B viruses more often than controls, nor found evidence to suggest, where the onset of symptoms had been within 1 year, that a viral infection had also occurred recently (unpublished data). Interpretation of single titres is difficult: for example, Coxsackie virus titres remain high for months or years after infection, and can be elevated by other infections with antigenically related enteroviruses[21]. The use of paired sera[19,20] failed to demonstrate a changing titre suggestive of recent or active infection. It is not surprising that, in a disease where the time of onset and clinical presentation are separated by an unknown period of time, tests to isolate virus or demonstrate a change in virus titres are unhelpful.

Acute myocarditis may have long term sequelae and some believe that this may represent at least one aetiological factor in congestive cardiomyopathy[24]. The majority recover completely, but instances of acute myocarditis progressing to a chronic heart disease have been documented[25,26]; whether this is in fact the same as congestive cardiomyopathy is still circumstantial.

Histological evidence is required first of all to confirm the presence of acute myocarditis rather than congestive cardiomyopathy brought to light by heart failure associated with, or precipitated by, an infection[27], and secondly to document the nature of the chronic histological changes, whether focal or diffuse, and the quantity and type of cellular infiltration. Animal studies[28,29] have shown that mice infected with Coxsackie B-3 virus develop acute myocarditis and the chronic histological changes are not dissimilar to those found in congestive cardiomyopathy apart from mineralization; in addition, virus could be isolated in the acute, but not the chronic, stage. However, congestive cardiac failure did not occur in any instance; whether this is a true model of the aetiology of congestive cardiomyopathy remains speculative.

Judging by the classical criteria for evidence of virus infection as a cause of a disease, an overwhelming case for its influence in the aetiology of congestive cardiomyopathy is wanting.

CELLULAR IMMUNITY AND CONGESTIVE CARDIOMYOPATHY

Antibodies and cell-mediated immunity are important protective mechanisms against infection. When these mechanisms themselves are responsible for tissue damage and destruction, this is known as hypersensitivity[30]. Antibody and cellular hypersensitivity can occur separately or together. Cell-mediated (or delayed) type of hypersensitivity usually involving T-lymphocytes and non-specific inflammatory cells is known as Type IV. Evidence for this type of reaction is obtained by delayed hypersensitivity skin testing with the suspected antigen[31]. It can be obtained by *in vitro* culture of peripheral blood lymphocytes in the presence of the antigen. Sensitized cells will undergo transformation into blast-like cells and increase their DNA synthesis in the process of cell replication[32]. They will also synthesize and release peptides with pharmacological activities called lymphokines. These are usually detected by their effect of inhibiting the spontaneous migration in tissue culture of macrophages or polymorphonuclear leukocytes[33].

Abnormalities of cellular immunity are known to occur in heart diseases. In rheumatic fever, marked cellular hypersensitivity has been demonstrated to streptococcal cell membranes, specifically to group A streptococci, which persists for 5 years after the acute attack[34]; patients with streptococcal sore throats do not demonstrate this reactivity[34]. In Chagas' disease (which presents a similar clinical picture to congestive cardiomyopathy in its chronic stage[35]) cytotoxic T-lymphocytes are directed to both the parasite, *Trypanosoma cruzi*, and to heart muscle cells[36]. Cellular hypersensitivity has also been demonstrated in ischaemic heart disease[37–39]. Whether these abnormalities are the result or cause of myocardial damage in these conditions is still unknown. Autosensitized lymphokine-producing or cytotoxic cells have been sought in congestive cardiomyopathy.

It has been suggested that in congestive cardiomyopathy the normal cell-mediated immune process may be deficient and allow virus damage that would not occur otherwise (as in subacute sclerosing panencephalitis). In studies by Das and his colleagues[40,41], 28%[40] and 42%[41] of congestive cardiomyopathy patients had abnormal cell-mediated responses compared with less than 11% normal controls; however, the mean values for each patient group studied showed that patients with other heart diseases had impaired cell-mediated responses and the mean values were not significantly different from the congestive cardiomyopathic group (Table 8.1.1). Similar-

Table 8.1.1   Lymphocyte transformation results*

Antigen or mitogen	Patient group	Result – ratio of counts of stimulated lymphocytes to unstimulated control (mean ± SEM)
Phytohaemagglutinin	Congestive cardiomyopathy	81.4 ± 25.9
	Other heart disease	94.3 ± 13.5
	Normal control group	220.0 ± 21.8
Heart antigen	Congestive cardiomyopathy	1.8 ± 0.71
	Other heart disease	1.5 ± 0.27
	Normal control group	1.0 ± 0.50

*From Das et al. (1980)[40]
SEM = standard error of the mean

ly, in tests by the same authors seeking prior cellular sensitization to human heart antigen, up to 25% of patients with congestive cardio-myopathy gave results suggesting such previous sensitization but up to 52% of patients with ischaemic heart disease showed a similar result[41]. This suggests that the abnormalities of cellular immunity found in congestive cardiomyopathy are not specific but may be secondary to cardiac damage rather than primarily involved in pathogenesis. It also emphasizes the importance of rigid exclusion of other causes of a dilated heart, such as ischaemic heart disease, when defining the cardiomyopathic group. Frances-chini et al[42], who claimed to show abnormal T-cell response, did not clarify whether coronary angiography had been undertaken in their patients with presumed cardiomyopathy, whilst their only control group consisted of healthy individuals. Sachs and Lanfranchi[43] reported two isolated cases of patients with congestive cardiomyopathy who showed impaired cellular responsiveness but without comparison with control patients. Other groups have failed to demonstrate any abnormality of cell-mediated immunity to environmental antigens or mitogens[44,45]. However, in our own laboratory, although we failed to demonstrate Type IV hypersensitivity to heart antigen in congestive cardiomyopathy as a whole, a subgroup of these patients was hypersensitive to heart antigen[45]. Although this was not specific to the cardiomyopathy group, it occurred more often in that group compared with other heart diseases and normal healthy controls. These results need to be interpreted with caution as there are other causes of leukocyte migration inhibition apart from inhibitory lymphokines. Cytotoxic antibody produced to a specific antigen will cause migration inhibition in the presence of the antigen[46]; leukocytes or macrophages can be passively sensitized with the cytophilic antibody and thus hinder cell migration[47]. A similar passive sensitization of macrophages by antigen–antibody complexes has been demonstrated[48]. Obviously anything which is toxic to the indicator cells will appear to cause migration inhibition; it is important that the antigen used in the test is not used in toxic concentrations[49] and it must be prepared with utmost care. The use of normal controls and other heart disease groups was an attempt to eliminate some of the other causes of migration inhibition. Test cells were washed to remove patient's serum and the procedure was carried out in buffer with 10% fetal calf serum, but it is otherwise difficult to completely exclude the possibility that antibody or immune complexes might be causing cell migration inhibition. Our own work[45], and that of others[40,41], would suggest that some patients with congestive cardio-myopathy may have cellular abnormalities. There is no evidence to clarify whether these abnormalities are primary or secondary, and these studies are open to the same erroneous interpretations that have marred the humoral work in the past.

Jacobs et al.[50] found cell-mediated cytotoxicity against cultured human myocardial cells in 30% of congestive cardiomyopathic patients, 24% of patients with other forms of heart disease, and 4% of normal individuals; these patients who demonstrated cytotoxicity could not be differentiated in any way from the rest of the group. The authors concluded that the findings indicated a secondary phenomenon of non-specific cardiac damage.

Loss of self-tolerance allows autoimmunity to develop and abnormalities of cells involved in immunoregulation have been found in patients with congestive cardiomyopathy.

Recently, information about the immunoregulatory function of T-lym-phocytes has been clarified[51]. There are two main subsets of T-lymphocytes present in the serum: helper T-cells which induce B-cell production of antibody, help T–T cell interactions and T–macrophage interactions, and suppressor T-cells which regulate (by suppression) the helper cells and have cytotoxic properties. The normal proportion of helper to suppressor T-cells is approximately 2:1; the different subsets can be identified by antibodies produced to the different cell-surface antigens. Alteration of this ratio results in an immunologically compromised host, for example, as is seen in acquired immunodeficiency syndrome (AIDS)[52]. Abnormalities of suppressor cells have been reported in congestive cardiomyopathy. Fowles et al.[53] found a failure of suppression by suppressor T-cells in patients with conges-tive cardiomyopathy. This finding, linked with the report[54] that six of 37 patients transplanted for congestive cardiomyopathy had developed lym-phoma (compared with none of 54 patients transplanted for ischaemic heart disease), prompted the suggestion that the increased risk of lymphoma in the cardiomyopathy group could be the result of impaired suppressor cell function and this may have a bearing on the aetiology of congestive cardiomyopathy. However, a deficiency of suppressor activity was demon-strated in only one of the six patients. Another group[55] confirmed the results of Fowles *et al.*, although the definition of their patient groups was far from ideal: there was no report of coronary angiography in the so-called congestive cardiomyopathy group. Also, unlike Fowles *et al.*, they did find low suppressor cell activity in some subjects in both control groups. Anderson *et al.*[56] failed to demonstrate any abnormality of suppressor T-cell function in patients with congestive cardiomyopathy; this group used similar methodology to that used in the other studies, but in addition eliminated bias by blinding the technicians. Our own group[45] has undertaken a small quantitative analysis of T-cells without investigating function and we have shown that the ratio of T helper to suppressor cells is normal in our patients with congestive cardiomyopathy.

Suppressor and helper T-lymphocytes are not the only cells involved in immunological regulation: natural killer cells appear to be important in this role too. Natural killer cells are non-T-lymphocytes which are cytotoxic to certain tumour cells. It has been suggested that deficiency in natural killer cell activity might allow progression of myocardial damage after an initiating insult such as viral infection; Anderson and colleagues[57] found that a subgroup of patients (50%) had low or undetectable natural killer cell activity in contrast to normal controls and a group with other heart disease. However, this finding could not be confirmed in a subsequent study by a different group[58].

To date, the work on cellular immunity has failed to demonstrate a uniform abnormality in congestive cardiomyopathy which might be implicated in aetiology. Subgroups of patients have shown abnormalities, but results are conflicting and may simply reflect secondary immunological abnormalities which occur as a result, rather than a cause, of congestive cardiomyopathy, and may be further confounded by lack of 'blindness', repeated observations and several observers in the experimental procedures employed.

The evidence that congestive cardiomyopathy is a disorder of cellular immunity and infection does not exist. Data suggesting that viruses may initiate the disease process are mostly speculative and circumstantial. Abnormalities of cellular immunity appear variable and inconclusive and may reflect secondary and non-specific changes. A link between the two, although apparently demonstrated in animals[59], has yet to be established in humans.

References

1. Goodwin, J.F. (1982). The frontiers of cardiomyopathy. *Br. Heart J.*, **48**, 1
2. Kawai, C., Matsumori, A., Kitaura, Y. and Takatsu, T. (1978). Viruses and the heart: viral myocarditis and cardiomyopathy. In Yu, P.N. and Goodwin, J.F. (eds.) *Progress in Cardiology.* pp. 141–62. (Philadelphia: Lea and Febiger)
3. Maisch, B., Deeg, P., Liebau, G. and Kochsiek, K. (1983). Diagnostic relevance of humoral and cytotoxic immune reactions in primary and secondary dilated cardiomyopathy. *Am. J. Cardiol.*, **52**, 1072
4. Das, S.K., Callen, J.P., Dodson, V.N. and Cassidy, J.T. (1971). Immunoglobulin binding in cardiomyopathic hearts. *Circulation*, **44**, 612

5. Bolte, H.-D. and Grothey, K. (1977). Cardiomyopathies related to immunological processes. In Riecker, G., Weber, A. and Goodwin, J.F. (eds.) *Myocardial Failure*, pp. 266–74. (Berlin, Heidelberg, New York: Springer)

6. Sanders, V. and Ritts, R.E. (1965). Ventricular localization of bound gamma globulin in idiopathic disease of the myocardium. *J. Am. Med. Assoc.*, **194**, 59

7. Zabriskie, J.B., Hsu, K.C. and Siegal, B.C. (1970). Heart-reactive antibody associated with rheumatic fever: characterization and diagnostic significance. *Clin. Exp. Immunol.*, 7, 147

8. Maisch, B., Berg, P.A. and Kochsiek, K. (1980). Immunological parameters in patients with congestive cardiomyopathy. *Basic Res. Cardiol.*, **75**, 221

9. Das, S.K., Dodson, V.N. and Willis, P.W. (1969). Antiheart immunoglobulins in cardiomyopathy, especially in hypertrophic muscular subaortic stenosis. (Abstr) *Am. J. Cardiol.*, **23**, 108

10. Das, S.K., Cassidy, J.T., Dodson, V.N. and Willis, P.W. III. (1973). Antiheart antibody in idiopathic hypertrophic subaortic stenosis. *Br. Heart J.*, **35**, 965

11. Kirsner, A.B., Hess, E.V. and Fowler, N.O. (1973). Immunologic findings in idiopathic cardiomyopathy: a prospective serial study. *Am. Heart J.*, **86**, 625

12. Camp, T.F., Hess, E.V., Conway, G. and Fowler, N.O. (1969). Immunologic findings in idiopathic cardiomyopathy. *Am. Heart J.*, **77**, 610

13. Trueman, T., Thompson, R.A. and Littler, W.A. (1981). Heart antibodies in cardiomyopathies. *Br. Heart J.*, **46**, 296

14. Lowry, P.J., Thompson, R.A. and Littler, W.A. (1983). Humoral immunity in cardiomyopathy. *Br. Heart J.*, **50**, 390

15. Lerner, A.M. and Wilson, F.M. (1973). Virus myocardiopathy. *Prog. Med. Virol.*, **15**, 63

16. Hibbs, R.G., Ferrans, V.J., Black, W.C., Walsh, J.J. and Burch, G.E. (1965). Virus-like particles in the heart of a patient with cardiomyopathy: an electron microscopic and histochemical study. *Am. Heart J.*, **69**, 327

17. Lowry, P.J., Edwards, C.W. and Nagle, R.E. (1982). Herpes-like virus particles in myocardium of patient progressing to congestive cardiomyopathy. *Br. Heart J.*, **48**, 501

18. Kawai, C. (1971). Idiopathic cardiomyopathy: a study on the infectious-immune theory as a cause of the disease. *Jpn. Circ. J.*, **35**, 765

19. Cambridge, G., MacArthur, C.G.C., Waterson, A.P., Goodwin, J.F. and Oakley, C.M. (1979). Antibodies to Coxsackie B viruses in congestive cardiomyopathy. *Br. Heart J.*, **41**, 692

20. Grist, N.R. and Bell, E.J. (1974). A six-year study of Coxsackie virus B infections in heart disease. *J. Hyg.*, **73**, 165

21. Fletcher, G.F., Coleman, M.T., Feorino, P.M., Marine, W.M. and Wenger, N.K. (1968). Viral antibodies in patients with primary myocardial disease. *Am. J. Cardiol.*, **21**, 6

22. Sanders, V. (1963). Viral myocarditis. *Am. Heart J.*, **66**, 707

23. McKay, E.H., Littler, W.A. and Sleight, P. (1978). Critical assessment of diagnostic value of endomyocardial biopsy. Assessment of cardiac biopsy. *Br. Heart J.*, **40**, 69

24. Abelman, W.H., Miklozek, C.L. and Modlin, J.F. (1981). The role of viruses in the aetiology of congestive cardiomyopathy. In Goodwin, J.F., Hjalmarson, A. and Olsen, E.G.J. (eds.) *Congestive Cardiomyopathy*. pp. 76–84. (Mölnar, Sweden: AB Hässle)

25. Smith, W.G. (1970). Coxsackie B myopericarditis in adults. *Am. Heart J.*, **80**, 34

26. Sainani, G.S., Krompotic, E. and Slodki, S.J. (1968). Adult heart disease due to the Coxsackie virus B infection. *Medicine*, **47**, 133

27. Leading article (1972). Acute myocarditis and its sequelae. *Br. Med. J.*, **2**, 783

28. Wilson, F.M., Miranda, Q.R., Chason, J.L. and Lerner, A.M. (1969). Residual pathologic changes following murine Coxsackie A and B myocarditis. *Am. J. Pathol.*, **55**, 253

29. Kawai, C. and Takatsu, T. (1975). Clinical and experimental studies on cardiomyopathy. *N. Engl. J. Med.*, **293**, 592

30. Coombs, R.R.A. and Gell, P.G.H. (1975). Classification of allergic reactions responsible for clinical hypersensitivity and disease. In Gell, P.G.H., Coombs, R.R.A. and Lachman, P. (eds.) *Clinical Aspects of Immunology*. pp. 761–81 (Oxford: Blackwell Scientific)

31. Brown, D.L. (1982). Interpretation of test of immune function. In Lachman, P.J. and Peters, D.K. (eds.) *Clinical Aspects of Immunology*. pp. 414–42. (Oxford: Blackwell Scientific)

32. Webster, A.D.B. (1977). Immunodeficiency. In Holborow, E.J. and Reeves, W.G. (eds.) *Immunology in Medicine: a Comprehensive Guide to Clinical Immunology*. pp. 478–9. (London: Academic Press)

33. Hamblin, A.S. (1981). The clinical measurement of lymphokines. In Thompson, R.A. (ed.) *Techniques in Clinical Immunology*. pp. 254–72. (Oxford, London, Edinburgh, Boston, Melbourne: Blackwell Scientific)

34. Read, S.E., Fischetti, V.A., Utermohlen, V., Falk, R.E. and Zabriskie, J.B. (1974). Cellular reactivity studies to streptococcal antigens: migration inhibition studies in patients with streptococcal infections and rheumatic fever. *J. Clin. Invest.*, **54**, 439

35. WHO (1960). Chagas' disease. *World Health Organization Tech. Rep. Ser.*, No. 202. (Geneva: WHO)

36. Teixeira, A.R.L., Teixeira, G., Macedo, V. and Prata, A. (1978). Trypanosoma Cruzi-sensitized T-lymphocytes mediated ^{51}Cr release from human heart cells in Chagas' disease. *Am. J. Trop. Med. Hyg.*, **27**, 1097

37. Wartenberg, J. and Brostoff, J. (1973). Leucocyte migration inhibition by heart extract and liver mitochondria in patients with myocardial infarction. *Br. Heart J.*, **35**, 845

38. Sharma, R.K., Ahuja, R.C., Tandon, O.P. and Chaturvedi, U.C. (1978). Leucocyte migration inhibition test in cases of ischaemic heart disease. *Br. Heart J.*, **40**, 541

39. Das, S.K., Stein, L.D., Thebert, P.J., Reynolds, R.T. and Cassidy, J.T. (1983). Inhibition of leucocyte migration by stimulated mononuclear cell supernatants from patients with ischaemic heart disease. *Br. Heart J.*, **49**, 381

40. Das, S.K., Petty, R.E., Meengs, W.A. and Tubergen, D.G. (1980). Studies of cell-mediated immunity in cardiomyopathy. In Sekiguchi, M. and Olsen, E.G.J. (eds.) *Cardiomyopathy*. pp. 375–7. (Tokyo and Baltimore: University of Tokyo Press)

41. Das, S.K., Stein, L.D., Reynolds, R.T., Thebert, P. and Cassidy, J.T. (1981). Immunological studies in cardiomyopathy and pathophysiological implications. In Goodwin, J.F., Hjalmarson, A. and Olsen, E.G.J. (eds.) *Congestive Cardiomyopathy*. pp. 87–93. (Mölnar, Sweden: AB Hässle)

42. Franceschini, R., Petillo, A., Corazza, M., Nizzo, M.C., Azzolini, A. and Gianrossi, R. (1983). Lymphocyte blastogenic response in dilated cardiomyopathy. *IRCS Med. Sci.*, **11**, 1019

43. Sachs, R.N. and Lanfranchi, J. (1978). Cardiomyopathies primitives et anomalies immunitaires. *Coeur Méd. Intern.*, **17**, 193

44. Retief, L., Hatchett, M., Haeney, M.R., Thompson, R.A. and Littler, W.A. (1980). Cell-mediated immunity in patients with cardiomyopathy. (Abstr.) *Clin. Sci.*, **59**, 17p

45. Lowry, P.J., Thompson, R.A. and Littler, W.A. (1984). Humoral and cellular mechanisms in congestive cardiomyopathy. (Abst.) *Br. Heart J.*, **51**, 109

46. Amos, H.E., Gurner, B.W., Olds, R.J. and Coombs, R.R.A. (1967). Passive sensitization of tissue cells. *Int. Arch. Allergy*, **32**, 496

47. Brostoff, J. (1974). Critique of present *in vitro* methods for the detection of cell-mediated immunity. *Proc. R. Soc. Med.*, **67**, 514

48. Spitler, L., Huber, H. and Fudenberg, H.H. (1969). Inhibition of capillary migration by antigen–antibody complexes. *J. Immunol.*, **102**, 404

49. Gorski, A.J. (1974). Superiority of corpuscular B.C.G. to soluble P.P.D. antigen in the leucocyte migration assay. *Clin. Exp. Immunol.*, **18**, 149

50. Jacobs, B., Matsuda, Y., Deodhar, S. and Shirey, E. (1979). Cell-mediated cytotoxicity to cardiac cells of lymphocytes from patients with primary myocardial disease. *Am. J. Pathol.*, **72**, 1

51. Reinherz, E.L. and Schlossman, S.F. (1980). Regulation of immune response-inducer and suppressor T-lymphocyte subsets in human beings. *N. Engl. J. Med.*, **303**, 370

52. Kornfeld, H., Stouwe, R.A.V., Lange, M., Reddy, M.M. and Grieco, M.H. (1982). T-lymphocyte subpopulations in homosexual men. *N. Engl. J. Med.*, **307**, 729

53. Fowles, R.E., Bieber, C.P. and Stinson, E.B. (1979). Defective *in vitro* suppressor cell function in idiopathic congestive cardiomyopathy. *Circulation*, **59**, 483

54. Anderson, J.L., Fowles, R.E., Bieber, C.P. and Stinson, E.B. (1978). Idiopathic cardiomyopathy, age, and suppressor-cell dysfunction as risk determinants of lymphoma after cardiac transplantation. *Lancet*, **2**, 1174

55. Eckstein, R., Mempel, W. and Bolte, H.-D. (1982). Reduced suppressor cell activity in congestive cardiomyopathy and in myocarditis. *Circulation*, **65**, 1224

56. Anderson, J.L., Greenwood, J.H. and Kawanishi, H. (1981). Evaluation of suppressor-immune regulatory function in idiopathic congestive cardiomyopathy and rheumatic heart disease. *Br. Heart J.*, **46**, 410

57. Anderson, J.L., Carlquist, J.F. and Hammond, E.H. (1982). Deficient natural killer cell activity in patients with idiopathic dilated cardiomyopathy. *Lancet*, **2**, 1124

58. Cambridge, G., Campbell-Blair, G., Wilmshurst, P., Coltart, D.J. and Stern, C.M.M. (1983). Deficient 'natural' cytotoxicity in patients with congestive cardiomyopathy. (Abstr.) *Br. Heart J.*, **49**, 623

59. Kawai, C., Matsumori, A., Kitaura, Y. and Tokatsu, T. (1978). Viruses and the heart: viral myocarditis and cardiomyopathy. In Yu, P.N. and Goodwin, J.F. (eds.) *Progress in Cardiology*. pp. 141–62. (Philadelphia: Lea and Febiger)

8.2
Dilated (congestive) cardiomyopathy – arguments for immunological relevance

H.-D. BOLTE

Autoantibodies reacting with heart have been found in several clinical conditions. These antibodies are found most consistently and in high titres in acute rheumatic fever[1] and postpericardiotomy syndrome[2] also postmyocardial infarction[3] and appear to correlate well with the acute phase of the illness. But the actual role in the pathogenesis is not essentially clear. On the other hand there is much evidence available that in rheumatic heart disease the cross-reactivity of antibodies against myocardial cellular walls and streptococcal membranes has a relevance for the pathogenesis. This conclusion has been drawn on the basis of a remarkable number of findings, including the therapeutic effectiveness of steroids in rheumatic carditis[1,4]. Despite that, it has to be stated in general: detecting autoantibodies in a particular disease does not prove that these antibodies contribute to the pathogenesis of the disorder in question. However, it is possible to devise general principles for deciding whether this is likely.

First, when autoantibodies have a specificity for target cells which are primarily involved in a disease process, this at least offers a plausible explanation for the tissue damage. In myasthenia gravis the primary lesion is the progressive loss of acetylcholine receptors in the motor end-plate, and these structures are the specific targets for the autoantibodies observed in this disorder. Since the appearance and pattern of autoantibodies can be correlated with the source of the disease, it is unlikely that these antibodies are simply an epiphenomenon. By contrast, the autoantibodies to heart muscle which appear transiently in patients with recent myocardial infarction or after periods of acute myocardial ischaema are unlikely to contribute to the course of disease[5].

According to the classification reported by the WHO/ISFC Task Force on the classification and definitions of myocardial disease[6], dilated cardiomyopathy is a disease in which a cause cannot be detected. In order to follow the framework of this definition the following contribution will report on relations between dilated cardiomyopathy and immunological data. The description of these data which should roughly be classified into

MYOCARDIAL IMMUNOFLUORESCENCE

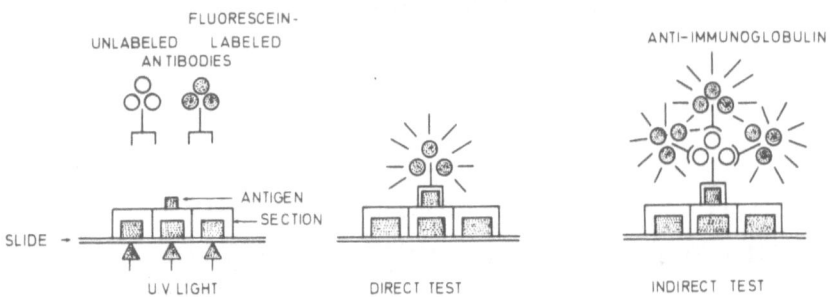

Figure 8.2.1   The principles of the direct and indirect immunofluorescence tests

humoral immunological processes and involvement of B- and T-lymphocytes will be discussed particularly in respect to their relevance, either
diagnostically or pathogenetically or otherwise.

HUMORAL IMMUNOLOGY

For many years techniques have been available to test the presence of
antibodies in the serum against tissue preparations, as for instance heart
muscle tissue of different species[7-11].

In these techniques myocardium (human heart muscle, guinea pig, rat)
serves as an antigen. Microscopic sections are covered with a patient's
serum containing the antibody in question. The bound globulins of the
serum are separated by rinsing the section with a phosphate-buffer medium.
In order to visualize antigen–antibody binding microscopically, conjugates
of antiglobulins with a fluorescent agent are used[7,8] (Figure 8.2.1). Indirect
immunofluorescence has been used with fluorescein-isothiocyanate-conju-
gated antihuman-globulins from rabbit (anti-IgG, anti-IgA, anti-GgM)
(Behring-Werke, Marburg) test to examine sera and direct test to examine
myocardial biopsies. The sera of the patients were diluted 1:5. The
conjugates were diluted 1:10, 1:30, up to 1:40. Results of the indirect
immunofluorescence test in patients with various forms of cardiomyopathy
are summarized in Figure 8.2.2.

In agreement with other investigations[9,12,13] we found humoral myocardial
antibodies (sarcolemmal localization) in postmyocardial infarction syndrome and in postcardiotomy syndrome. These results were important for
the diagnosis of the disease and influenced the therapy. In addition to positive
results in patients with congestive cardiomyopathy of unknown aetiology,
the immunofluorescence test was positive in ten (41%) of 24 patients, i.e.
eight sarcolemmal type and two intermyofibrillar type. In the controls (30
clinically healthy persons), only one (3%) positive immunofluorescence test
was observed.

More quantitatively we demonstrated the same results by the antiglobulin

EVIDENCE AGAINST IMMUNOPATHOGENESIS

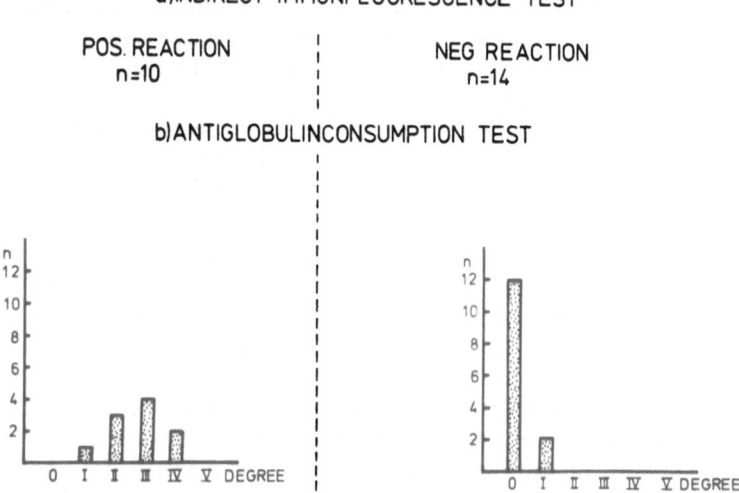

Figure 8.2.2 Determinations of myocardial antibodies in 24 patients with primary cardio-myopathy by the indirect immunofluorescence test and the indirect antiglobulin consumption test. Ten patients showed the positive reaction in the immunofluorescence test; the titres in the antiglobulin consumption test correspond to degree I–IV. In 12 of the 14 negative sera (immunofluorescence) no antibodies in the antiglobulin consumption test were detectable

consumption test which yielded an increased antiglobulin consumption directly proportional to concentration. The antiglobulin consumption test yielded titre decrease for congestive cardiomyopathy greater than that for controls by more than one step in 12 (50%). In the controls only two (10%) showed a titre decrease of only step[14,8]. The positive antibody results coincided with more severe symptoms of congestive heart failure; those patients with negative antibody results did not have symptoms of congestive heart failure to the same extent. Furthermore the longer the duration of clinical symptoms, the higher the percentage of antibody coincidence: 36% in duration 0–5 years and 100% in duration 5–10 years[8].

Several groups have researched circulating heart antibody. Robinson and co-workers noted an 11% incidence of heart reactive antibody[4]. Using an indirect immunofluorescence method Das and co-workers[9] found heart reactive antibodies in six of 35 patients (17%) with idiopathic cardiomegaly and in one of 43 control subjects. A similar coincidence of positive test result has been found in a study of 33 patients (12% of heart reactive antibodies[13]) and in a study of 68 patients, 60 of whom demonstrated antibodies against heart muscle sarcolemma[12]. These results indicate that immunological evaluation is relevant for following the disease.

Recently modifications of the mentioned tests have been reported. So an attempt has been made to produce a differentiation between antimyolemmal and antisarcolemmal antibodies in rat cardiocytes, which have been prepared by a special technique with collagenase, to remove the sarcolemmal part of the membrane, leaving only the myolemma in these preparations.

In the same preparation it could be shown that antimyolemmal antibodies could have a cytolytic effect. This can be taken as an indicator that antimyolemmal antibodies could be cytotoxic and, to that extent, could have pathogenetic relevance[15].

However, it has not yet been decided whether the immune phenomena in cardiomyopathies of unknown aetiology have diagnostic significance only, or if they can serve also as indicators of the underlying pathogenetic mechanism. In this regard, it is also remarkable that in 22 patients with cardiomyopathy due to chronic alcoholism a negative myocardial antibody test has been observed; but in 95%, the IgA value was increased by 100% on the average. The simultaneous existence of a congestive heart failure as the correlate to cardiomyopathy and the further symptoms of a negative immunofluorescence test and increased IgA value can serve as a guide to the diagnosis of cardiomyopathy due to chronic alcoholism. In the patients examined, there was no evidence for hepatic cirrhosis[16,17,8]. Furthermore, humoral myocardial antibodies could be detected in none of 21 patients with the characteristic symptoms of hypertrophic obstructive cardiomyopathy. All of the patients were examined clinically and by heart catheterization (ref. 18; and Bolte and von Geldern, unpublished results, 1977). We determined the typical intraventricular pressure gradient and, by angiography, the septal hypertrophy and outflow tract obstruction[18-20]. These data mean in general that there is a distinct difference in the existence of myocardial antibodies in different myocardial diseases. So this difference and the higher incidence of myocardial antibodies in this case make it possible to suggest that myocardial antibodies of the sarcolemmal type against the myocardium play a pathogenetic role as well as a diagnostic one.

This suggestion is substantiated by an additional finding, as follows. In a total of 24 patients with dilated cardiomyopathy of unknown aetiology binding of immunoglobulin G was found in a high percentage. Since the ejection fraction is one of the most reliable measurements of pump function we separated these patients into one group with ejection fraction below 30% and another group above 30%. The positive reaction was plotted as a percentage of the total number of patients. Figure 8.2.3 shows that in the group with lower ejection fractions immunoglobulin binding of IgG is remarkably higher than in the group with higher ejection fractions. In order to underline this correlation a third group was correlated with myocardial diseases of different aetiology. This group with different aetiology included coronary heart disease with normal ejection fraction and some patients with cardiomyopathy possibly on account of electrocardiographically documented abnormalities. The plot shows an inverse correlation with ejection fraction showing that, with low ejection fractions, immunoglobulin G is bound in a high percentage and is lowest in the group with high ejection fractions[20].

The high percentages of myocardium-bound immunoglobulins observed are in agreement with the findings reported by Das et al.[21]. This group of

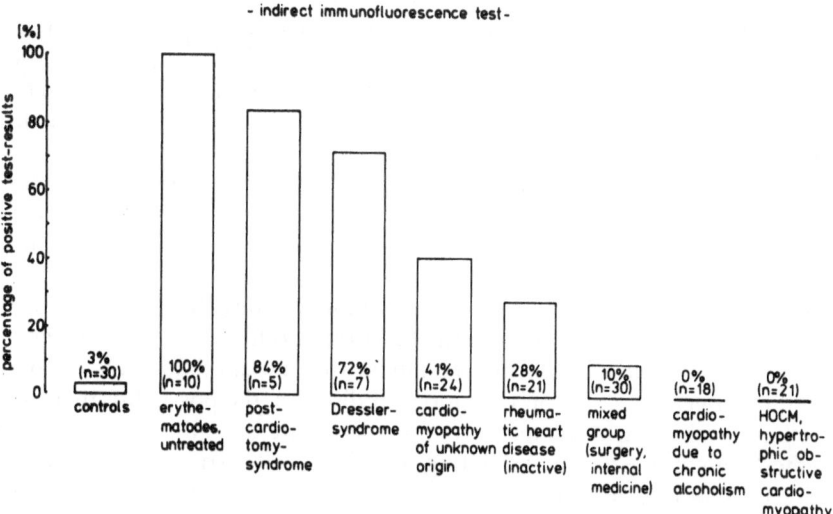

HUMORAL MYOCARDIAL ANTIBODIES

- indirect immunofluorescence test -

Figure 8.2.3 Myocardial antibodies (indirect immunofluorescence test) in various myocardial diseases. The non-existence of myocardial antibodies in alcoholic cardiomyopathy and in hypertrophic obstructive cardiomyopathy is remarkable

workers demonstrated bound γ-globulin in the explanted heart of patients with congestive cardiomyopathy who had undergone cardiac transplantation. The results indicate that the heart muscles in patients with congestive cardiomyopathy bind IgG and IgA, a finding of great importance in those cases in which morphological diagnosis does not suggest established congestive cardiomyopathy. The results have also shown that the presence of immunoglobulin binding correlates well with the haemodynamic findings. At present the pathophysiological implications are not clear, but during the development of congestive cardiomyopathy there appears to be, in a number of cases, an association between the immunoglobulin-binding of the myocardium and the existence of humoral antibodies against the myocardium. The possible functions of the antibody, either bound to sarcolemmal structures in the myocardium of the diseased patients or demonstrable as a humoral antibody in the serum of patients with heart disease, include: (1) the antibody is a phenomenon which may be of diagnostic importance but which does not play a direct pathogenic role, (2) the antibody itself may be cytotoxic to heart cells, (3) the antibody, by adhering to heart sarcolemmal structures, may induce an antibody-dependent, lymphocyte-mediated cytotoxicity and (4) the antibody may mask the antigenic sites of the heart cells, thereby protecting the cells from the cytotoxic effect of sensitized lymphocytes. In so far as complement is bound, the role of bound immunoglobulin can be assumed to be cytotoxic.

The adenine nucleotide translocator is an intrinsic hydrophobic protein located in the inner mitochondrial membrane. Since this membrane is *a priori* impermeable to hydrophilic metabolites the transfer to ATP to cytosol with its energy-consuming processes and the return of ADP to the inner mitochondrial space for regeneration by oxidative phosphorylation requires a particular transport catalysis. The ADP/ATP shuttle being the only active nucleotide transport system in mitochondria, is highly specific and corresponds exactly to the requirements of the ATP production in aerobic cells.

Interestingly enough, it is in a similar manner as already reported in the last chapter that the antibody activity against mitochondrial proteins (ANT) is negatively correlated to ejection fraction: the low ejection fraction is the higher is the antibody activity.

As already mentioned, antireceptor autoimmune diseases – for instance myasthenia gravis – can modulate the function of cell surface receptors and their function. Since it is difficult to establish that autoantibodies play a role in the pathogenesis of autoimmunological diseases, the possibility that the blocking antibodies in dilated cardiomyopathy are actually impairing the haemodynamic function by inhibiting the ADP/ATP carrier in the myocardial cell cannot be yet ruled out. Although there are some indications that antibodies might penetrate into living cells there is as yet no proof about the function and integrity of these antibodies intracellularly[22,23].

SPECIFIC ANTIBODIES AGAINST MITOCHONDRIAL PROTEINS

Recently, using immunological techniques the adenine nucleotide translocator (ANT) could be identified as an intrinsic protein of the inner mitochondrial membrane. This antigen has been shown as existing in dilated cardiomyopathy. Further immunochemical characterization by crossed immunoelectrophoresis, indirect solid phase radioimmunoassay and immunoabsorption studies on the isolated translocator protein and mitochondria from heart, kidney and liver showed the existence of organ-specific antigenic determinants although partial cross-reactivity between the three proteins was observed. Sera from 18 patients with histologically proven dilated cardiomyopathy were studied for their capacity to bind to the translocator protein. Seventeen of 18 patients showed a significant binding, while in the sera of patients with coronary heart disease, suspected alcoholic heart disease or healthy blood donors no anti-ANT antibodies were observed. Further studies showed organ-specific and functional active autoantibodies, inhibiting the ADP/ATP exchange rate from heart mitochondria. A close correlation was found between the antibody titre and the haemodynamic function. These results give new evidence for autoimmunological events in dilated cardiomyopathy[24].

CELLULAR IMMUNOLOGY

B-lymphocytes synthesize humoral antibodies, which are found in the serum. Helper and suppressor T-cells modify this activity quantitatively. As a consequence of a diminished suppressor T-cell function, the physiological

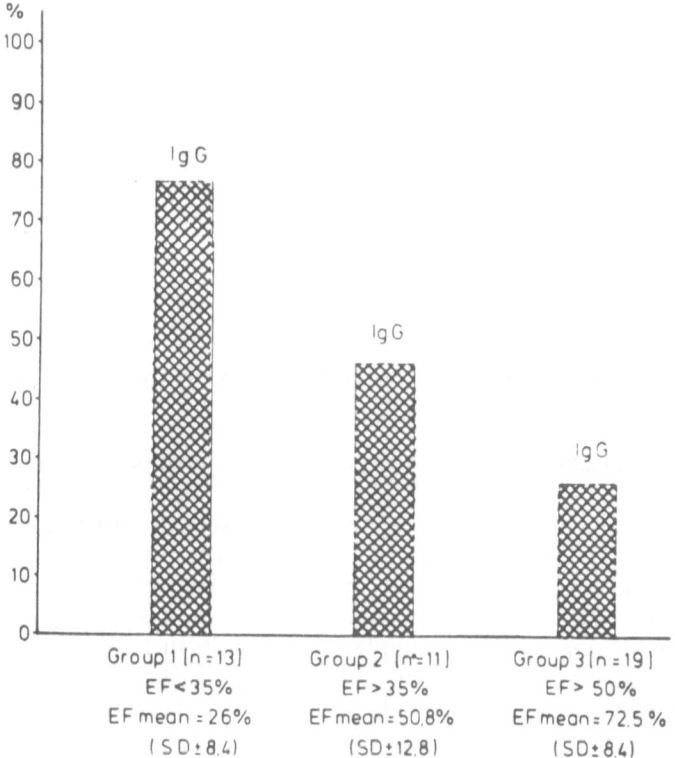

Figure 8.2.4 Binding of IgG in myocardial biopsies. Note the different incidence of binding in different groups of ejection fraction

control of the antibody synthesis may be disturbed. Subsequently, specifically acting pathological agents may cause an excessive production of cardiotoxic antibodies, which then bind to myocardial structures.

In studies employing [³H]thymidine incorporation into the DNA of stimulated lymphocytes in the presence of concanavalin-A-treated peripheral blood mononuclear cells, Fowles et al.[25] found depressed suppressor cell function in patients with dilated cardiomyopathy. These results could be confirmed although there were differences in the experimental design, experimental controls and methods of calculation, and in addition a low suppressor cell activity in patients with myocarditis (MC) and in some healthy controls could be detected[26].

Recently, a high percentage of patients in the acute phase of viral carditis were found by methods employing indirect immunofluorescence to have myocardial antibodies. Nuclear bound IgM antiglobulin was found in all of these patients[6,11,27]. A high percentage of bound immunoglobulins could be detected in myocardial biopsy tissue from patients with dilated cardiomyopathies (Figure 8.2.4). IgG was most often demonstrated in sarcolemmal structures from patients with low ejection fractions (<35%); in patients

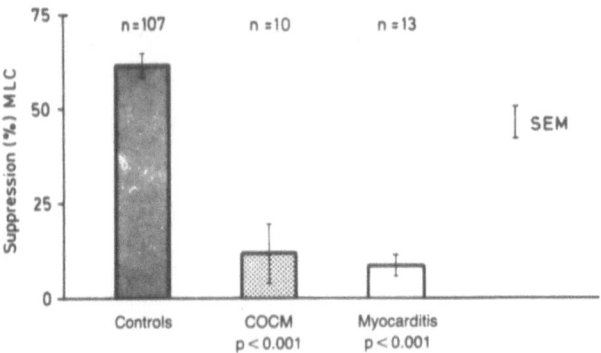

Figure 8.2.5 Suppressor cell activity in myocarditis and congestive cardiomyopathy. Note the low T-cell suppressor activity in congestive cardiomyopathy

with higher ejection fractions, the percentage of binding was considerably lower[20].

Several explanations for the reduced suppressor cell activity are possible (Figure 8.2.5). The suppressor cell compartment may be quantitatively reduced. The suppressor cells may be defective but unreduced in number, or there may be a combination of reduced numbers and defective functioning. In lupus erythematosus, for example, serum factors such as antilymphocytic auto-antibodies can attack suppressor T-lymphocytes and, by cell injury and destruction, can lead to a reduced function of the suppressor compartment. Cells from quantitatively and functionally normal compartments could also be inhibited by such serum factors. Otherwise, a low suppressor cell activity could be genetically determined as a normal variation of the immune system.

In this respect it has to be taken into account that suppressor cell activity may be determined by genes of the major histocompatibility complex of chromosome 6[28]. So a certain trend towards an increase in the number of HLA genes A11, A28, A29, B12, B15, B16 and B17 occurring in persons with low suppressor cell activity, especially in patients with myocarditis and dilated cardiomyopathy, has been observed[29]. Some of these genes show a positive relation to low suppressor cell activity which has been detected in healthy controls, myocarditis and dilated cardiomyopathy. This could mean that persons with these genes more often have low suppressor cell activity and therefore probably run a higher risk of developing myocarditis or dilated cardiomyopathy. Furthermore, it is remarkable that those genes are more often combined in individuals from the pathological groups than in unselected healthy controls. The relative risk (rR) for persons with these gene combinations is 3.61 for myocarditis (comparable to the risk of someone with the gene DRw4 developing rheumatoid arthritis) and 7.22 for dilated cardiomyopathy (comparable to the risk of someone with the gene DRw3 developing chronic active hepatitis)[30].

As the relative risk of dilated cardiomyopathy is distinctly higher, patients with myocarditis, relevant gene combinations, and low suppressor cell

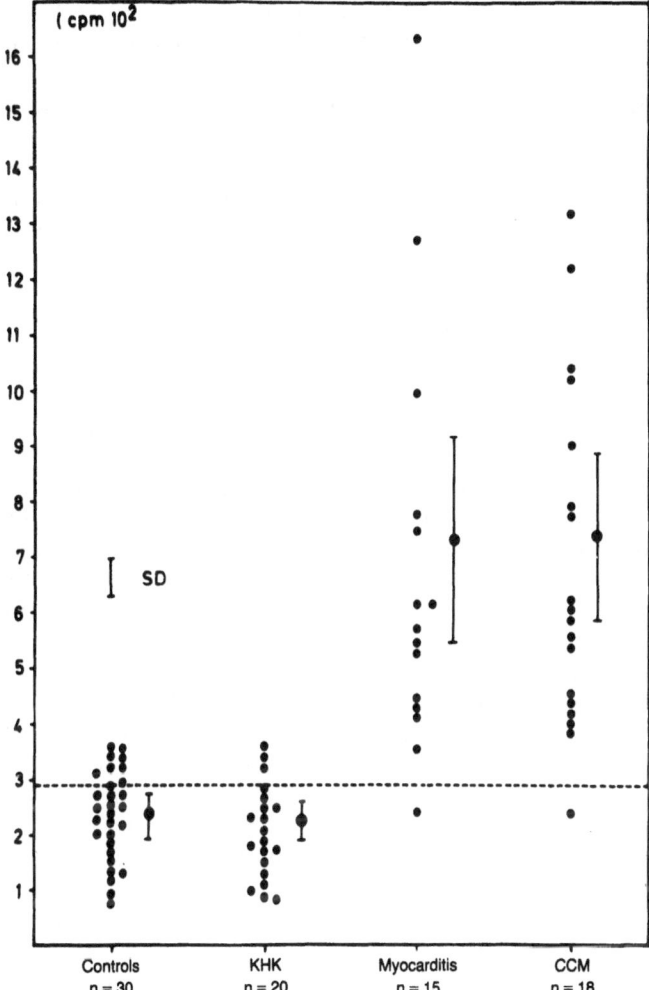

Figure 8.2.6 Mitochondrial antibodies against the myocardial ADP/ATP translocator protein in patients with coronary artery disease, myocarditis and dilated cardiomyopathy, compared to healthy controls. Note that in myocarditis and in dilated cardiomyopathy an increased amount of antibody activity has been documented. These results indicate that both diseases can be regarded as different stages of the same entity

activity may be the recruiting collective for the dilated cardiomyopathies. And these myocarditis patients may well stem from a group of healthy individuals with certain HLA gene combinations and low suppressor cell activity. Therefore, reduced suppressor cell activity may indicate a genetically determined variation of the immune system. This variation, either alone or together with other components of immune function, coincidental with specifically acting pathological agents such as viruses, and possibly with disturbed control of the B-cell antibody synthesis, may lead to apparent or inapparent myocarditis and subsequently to dilative cardiomyopathy, as well as to other autoaggressive disorders. Patients with dilative cardiomyopathy were found to have higher Coxsackie virus titres than controls[31,32].

This incidence assumes that there could be a common cause for myocarditis and cardiomyopathy, and that myocarditis could be seen as an early stage of dilated cardiomyopathy. Our results support this concept[33]. Reduced suppressor cell activity, probably determined by genes of the major histocompatibility complex of chromosome 6, may well be the common important predisposing condition for both myocarditis and dilative cardiomyopathy. Thus this group of dilated cardiomyopathy patients should be distinguished as a separate entity from those with dilated cardiomyopathies of unknown origin (Figure 8.2.6).

SUMMARY AND CONCLUSIONS

The data and investigations reported and discussed above give evidence that immunological processes play an important role in dilated cardiomyopathy. Despite the arguable fact that in some cases immunological symptoms, for example humoral antibodies against the myocardium, are epiphenomena, it nevertheless has to be kept in mind that dilated cardiomyopathy can be regarded in a remarkable number of cases as an immunological end-point of a genetically determined disposition to that disease. This immunologically determined disposition includes an increased susceptibility to viral infections, so these highly relevant findings have additional support. Myocarditis of viral origin can be regarded as an early stage of subsequently developing dilated cardiomyopathy or dilated myocardial disease in a special group of patients which has been regarded up to now only as comprising cases of dilated cardiomyopathy without detectable origin.

These conclusions are based on

(1) the detection of humoral antibodies against myocardial cell walls and against special proteins of cell organelles such as mitochondria,
(2) the evidence of cytotoxicity in animal models of cardiac rat myocites,
(3) the increased binding incidence of immunoglobulins in myocardial biopsy tissues in relation to the decrease of myocardial pump function,
(4) the existence of specific antibodies against a virologically very important protein, related to the specific ADP/ATP transporting mitochondrial system,
(5) a low T-cell suppressor activity which could be assessed in dilated cardiomyopathy, myocarditis and a special group of healthy controls.

Regarding measurements of HLA-genes the T-cell suppressor activity has to be attributed to a special group of genes which shows the close relation to the histocompatibility complex.

Further evidence for the genetically determined influences of the immunological system can be drawn from observations of an increased incidence of dilated cardiomyopathy in siblings, very recently reported[34]. Furthermore, it is in the same sense convincing that, in two families with dilated cardiomyopathy, clinical and pathological findings of myocarditis could be detected[35].

References

1. Zabriskie, J.B., Read, S.E. and Ellis, R.J. (1971). Cellular and humoral studies of diseases with heart reactive antibodies. In Amos, B. (ed.) *Progress in Immunology.* (New York: Academic Press)
2. Engle M.A., McCabe, J.C., Ebert, P.A. and Zabrinskie, J. (1974). The postpericardiotomy syndrome and antiheart antibodies. *Circulation*, 49, 401
3. Van der Geld, H. (1964). Antibodies in the postpericardiotomy- and post-myocardial-infarction-syndromes. *Lancet*, 2, 618
4. Robinson, J., Anderson, T. and Grieble, H. (1966). Serologic anomalies in idiopathic myocardial disease. *Clin. Res.*, 14, 335
5. Agrawal, C.G., Gupta, S.P., Chaturvedi, U.C., Mitra, M.K., Gupta, N.N. and Gupa, S. (1978). T lymphocytes and anticardiac antibodies in patients with ischemic heart diseases. *Int. Arch. Allergy Appl. Immunol.*, 57, 246–52
6. Report of the WHO/ISFC Task Force on the definition and classification of cardio-myopathies (1980). *Br. Heart J.*, 44, 672
7. Coons, A.H., Creech, H.J. and Jones, R.N. (1941). Immunological properties of an antibody containing a fluorescent group. *Proc. Soc. Exp. Biol. Med.*, 47, 200
8. Bolte, H.D. and Grothey, K. (1977). Cardiomyopathies related to immunological proces-ses. In Riecker, G., Weber, A. and Goodwin, J.F. (eds.) *Myocardial Failure.* p. 266. (New York, Heidelberg, Berlin: Springer)
9. Das, S.K., Cassidy, J.T. and Petty, R.E. (1970). Antibodies against heart muscle and nuclear constituents in cardiomyopathy. *Am. J. Cardiol.*, 25, 91
10. Lessof, H. (ed.) (1981). *Immunology of Cardiovascular Disease.* (New York, Basel: Dekker)
11. Bolte, H.-D. and Schultheiss, P. (1978). Immunological results in myocardial diseases. *Postgrad. Med. J.*, 54, 500–3
12. Sack, W., Sebening, H. and Wachsmut, E.D. (1975). Auto-Antikörper gegen Herzmuskel-sarkolemm im Serum von Patienten mit primärer Cardiomyopathie. *Klin. Wochenschr.,* 35, 103
13. Camp, T.F., Hess, E.V., Conway, G. and Fowler, N.O. (1969). Immunologic findings in idiopathic cardiomyopathy. *Am. Heart J.*, 77, 610
14. Oevermann, W., Bolte, H.-D., and Zwehl, W. (1973). Indirekter Immunfluoreszenztest und indirekter Antiglobulinkonsumptionstest in der Diagnostik primärer Kardio-myopathien. *Verh. Dtsch. Ges. Inn. Med.*, 79, 1121
15. Maisch, B., Deeg, P., Liebau, G. and Kochsiek, K. (1983). Diagnostic relevance of humoral and cytotoxic immune reactions in primary and secondary dilated cardiomyopathy. *Am. J. Cardiol.*, 52, 1072–8
16. Bolte, H.-D. (1976). Alkoholkardiomyopathie. *Münch. Med. Wochenschr.*, 118, 355
17. Bolte, H.-D., Milstry, H.R., Tebbe, U. and Rahlf, G. (1974). Neurere Aspekte zur klinischen Diagnostik der Alkoholkardiomyopathie. *Verh. Dtsch. Ges. Inn. Med.*, 80, 1206
18. Von Geldern, S. (1975). *Immunologische Untersuchungen bei hypertrophischer obstruk-tiver Kardiomyopathie.* Thesis, University of Göttingen
19. Bolte, H.-D. (1978). Immunologic investigations in patients with cardiomyopathies. In Kaltenbach, M., Loogen, F. and Olsen, E.G.J. (eds.) *Cardiomyopathy and Myocardial Biopsy.* p. 251. (Berlin, Heidelberg, New York: Springer)
20. Bolte, H.-D., Schultheiss, P., Cyran, J. and Goss, F. (1980). Binding of immunoglobulins in the myocardium (biopsies). In Bolte, H.H.D. (ed.) *Myocardial Biopsy – Diagnostic Significance.* p. 85. (Berlin, Heidelberg, New York: Springer)

21. Das, S.K., Callen, J.P., Dodson, V.N. and Cassidy, J.T. (1971). Immunoglobulin binding in cardiomyopathic hearts. *Circulation*, **44**, 612
22. Alarcon-Segovia, D. (1981). Penetration of antinuclear antibodies into immunoregulatory T cells: pathogenic role in the connective tissue disease. *Clin. Immunol. Allergy*, **1**, 117–26
23. Alarcon-Segovia, D., Ruiz-Arguelles, A. and Fishbein, E. (1979). Antibody penetration into living cells. I. Intranuclear immunoglobulin in peripheral blood mononuclear cells in mixed connective tissue disease and systemic lupus erythematosus. *Clin. Exp. Immunol.*, **35**, 364–75
24. Schultheiss, H.P. and Bolte, H.-D. (1985). Immunological analysis of auto-antibodies against the adenine nucleotide translocator in dilated cardiomyopathy. *J. Mol. Biol. Med.* (In press)
25. Fowles, R.E., Bieber, C.P. and Stinson, E.B. (1979). Defective in vitro suppressor cell function in idiopathic congestive cardiomyopathy. *Circulation*, **59**, 483–91
26. Eckstein, R., Mempel, W. and Bolte, H.-D. (1982). Reduced suppressor cell activity in congestive cardiomyopathy and in myocarditis. *Circulation*, **65**, 1224–9
27. Bolte, H.-D., Ludwig, B. and Schultheiss, H.P. (1983). Virusmyokarditis: Symptomatologie, klinische Diagnostik und Hämodynamik. *Verh. Dtsch. Ges. Herz- und Kreislaufforsch*, **49**, 131–40.
28. Benacerraf, B. (1981). Role of MHC gene products in immune regulation. *Science*, **21**
29. Eckstein, R., Mempel, W., Heim, M. and Bolte, H.-D. (1984). The role of human leucocyte antigen genes and low suppressor cell activity in the pathogenesis of myocarditis and dilated cardiomyopathies. In Bolte, H.-D. (ed.) *Viral Heart Disease.* p. 151 ff. (Berlin, Heidelberg, New York: Springer)
30. Mayr, W.R. (1980) Die klinische Bedeutung der Leukozytenalloantigene. *Lab. Med.*, **4**, 193–7
31. Waterson, A.P. (1978). Virological investigations in congestive cardiomyopathy. *Postgrad. Med. J.*, **54**, 505–7
32. Cambridge, G., MacArthur, C.G., Waterson, A.P., Goodwin, J.F. and Oakley, C.M. (1979). Antibodies to Coxsackie B viruses in congestive cardiomyopathy. *Br. Heart J.*, **41**, 692–6
33. Bolte, H.D. and Ludwig, B. (1984). Viral myocarditis: symptomatology, clinical diagnosis and hemodynamics. In Bolte, H.D. (ed.) *Viral Heart Disease.* (Berlin, Heidelberg, New York: Springer)
34. Shapiro, H.M., Rozkovec, A., Cambridge, G., Hallidie-Smithe, K.A. and Goodwin, J.F. (1983). Myocarditis in siblings leading to chronic heart failure. *Eur. Heart J.*, **4**, 742–6
35. O'Connell, J.B., Fowles, R.E., Robinson, J.A., Subramanian, R., Henkin, R.E. and Gunnar, R.M. (1983). Clinical and pathologic findings of myocarditis in two families with dilated cardiomyopathy. *Am. Heart J.*, **107**, 127

Index